Wrist Functional Anatomy and Therapy

Grégory Mesplié
Editor

Wrist Functional Anatomy and Therapy

Springer

Editor
Grégory Mesplié
ISAMMS
Biarritz, France

ISBN 978-3-031-42878-4 ISBN 978-3-031-42879-1 (eBook)
https://doi.org/10.1007/978-3-031-42879-1

Translation from the French language edition: "Thérapie de la main: anatomie fonctionnelle et thérapie des pathologies du poignet" by Grégory Mesplié, © Sauramps medical 2023. Published by Sauramps medical. All Rights Reserved.

This Springer imprint is published by the registered company Springer Nature Switzerland AG
The registered company address is: Gewerbestrasse 11, 6330 Cham, Switzerland

Paper in this product is recyclable.

To my mother, the illustrator, for her incredible work and kindness.

To my family and closed ones for their support, this book is also yours.

To the whole team at the Institut Sud Aquitain de la Main et du Membre Supérieur, without whom these books wouldn't exist.

Foreword

On the very first day of the very first outpatient clinic of my residency in hand surgery, I was entirely unprepared for anything related to nonsurgical management of hand and wrist pain, as well was flabbergasted by the difficulty in performing a concise, clinical assessment while listening to a patient's history and description of symptoms. No matter how hard I tried to study the anatomy of the wrist, repeating mnemonics of carpal bones, I could not comprehend the complexity of correlating anatomy to symptoms to patient experience, let alone find a reliable solution to treat.

One of the most frustrating cases of that challenging morning in early June 2001 was a patient that had come for cast removal 6 weeks after an open TFCC repair. With me in the room was a hand therapist who asked how I would like to proceed with the rehabilitation and possible splinting. As she saw my puzzled expression, she quickly added, "Doctor, we follow protocol as per usual, I assume?," saving not only my face but adding a sense of comfort and security to the patient in need of further care.

The name of the hand therapist was Ami Rosenqvist. She exuded calmness and confidence that undoubtedly had a healing effect on our patients. And after that day in the clinic, she proceeded to guide me as a future hand surgeon in the principles of hand therapy and the important relationship between surgeon and therapist, using her 30+ years of experience to explain how edema affects movement, how pain limits progress, and how splints can both be an aid and a hindrance if not used correctly.

Since that day, I have always taken great care in cherishing the collaboration with my hand therapists, realizing that—undoubtedly—their treatments provide our patients with an outcome that supersedes anything I could accomplish on my own. Although the saying goes, "It takes two to tango," in hand and wrist disorders it takes three—the surgeon, the therapist, and the patient.

This book on Hand and Wrist Therapy is a collation of information that is of essence not just to the physiotherapist or occupational therapist dealing with hand and wrist disorders but also an important source of information for any surgeon in the field. The second volume of this book series is a review of pertinent bony, ligamentous, and tendinous wrist anatomy and physiology, as well as relevant diagnostics and treatments, both conservative and postoperative.

In short—a reference work in our daily care of our patients with wrist pain or injuries.

Enjoy!

Elisabet Hagert
Hand and Wrist Surgery
Aspetar Orthopedic and Sports
Medicine Hospital, Doha, Qatar

Karolinska Institutet, Stockholm, Sweden

Contents

Editors and Contributors

About the Editor

Grégory Mesplié ISAMMS, Biarritz, France

Contributors

Nicolas Christiaens Institut Sud Aquitain de la Main et du Membre Supérieur, Biarritz, France

Thomas Everaere Institut Sud Aquitain de la Main et du Membre Supérieur, Biarritz, France

Amélie Faraud Institut Sud Aquitain de la Main et du Membre Supérieur, Biarritz, France

Vincent Grelet Institut Sud Aquitain de la Main et du Membre Supérieur, Biarritz, France

Olivier Léger Institut Sud Aquitain de la Main et du Membre Supérieur, Biarritz, France

Cédric Le Petit Institut Sud Aquitain de la Main et du Membre Supérieur, Biarritz, France

1 Functional and Biomechanical Anatomy of the Radioulnar Unity and the Wrist

Grégory Mesplié

The wrist and the radioulnar unity are a joint complex that play a key role in the orientation and stabilization of the hand, both essential qualities for optimal prehensions. The understanding of their functioning has increased in recent years thanks to modern imaging techniques.

Osseous Elements

Radius and Ulna

Proximal extremities

The part we will talk about only concerns the radioulnar unity, so the radial head and the radial notch of the ulna.

- *Radial head*

It is an irregular cylinder slightly ovoid at the end of the radial neck. It is about 4 mm larger than the radial neck. The axis of the neck is the same as the radial axis in the sagittal plane but forms an angle of 165° outwards in the frontal plane (Fig. 1.1).

Thanks to this conformation, the radial head is positioned in the frontal plane. Its sponge-like structure makes it fragile, but it is reinforced by bone trabeculae whose homogeneous distribution

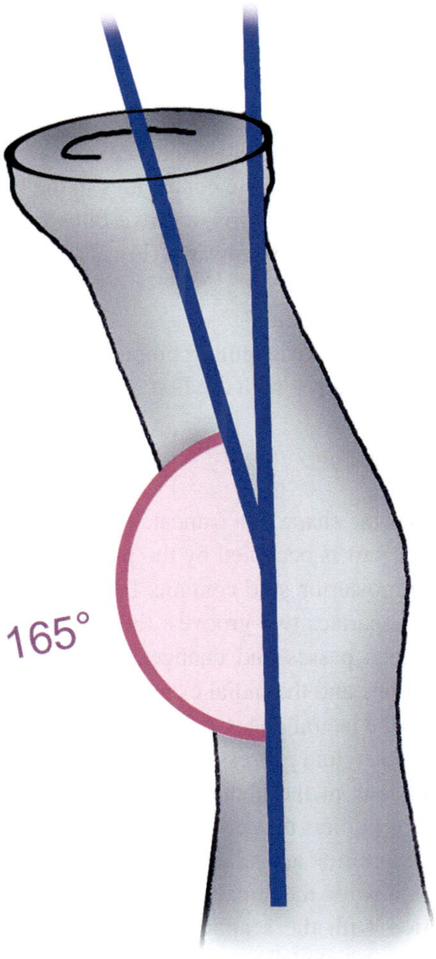

Fig. 1.1 The radial head forms an angle of 165° with the radial neck axis

G. Mesplié (✉)
ISAMMS, Biarritz, France

G. Mesplié (ed.), *Wrist Functional Anatomy and Therapy*,
https://doi.org/10.1007/978-3-031-42879-1_1

avoids the formation of areas more fragile than others.

In supination, the ovoid axis is oriented inwards and frontwards and the radial tuberosity is oriented inwards. The radial head tilts so that its internal part is higher than its external part.

- *Lesser sigmoid cavity (or radial notch)*

It is a small cavity with a cartilaginous "crust" located under the greater sigmoid cavity (or trochlear notch). Both notches are separated by an anteroposterior ridge.

Diaphyses

The radial and ulnar diaphyses have special curvatures that allow important mobility in pronosupination.

In supination, the two bones are concave anteriorly but have opposite concavities in the frontal plane, where the ulna is concave outwards, and the radius is concave inwards (Fig. 1.2).

Distal Extremities

Along with the triangular complex, they form a set that interfaces with the first carpal row.

- *Radial epiphysis*

It has the shape of a truncated pyramid whose anterior part is occupied by the pronator quadratus. Its posterior side contains Lister's tubercle, which separates two grooves: the extensor pollicis longus passes and changes direction in the medial one and the radial extensors of the carpus pass in the lateral one. On its lateral side, there is the radial styloid process, in front of which passes the tendons of the abductor pollicis longus and extensor pollicis brevis.

The inferior articular side has a medial part (relation with the lunate) and an external part (relation with the scaphoid). It is concave and globally oriented frontwards (10°) and inwards (25°) (Fig. 1.3).

The internal side receives the radial notch of the ulna (trochoid joint).

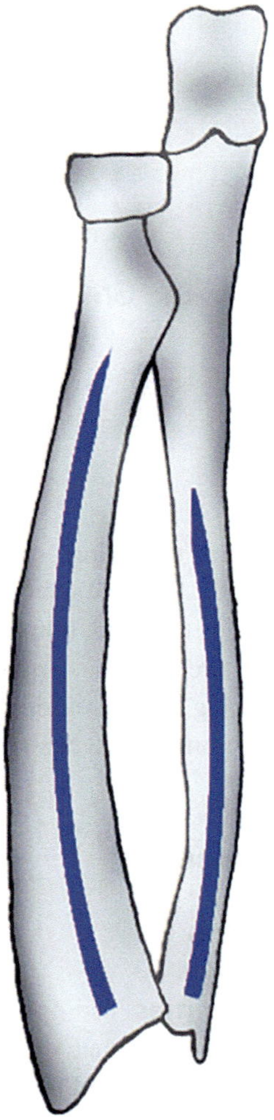

Fig. 1.2 The diaphysis of the two bones of the forearm have inverted concavities in the frontal plane, which allows their "winding" in pronation

Mechanically, the radius absorbs 80% of the axial constraints transmitted by the carpus. A 2-mm shortening is enough to transfer 40% more load on the ulnar compartment (Markolf et al. 2005).

- *Ulnar epiphysis*

Thinner than the radial epiphysis, it contacts with the radius by its external convex side to form the distal radioulnar joint.

Its inferior side has to do with the triangular complex, which articulates with the first carpal row.

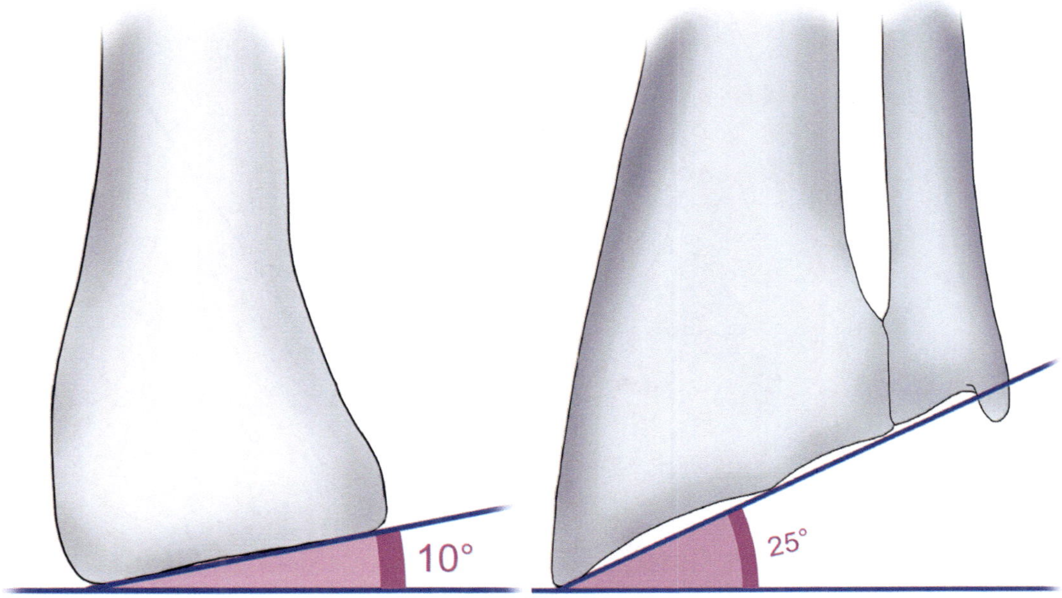

Fig. 1.3 Orientation of the radial socket downwards, frontwards, and inwards

First Carpal Row (Fig. 1.4)

The mobility between the bones of the first carpal row is complex and gives it a huge adaptive capacity allowing it to absorb part of the constraints imposed on it. From lateral to medial, it is made of:

Scaphoid

The word "scaphoid" comes from the Greek "skaphê": "boat". However, it has more of a "bean" shape. It is the most lateral bone of the first carpal row. There is an angle of 30° between the distal and proximal parts viewed from the side, and an angle of 40° viewed from the front (Fig. 1.5).

More than 80% of its surface is covered by cartilage, the remainder with ligamentous insertions.

It is the most voluminous bone of the first carpal row and the closest to the thumb, between the radius and the trapezo-trapezoidal joint.

Like for the lunate and triquetrum, there are no tendon insertion on it, but it is strongly attached to the radius and carpus by powerful ligaments.

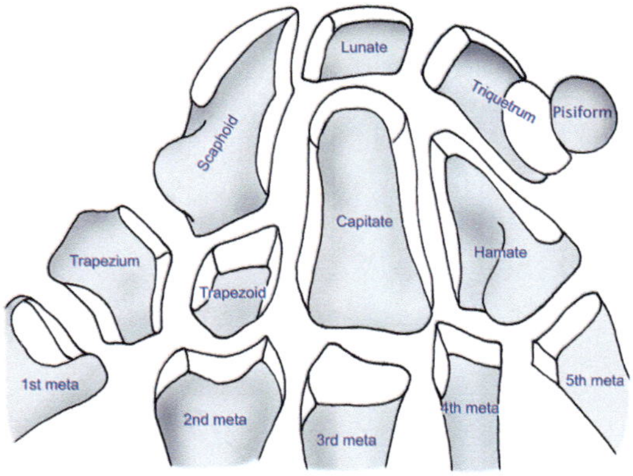

Fig. 1.4 Carpal bones

It forms a 45° angle with the radial axis in the frontal and sagittal plane. This orientation is the key element of the natural thumb opposition, essential in prehensions (Fig. 1.6).

It is made of three parts (Fig. 1.7):

- The proximal part is round, covered in cartilage, and articulates with the lunate (plane joint). This joint forms the lateral part of the carpal condyle. The superior side of the proximal part articulates with the radius. It can be

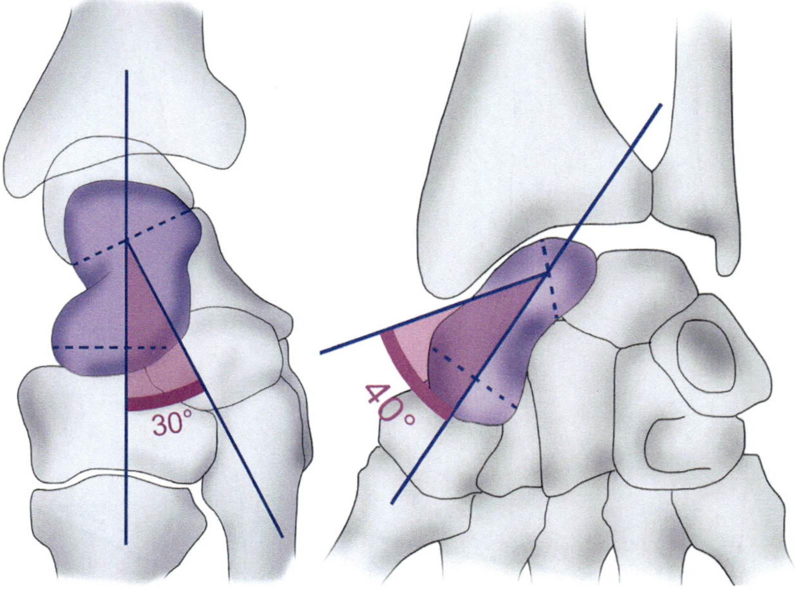

Fig. 1.5 Intra-scaphoidal angles

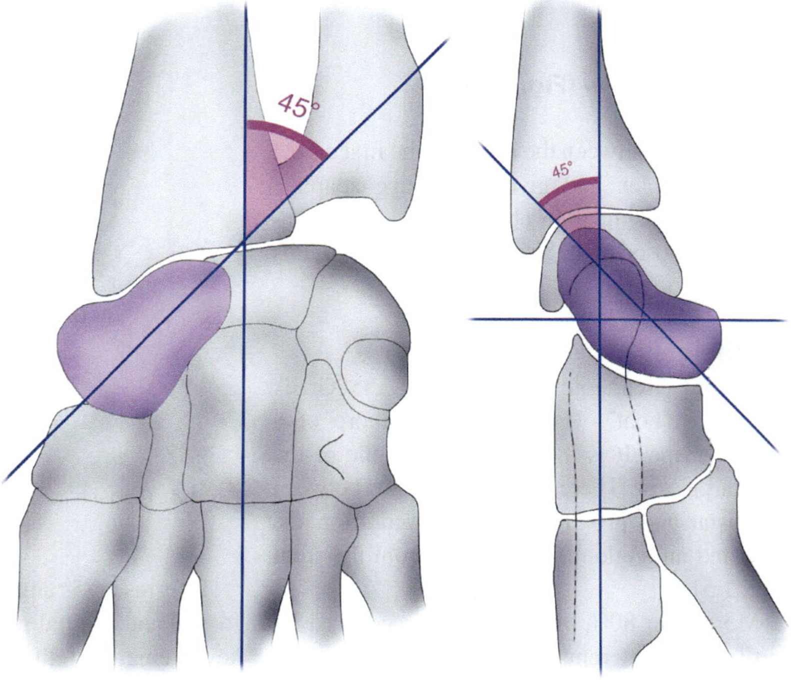

Fig. 1.6 Orientation of the scaphoid frontwards and outwards with respect to the radial axis

palpated in wrist flexion when it dorsally peeks out from the radio-carpal groove in the Lister's tubercle axis.

- The neck is the narrowest part of the bone (6 mm width). Its medial part articulates with the capitate. Its lateral part contacts with the radial artery and corresponds to the floor of the anatomical snuffbox.
- The base articulates with the trapezium and trapezoid distally. It is anteriorly prolonged by the scaphoid's tubercle. On this tubercle are inserted the flexors retinaculum and the

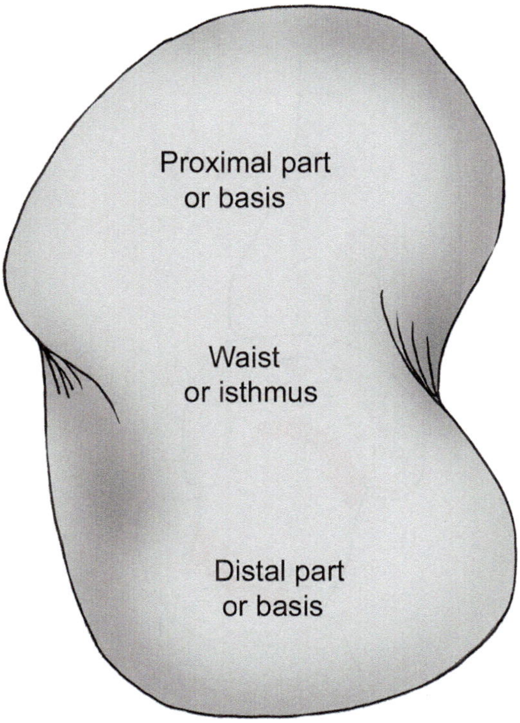

Fig. 1.7 The 3 parts of the scaphoid

abductor pollicis brevis. There is a medial groove where the flexor carpi radialis passes. This muscle then ends on the scapho-trapezo-trapezoidal joint and on the bases of the second and third metacarpals. It is easily palpable in wrist extension.

Its vascularization is ensured by the branches of the radial artery, in two groups:

- The dorsal group enters the scaphoid's neck and takes care of 70% of the vascularization.
- The distal palmar group enters the scaphoid's tubercle and takes care of 30% of the vascularization (Gelberman and Menon 1980) (Fig. 1.8).

There are no vessels entering the proximal part, which explains why there is an important risk of pseudoarthrosis and necrosis in case of fractures at this level.

The scaphoid is "stuck" between the radius and the trapezo-trapezoidal joint and is under

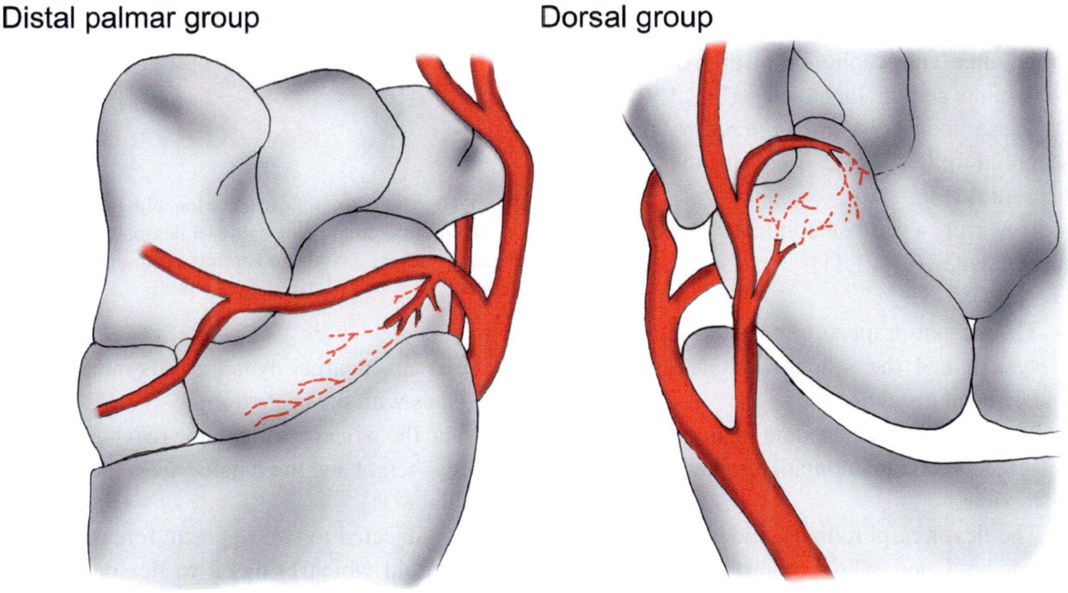

Fig. 1.8 The vascularization of the scaphoid is ensured by two groups given off by the radial artery. The proximal group enters by the waist and represents 70% of this vascularization. There are no vessels that directly enter the head of the scaphoid

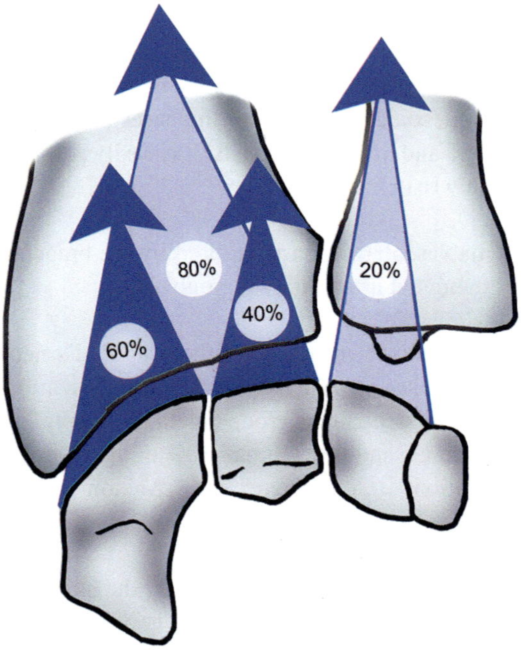

Fig. 1.9 The radius bears 80% of the longitudinal forces coming from the carpus. The scaphoid transmits 60% of these forces to the radius

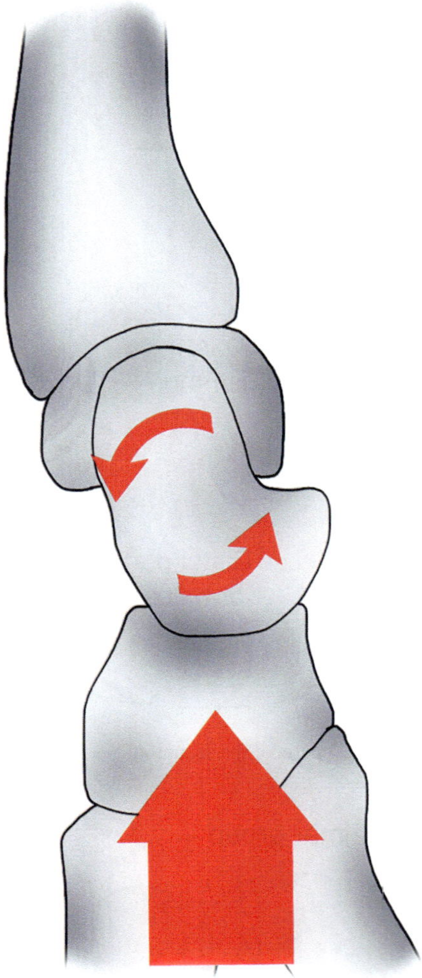

Fig. 1.10 The scaphoid's orientation with respect to the radius in the sagittal plane causes a flexion of the radius because of the axial constraints coming from the carpus

important compressive constraints as 80% of the carpus load is transmitted to the radius and 20% to the ulna. The scaphoid transmits 60% of these constraints and the lunate 40% (Fig. 1.9).

These axial constraints tend to bring the scaphoid to flexion because of its 45° angle with the radius (Fig. 1.10).

However, several anatomical elements oppose this tendency (Fig. 1.11):

- The scapho-trapezo-trapezoidal ligamentous system and the scapho-capitate ligament: a powerful distal anchor.
- The radio-scapho-capitate ligament makes the scaphoid do an automatic pronation during its flexion.
- The flexor carpi radialis, slides in front of the scaphoid and whose contraction brings the distal part of the scaphoid backwards.

Lunate

It has the shape of an irregular lunar crescent with a distal concavity articulated with the capitate. Its anterior horn is bigger than the posterior one. Its lateral side articulates with the scaphoid: this is the key pair in carpal dynamics. Its internal side articulates with the triquetrum.

When the wrist is straight, the two horns are at the same height and the lunate axis is the same as the radial axis.

It is subjected to two opposite forces through the scaphoid which brings it to flexion and the triquetrum and capitate, which bring it to extension (Fig. 1.12).

Triquetrum

It is the most internal bone of the first carpal row, in the shape of a pyramid lying down with an external base and an internal top.

Its superior part is convex in every way and forms the carpal condyle with the lunate and scaphoid. The external side (2/3) of its inferior part is concave and the internal side (1/3) is convex, to harmoniously articulate with the hamate.

Pisiform

It is a sesamoid bone, so it is not really a part of the first carpal row. It is a sort of "patella" for the flexor carpi ulnaris; it helps the muscle be more efficient in the sagittal plane by improving its tendinous angle.

Its deep surface articulates with the triquetrum.

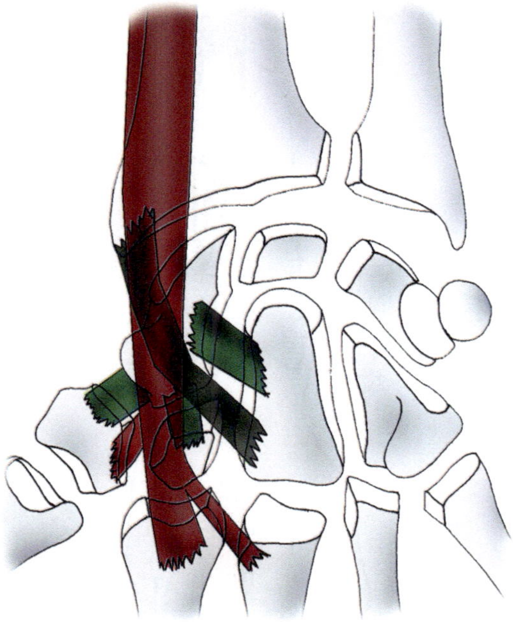

Fig. 1.11 Ligamentary (scapho-trapezo-trapezoidal system, scapho-capitate ligament, radio-scapho-capitate ligament) and muscular (flexor carpi radialis) elements opposing the flexion of the scaphoid

Second Carpal Row

It is a lot less mobile than the first carpal row and made from lateral to medial of:

Trapezium

It is cubical and articulates proximally with the scaphoid and distally with the first metacarpal. Its internal side articulates with the trapezoid (superior part) and second metacarpal (inferior part).

Its external face is not involved in any joint but is pierced with many vascular holes.

The anterior retinacular ligament, the superficial bundle of the flexor pollicis brevis and the opponens pollicis insert on its palmar side: it is the trapezium ridge, oblique downwards and outwards.

Trapezoid

It articulates proximally with the scaphoid and distally with the second metacarpal. Its external part articulates with the internal part of the trapezium and its internal part with the external part of the capitate. The deep bundle of the flexor pollicis brevis and a few fibres of the adductor pollicis insert on its palmar side.

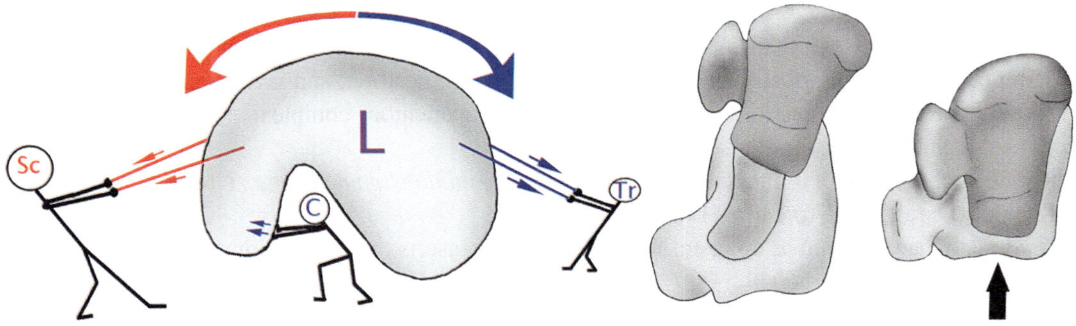

Fig. 1.12 The lunate bone is under opposite constraints; the scaphoid brings it in flexion with the scapholunate ligament, the triquetrum brings it in extension with the lunotriquetral ligament because of the hamate's pressure (2), and the capitate pressing on its posterior part brings it in extension

Capitate

It is the biggest and central carpal bone. It articulates with every other carpal bone, except for the triquetrum. Parts of the deep bundle of the flexor pollicis brevis and adductor pollicis insert on its anterior part.

Hamate

It is prism shaped and articulates proximally with the triquetrum, and distally with the fourth metacarpal (external part) and fifth metacarpal (internal part).

Its external part articulates with the capitate.

The flexor digiti minimi and opponens digiti minimi insert on the hamulus on its anterior part.

Joint Anatomy and Physiology

Radioulnar Joints

They stabilize and mobilize to efficiently direct the hand in pronosupination.

The amplitudes vary from one individual to the other, but it is usually 90° of supination and 60° of pronation.

The pronosupination range of motion is always measured with the elbow against the trunk, with 90° of flexion to prevent the shoulder from participating in the movement.

Some authors (Soubeyrand et al. 2007, 2011) have recently proposed the concept of "radioulnar unity", made of the distal and proximal radioulnar joints, as well as a third part: the interosseous membrane and the ulnar and radial diaphyses (middle lock).

This concept allows us to understand the functioning of the forearm globally, each component depending on the two others.

The three radioulnar joints are complementary and inseparable "locks". If one lock is blocked, it will block the rest of the forearm. However, instability in only one lock can be compensated by the two others.

Therefore, we cannot treat one of the radioulnar locks without checking the two others (Fig. 1.13).

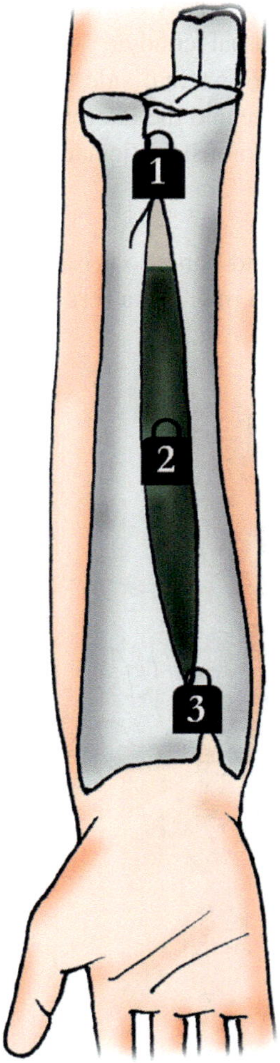

Fig. 1.13 The three locks of the radioulnar unity

Proximal Radioulnar Joint or Proximal Lock

It is a trochoid joint with only one degree of movement. Its congruence is maximal in an intermediate position, and it is stabilized by a powerful ligamentous complex:

- *Annular ligament* (Fig. 1.14)

It inserts on the anterior and posterior parts of the radial notch of the ulna and surrounds the radial head with its internal face that is covered with cartilage. Therefore, it plays de role of a joint surface as well as of a ligament.

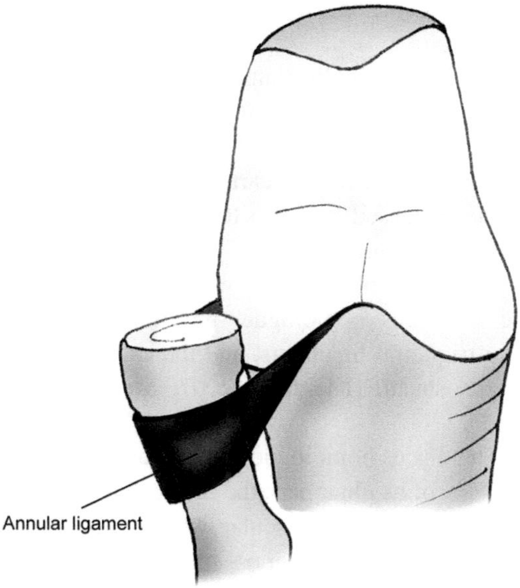

Fig. 1.14 The annular ligament surrounds the radial head. It is a predominant element in the proximal radioulnar stability

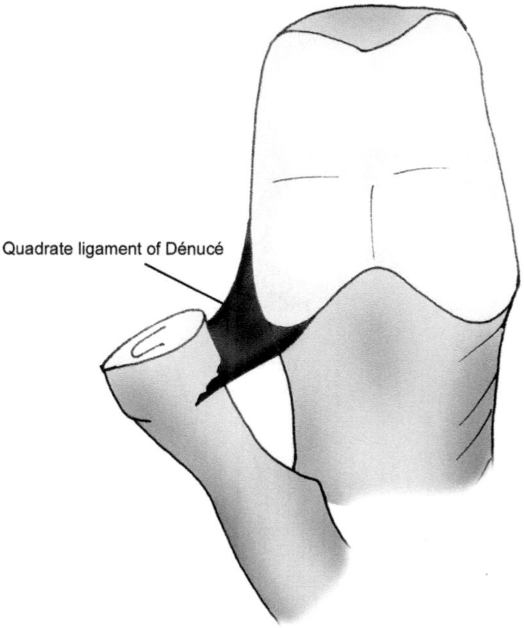

Fig. 1.15 The quadrate ligament is tensed between the radial notch of the ulna and the radial head

- *Quadrate ligament or ligament of Dénucé* (Fig. 1.15)

It inserts on the inferior part of the radial notch of the ulna and ends just below the radial head, above the radial tuberosity.

Its most anterior and posterior fibres mix with the most distal fibres of the annular ligament.

It is tensed in pronation because of its anterior fibres and in supination because of its posterior fibres.

Interosseous Membrane or Intermediate Radioulnar Joint

The middle lock is composed of the interosseous membrane and the two forearm bones described in the paragraph *"Osseous elements"*.

It is tensed on about 10 cm between the radius and the ulna. It is made of crossed connective fibres (collagen and elastin) that form a "network" efficiently opposed to the multidirectional constraints imposed on it:

- *Fibres oriented upwards from the ulna towards the radius (upwards and outwards)*

They form two "membranous" parts, one distal and one proximal, and a middle "ligamentous" part that is thicker and more resistant.

They are the most important, as their orientation allows them to transfer part of the constraints imposed on the radius towards the ulna.

In fact, 80% of the axial constraints are transmitted on the radius through the carpus, but in the elbow 70% of the constraints pass through the humeroulnar joint: the load transfer distribution is inverted between the elbow and the wrist (Fig. 1.16).

The triangular complex participates in this phenomenon at the distal level.

The interest of this load transfer is that the radial head is too fragile to bear 80% of the constraints coming from the carpus, while the coronoid process can do it.

- *Fibre oriented downwards from the ulna towards the radius (downwards and outwards)*

They form two individualized structures: the oblique cord and the proximal band.

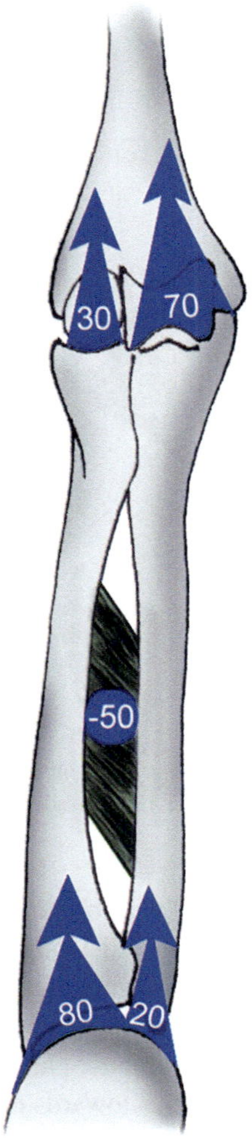

Fig. 1.16 The interosseous membrane transmits part of the longitudinal forces from the radius to the ulna, avoiding any excessive constraints on the radial head that is a fragile spongy bone

- *Tensioning*

The interosseous membrane is always tensed during pronosupination: the proximal part is tensed in pronation, the middle part in a neutral position and the distal part in supination (Soubeyrand et al. 2007) (Fig. 1.17).

Distal Radioulnar Joint or Distal Lock

It is a trochoid joint that is neither concordant, nor congruent (Fig. 1.18), which makes it particularly unstable, especially in pronation and supination (Fig. 1.19). The intermediary position is the most stable one, as in the proximal radioulnar joint.

It is the radioulnar unity's distal lock, stabilized by a powerful ligamentous complex called the triangular complex.

This biconcave fibrocartilage is covered with cartilage, tensed between the ulnar styloid process and the internal side of the radial epiphysis.

It is made of the distal radioulnar ligaments, the meniscus homologue, the ulno-lunar and ulno-triquetral ligaments, and the extensor carpi ulnaris sheath (Kleinman 2007; Mesplie et al. 2017).

The discus homologue is only vascularized in 10–40% of its ulnar part, the centre and the radial part being totally avascular which makes their spontaneous healing impossible.

It can have a hole in the middle, without any traumatic origin.

It stabilizes the distal radioulnar joint, but it is also a meniscus hanging between the two forearm bones and the carpus (Mesplie et al. 2017).

Because of this, it is under important multidirectional constraints. It opposes these constraints in different ways:

- Cushioning the longitudinal constraints, as 20% of the axial constraints of the wrist are transferred towards the ulna. It also participates in the transfer of the longitudinal forces from the radius towards the ulna, along with the interosseous membrane.
- Limiting pronosupination, putting in tension the anterior fibres of the superficial plane and the posterior fibres of the deep plane in supination, and the posterior fibres of the superficial plane and the anterior fibres of the deep plane in pronation (Fig. 1.20).
- Preventing the radius and the ulna from moving away from each other, especially when clamping (which causes the capitate to go upwards, leading to constraints on the distal radioulnar joint).

Biomechanics of the Radioulnar Unity

The pronosupination biomechanics depends on the conformation of the two forearm bones and the functional coupling of the radioulnar joints.

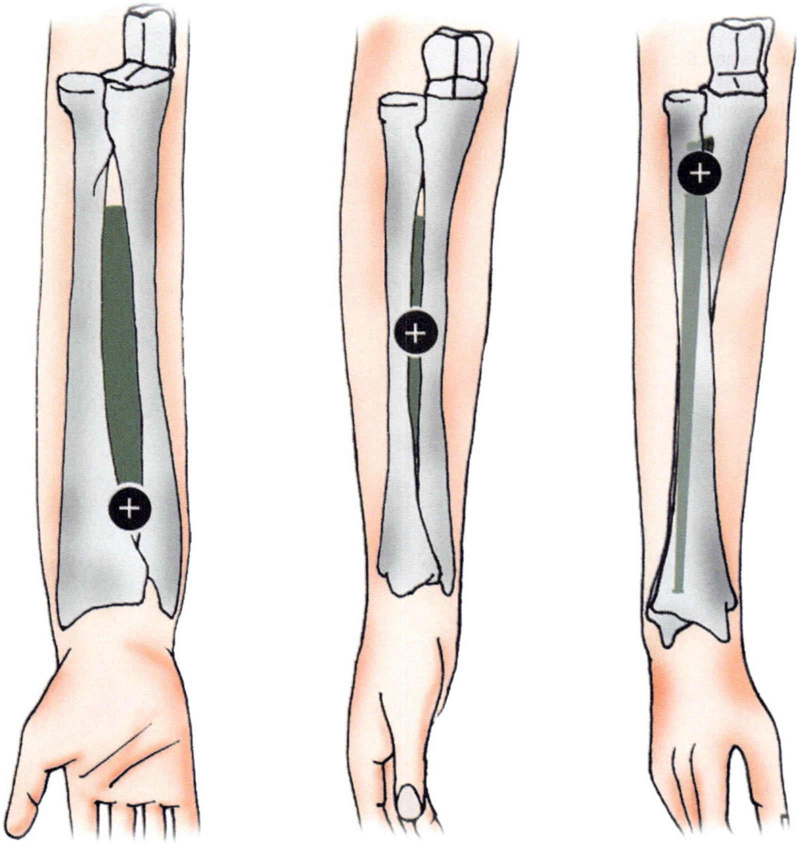

Fig. 1.17 The interosseous membrane is always tensed during pronosupination: its distal part during supination, its middle part during the intermediary position and its proximal part during pronation

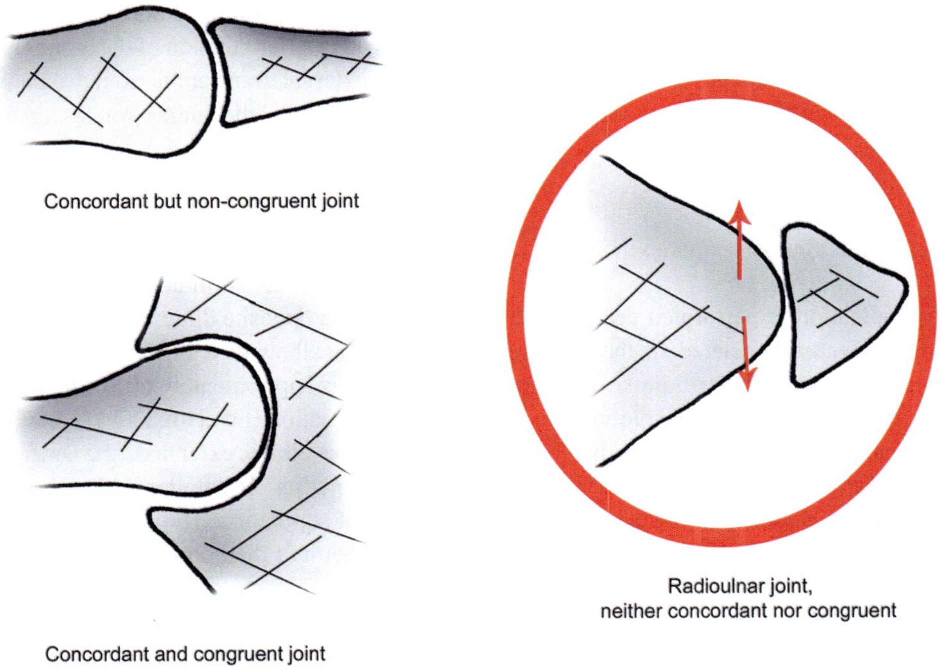

Fig. 1.18 The distal radioulnar joint is neither congruent (the bony elements do not "fit" together) nor concordant. This leads to joint instability

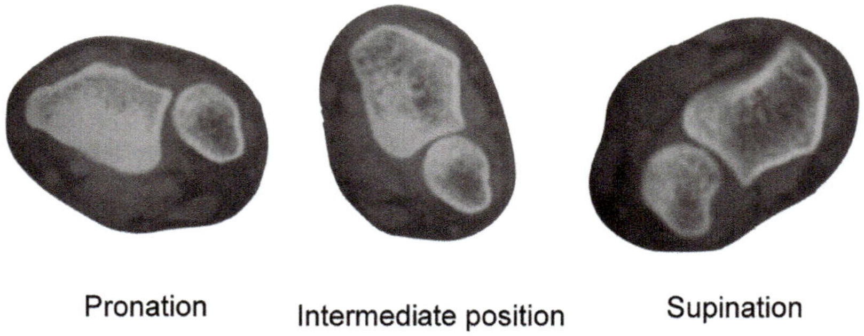

Fig. 1.19 The contact surface between the radius and the ulna is maximal in the intermediate position, which makes it the stability position for this joint

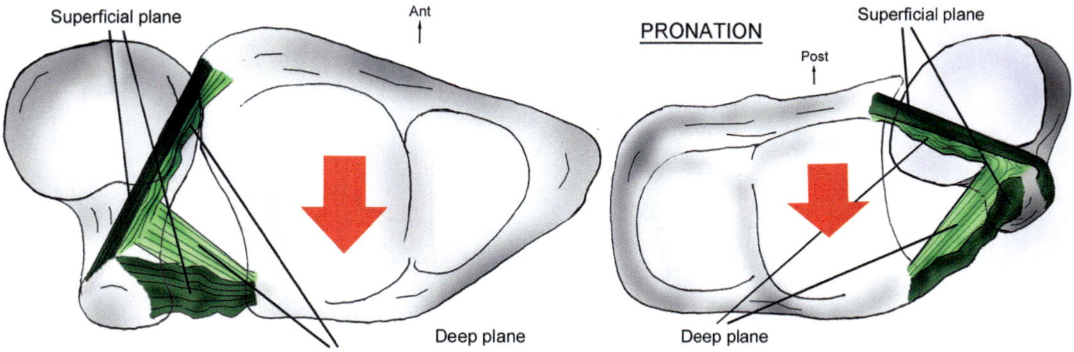

Fig. 1.20 The distal radioulnar ligaments stabilize the distal radioulnar joint by tensioning the anterior fibres of the superficial plane and the posterior fibres of the deep plane in supination (1), and the posterior fibres of the superficial plane and the anterior fibres of the deep plane in pronation (2)

- *Opposite concavity*

It is essential to maintain a normal pronation as it avoids the early block that would appear in pronation if the two bones were straight (Fig. 1.21).

- *Pronosupination biomechanics*

Pronosupination is performed according to a harmonious dynamics related to the functional coupling of the radioulnar joints. It happens around a non-materialized evolutionary axis passing near the radial and ulnar heads.

Even though the displacement of the radius is a lot less important than the one of the ulna, it does not stay still, and the two bones of the forearm perform a complex movement of circumduction, in opposite directions. The humerus participates in the movement in two different ways depending on the elbow's position (flexed or extended).

In pronation with the elbow in 90° of flexion, there is an external rotation of the humerus inducing an external translation of the ulna via the olecranon, while the radius rotates on its own axis (Fig. 1.22).

In supination with the elbow in 90° of flexion, we observe the opposite movement: an internal rotation of the humerus combined with an internal translation of the ulna and a rotation of the radius in the opposite direction (Fig. 1.23).

With the elbow flexed (90°), the normal range of motion is approximately 60° of pronation and 95° of supination (Fu et al. 2009).

With the elbow extended, the amplitude of pronosupination is smaller (40° of pronation and 90° of supination) (Fu et al. 2009), because of the tension of the humeroulnar ligaments and the loss of efficiency of the biceps and pronator teres placed in external race. However, this loss is largely compensated by the humeral internal rotation in pronation and the humeral external

Fig. 1.21 The opposite concavity of the two forearm bones avoids an early stop in pronation

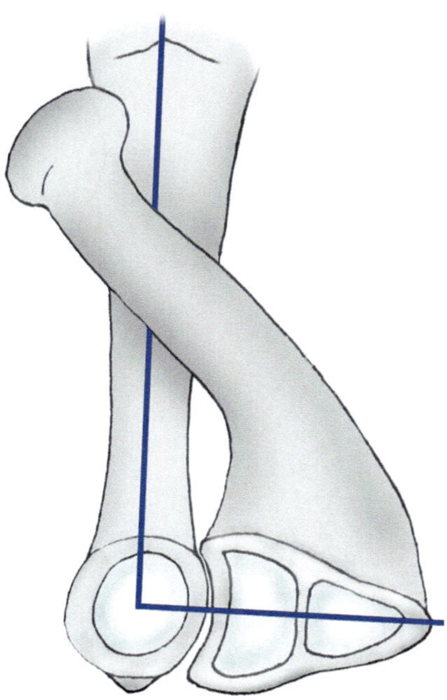

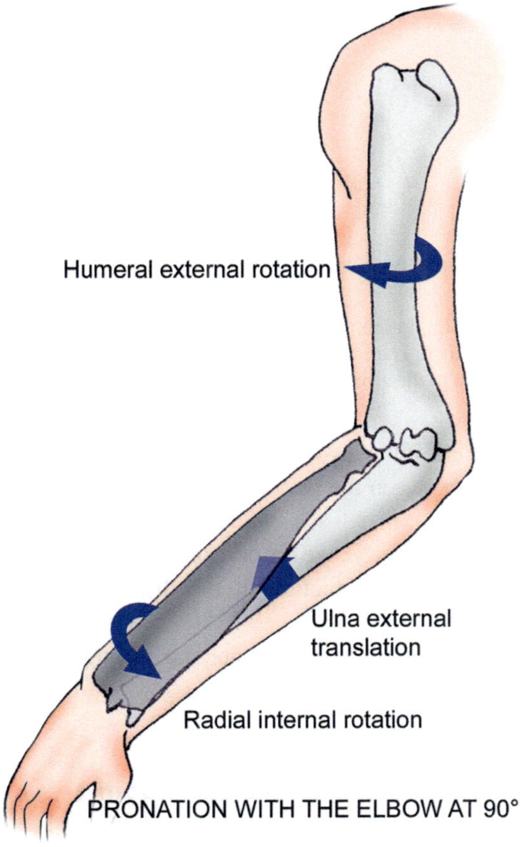

Fig. 1.22 In elbow flexion, the pronation is combined with an external rotation of the humerus

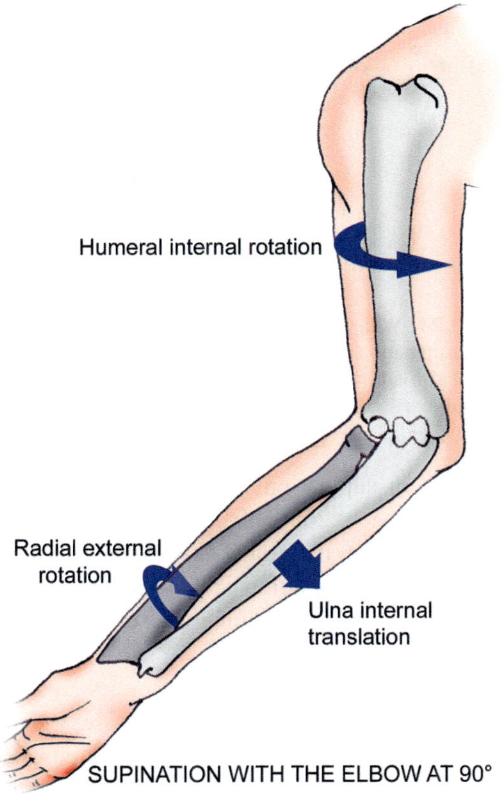

Fig. 1.23 In elbow flexion, the supination is combined with an internal rotation of the humerus

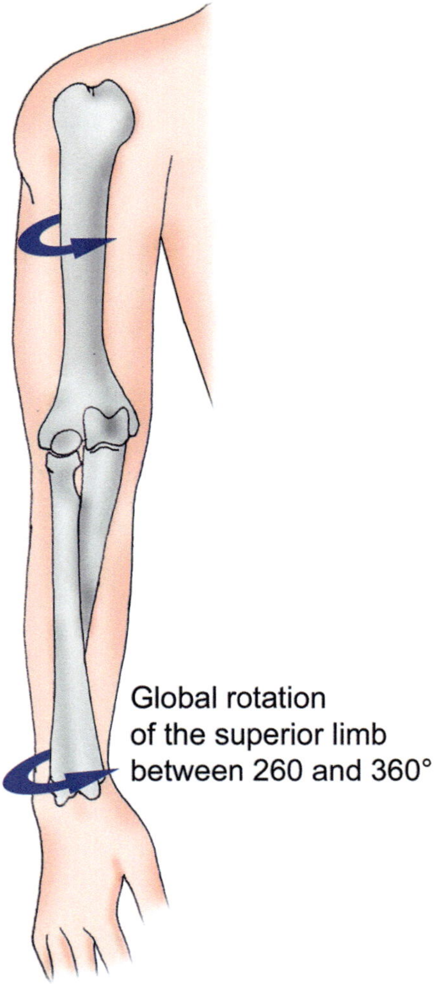

Fig. 1.24 With the elbow extended, the amplitudes of pronosupination and humeral rotation are added and allow a global rotation between 260° and 360°, depending on the authors

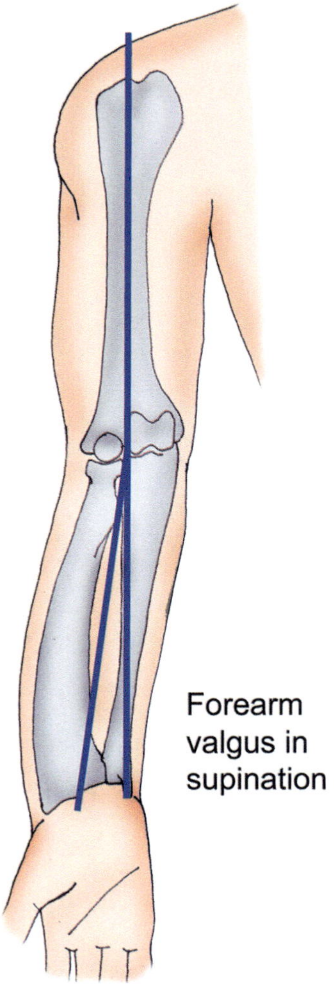

Fig. 1.25 In elbow extension with the palm towards the front, there is a physiological valgus of the forearm with respect to the arm

rotation in supination, which allow the whole limb to reach 260–360° (Fig. 1.24). In this elbow position, the global axis of the forearm is in valgus in supination and considered as the extension of the humerus in pronation (Fig. 1.25).

During pronation, the radius goes upwards with respect to the ulna, which increases the distal radioulnar index and the axial constraints on the radial head. The radial head moves forward with respect to the capitulum.

In pronation, the radial fovea presents its great axis, which leads to the radius moving apart from the ulna, allowing the passage of the radial tuberosity between the two bones (Arnold-peter et al. 1992).

In supination, we observe the opposite mechanism with a reduction of the distal radioulnar index.

The radioulnar joints are most congruent in the intermediate position.

Radio-carpal and Midcarpal Joints

The radio-carpal joint brings together the receiving cavity (radial epiphysis and triangular com-

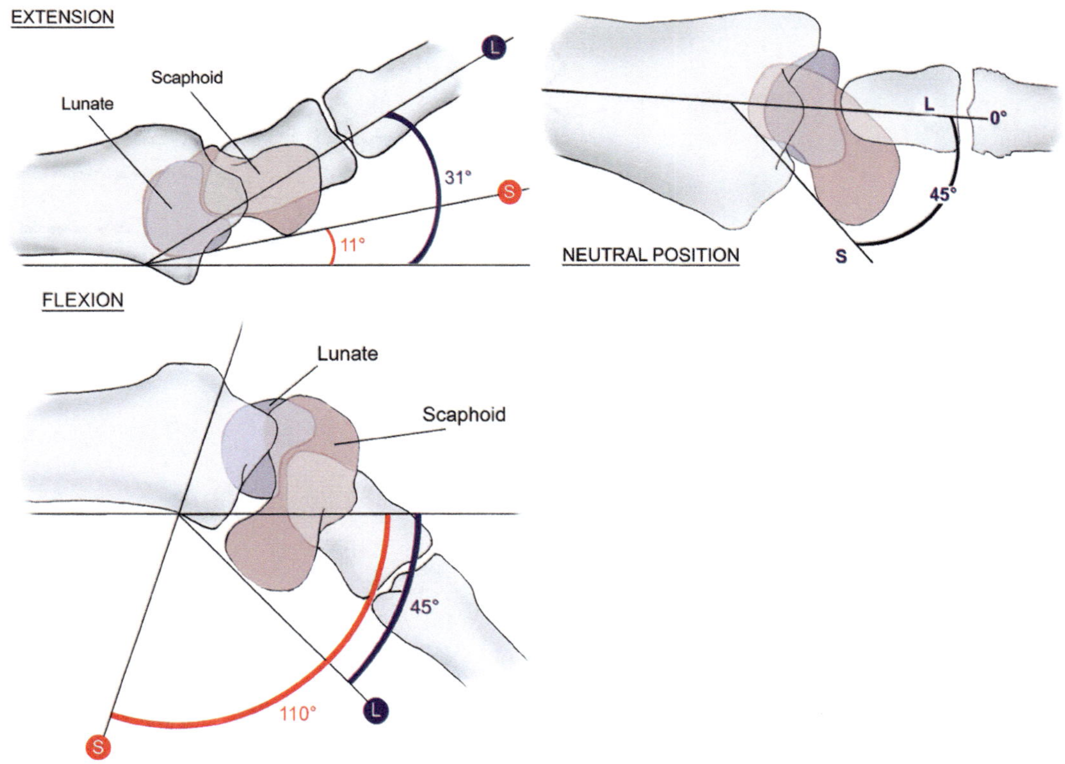

Fig. 1.26 The differential movement between the scaphoid and the lunate in the radio-carpal and midcarpal joints induces a rotation between those two bones. In extension, the scaphoid moves towards a 56° extension and the lunate towards a 31° extension with respect to the radius (1). In a neutral position, the lunate is aligned with the radius while the scaphoid is oriented in a 45° flexion (2). In flexion, the scaphoid moves towards a 65° flexion and the lunate towards a 45° flexion with respect to the radius (3)

plex) with the carpal condyle. It is neither concordant nor congruent.

The midcarpal joint is extremely complex and would be a plane joint for its lateral part, but rather a condyloid for its medial part. However, the opinions differ, and it seems that it works more like a screw thread allowing screwing and unscrewing the first and second carpal rows around the capitate.

Together, these two joints participate in global wrist mobility which is normally 45° of ulnar inclination, 15° of radial inclination, and 90° of flexion/extension—those numbers vary a lot from one person to the other (Kapandji 2005). At the level of the central column (lunate and capitate), 2/3 of the movements are performed in the midcarpal joint in extension and 1/3 in flexion. On the other hand, in the radial column (scaphoid, trapezium, and trapezoid), 2/3 of the movements are performed in the radio-carpal joint in flexion and extension (Kaufmann et al. 2006). This asynchrony explains the important rotations observed between the lunate and the scaphoid in wrist flexion, extension, and inclinations (Fig. 1.26).

There are no extrinsic tendinous insertions on the carpus except on the pisiform (flexor carpi ulnaris). This anatomical data helps us understand that with each extrinsic muscular contraction, the first carpal row is under compressive constraints to which it will have to adapt.

The ligamentous system of the wrist is made of deep and superficial palmar ligaments, and dorsal ligaments.

Extrinsic Ligaments of the Wrist

The extrinsic ligamentous system is composed of ligaments tensed between the radius and the first

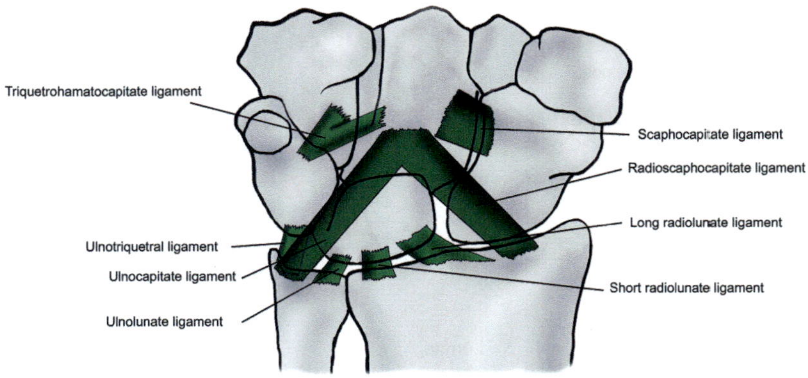

Fig. 1.27 Main superficial volar ligaments of the wrist

carpal row, between the first and the second carpal rows, and between the radius and the second carpal row. This complex system stabilizes the carpus along with the intrinsic ligaments and allows it to adapt to the constraints imposed on it.

The palmar ligaments are histologically stronger than the dorsal ones, which are more innervated (Hagert et al. 2007).

- *Essential ligaments* (Fig. 1.27)

Those ligaments play an important role in the carpal stability. On the palmar side, they are:

- The radio-scapho-capitate ligament
- The long radio-lunate ligament
- The short radio-lunate ligament
- The ulno-capitate ligament
- The scapho-capitate ligament
- The ulno-lunate ligament
- The ulno-triquetral ligament
- The triquetro-hamato-capitate ligament

On the dorsal side, the ligamentous system is less extensive and includes (Fig. 1.30) (Soubeyrand et al. 2007):

- The dorsal radio-carpal ligament (or dorsal radio-triquetral ligament)
- The dorsal intercarpal ligament (Viegas et al. 1999) (Fig. 1.28)
- The dorsal scapho-triquetral ligament
- The dorsal capsule-scapholunate septum (DCSS)

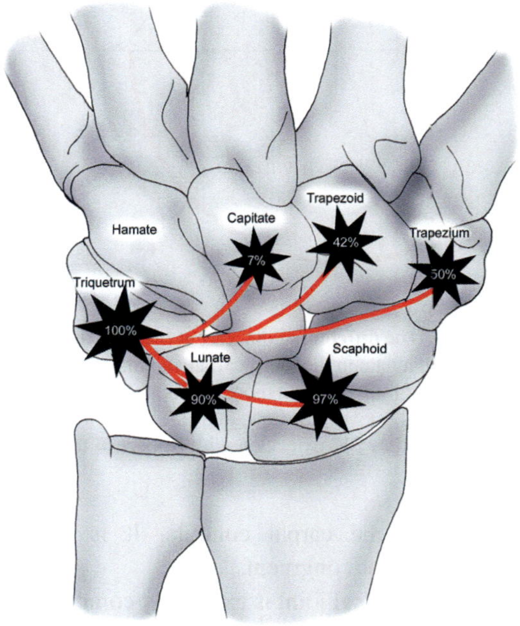

Fig. 1.28 Possible trajectories for the dorsal intercarpal ligament, and frequencies of its various insertions (according to Viegas—1999)

- *Roles in the frontal plane*

In the frontal plane, the palmar system must oppose the anterior pressure of the carpus related to the radial slope (oblique downwards and backwards).

There is a powerful palmar and dorsal anchor point at the level of the triquetrum, fighting against the tendency of the first carpal row to slide towards the ulnar side because of the radial

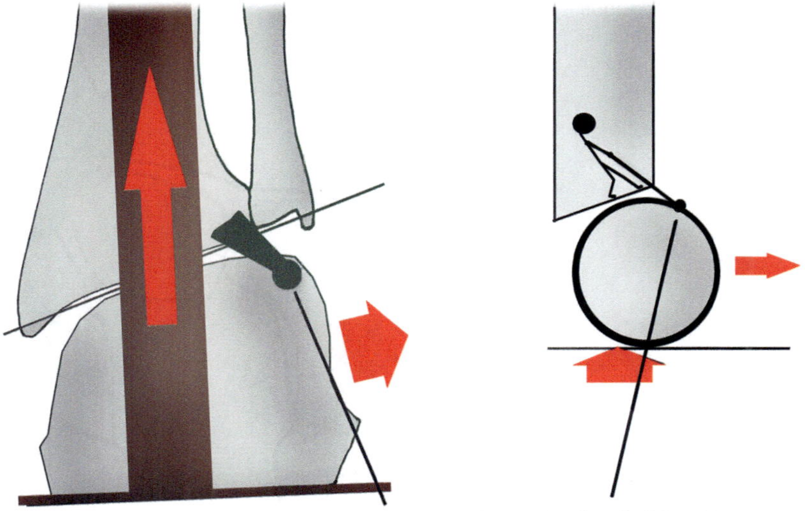

Fig. 1.29 The ulnar ligamentary anchor opposes the carpal physiological gliding occurring because of the longitudinal constraints and radial slope

slope (oblique downward and outwards) and the longitudinal muscle forces (Fig. 1.29).

This "pyramidal sling" is made of the anterior and posterior radio-triquetral ligaments, reinforced by the ulno-triquetral ligament, the dorsal intercarpal ligament, the dorsal scapho-triquetral ligament, and the triquetro-hamato-capitate ligament (Fig. 1.30).

This tendency of the first carpal row to slide towards the ulnar slide is increased in radial inclination, which is a naturally unstable position. It is cancelled in ulnar inclination, which is a natural functional and stable wrist position, as the first row is centred and coapted by the contraction of the longitudinal muscles that are perpendicular to the radial slope in this position (Fig. 1.31).

The radio-scapho-capitate ligament acts as a pivot imposing an automatic pronation on the scaphoid when the bone goes towards flexion (Fig. 1.32).

The radio-scapho-lunate ligament has a poor mechanical resistance but carries radio-carpal vessels (Fig. 1.33).

- *Roles in the sagittal plane*

In the sagittal plane, the wrist is stable when it is straight as the anterior and posterior ligamentous systems are equally tensed.

At 10° of flexion, the wrist is in its most stable position as the lunate is centred under the radial epiphysis that is oriented downwards and frontwards, and coapted by the longitudinal muscles.

However, in extension, the lunate slides frontwards along the radial slope and the longitudinal muscles increase this displacement. The anterior ligaments are important stabilizers and get tensed proportionally to the degree of extension to oppose this gliding (Fig. 1.34).

Therefore, the most stable position is in a 10° flexion and a 25° ulnar inclination.

Interosseous Ligaments

- *First carpal row*

They are particularly and allow transmitting the sagittal movements from one bone to the other.

The scapholunate ligament is made of three bundles with different mechanical resistances as the palmar portion has a resistance of 150 Newtons while the dorsal portion has a resistance of 300 Newtons.

Its elasticity allows a wide amplitude of movement between the scaphoid and the lunate, essential for the good functioning of the scapholunate pair.

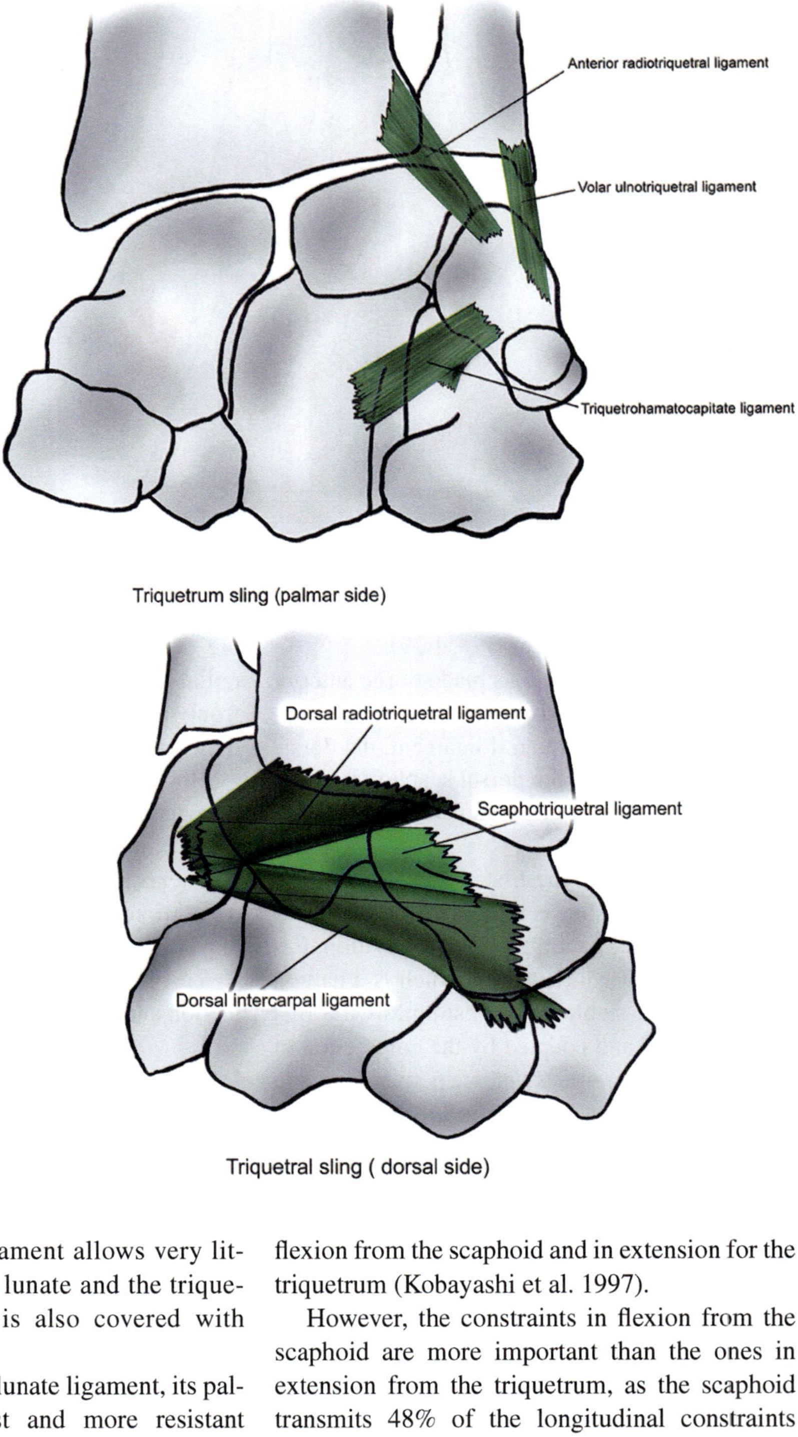

Fig. 1.30 Composition of the triquetral sling on the volar side (1) and on the dorsal side (2)

The lunotriquetral ligament allows very little mobility between the lunate and the triquetrum. Its superior part is also covered with cartilage.

Contrary to the scapholunate ligament, its palmar part is the thickest and more resistant (approximately 300 Newtons) than its dorsal part (150 Newtons).

The lunate hangs between the scaphoid and the triquetrum that have ligaments with equivalent resistances transmitting antagonist forces: in flexion from the scaphoid and in extension for the triquetrum (Kobayashi et al. 1997).

However, the constraints in flexion from the scaphoid are more important than the ones in extension from the triquetrum, as the scaphoid transmits 48% of the longitudinal constraints from the second carpal row while the triquetrum only transmits 20%.

Balance is maintained by the axial pressure of the capitate that brings the lunate in extension (Fig. 1.35).

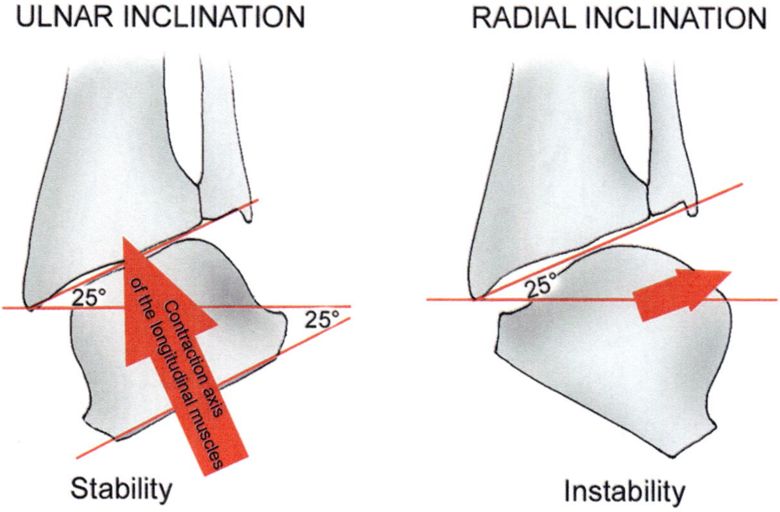

Fig. 1.31 In the frontal plane, the carpus is more stable in ulnar inclination as the ulnar gliding is null in this position. It is the opposite in radial inclination as the ulnar gliding is majored in this position

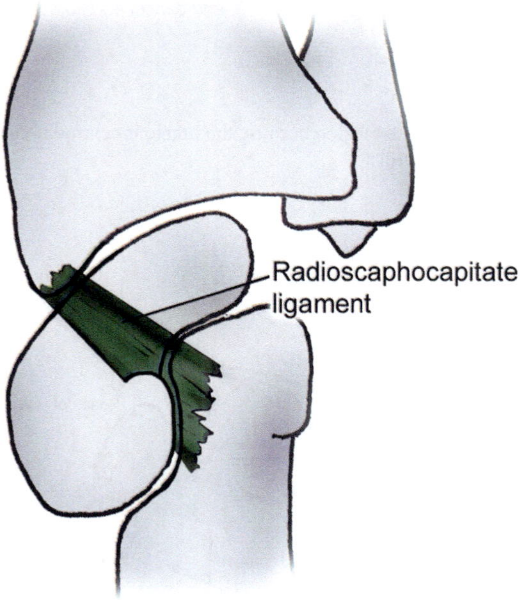

Fig. 1.32 The radioscapho-capitate ligament is a powerful anti-flexion stabilizer of the scaphoid

- *At the midcarpal level*

Ligaments are in the lateral and medial parts of the joint but are absent between the lunate and capitate.

Laterally, the distal scaphoid ligaments transmit the constraints from the second carpal row on the scaphoid and stabilize its distal pole.

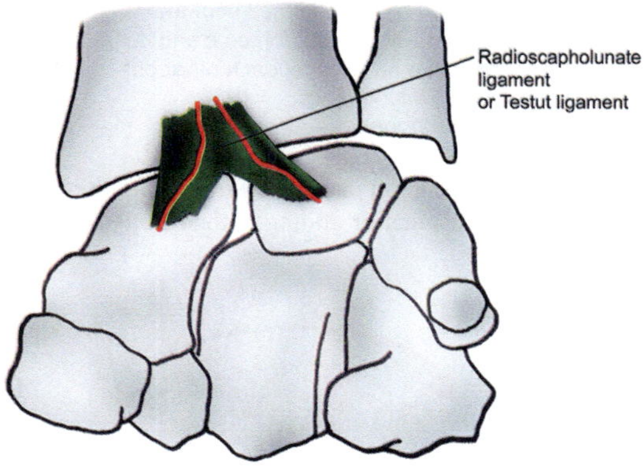

Fig. 1.33 The radioscapholunate ligament plays a vessel carrier role. Its mechanical action is very limited

Medially, the triquetro-hamatal system transmits the constraints from the second row to the first row and stabilizes the triquetro-hamatal space.

The arched ligament is made of the scapho-capital and triquetro-capital ligaments. It forms a central midcarpal lock essential in stability if we consider the fragility area created by the lack of luno-capital ligament (space of Poirier) (Fig. 1.36).

- *In the second row*

Ligaments lock the four distal carpal bones so that they biomechanically act like a monolithic block.

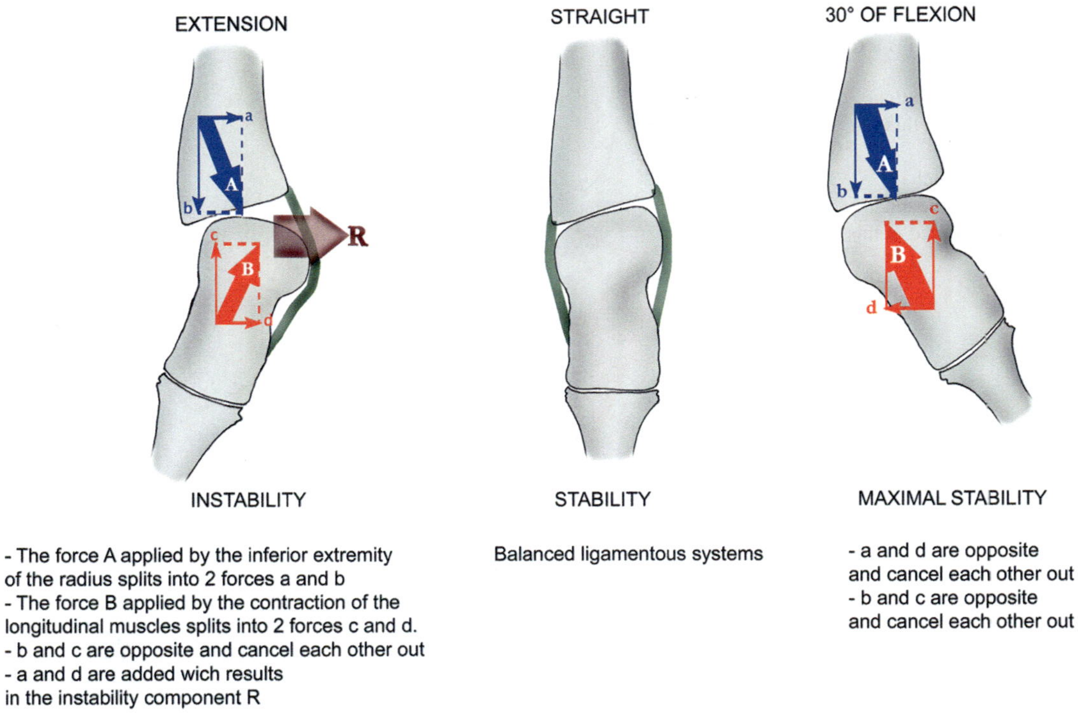

Fig. 1.34 In the sagittal plane, the carpus is more stable in flexion than in extension because the lunate is centred under the radius and the anterior gliding of the carpus along the radial slope is null

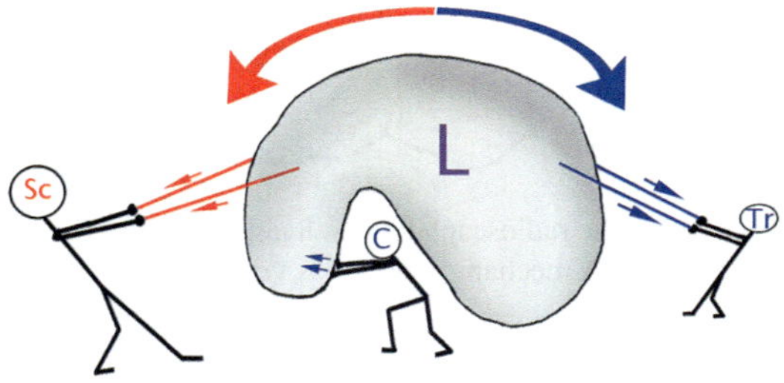

Fig. 1.35 The lunate bone is under opposite constraints; the scaphoid brings it in flexion while the capitate and the triquetrum bring it in extension

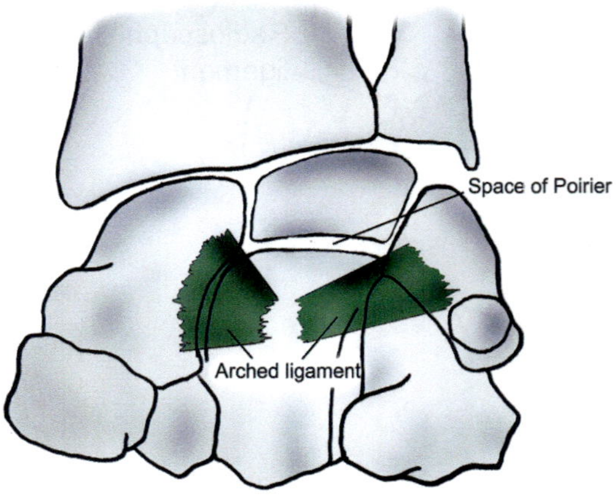

Fig. 1.36 The arched ligament stabilizes the midcarpal joint, which fragility zone is the space of Poirier between the lunate and capitate

Organization in "V"

Various ligamentous systems have this type of organization:

- *Proximal palmar "V"*: radio-lunate and ulno-lunate ligaments.
- *Distal palmar "V"*: scapho-capitate and triquetro-capitate ligaments (those two ligaments make the arched ligament) (Fig. 1.37).
- *Palmar triquetral "V"*: palmar radio-triquetral and triquetro-hamato-capital ligaments (Fig. 1.37).
- *Dorsal triquetral "V"*: dorsal intercarpal ligament (tense in ulnar inclination) and dorsal radio-triquetral ligament (tense in radial inclination) (Fig. 1.38).

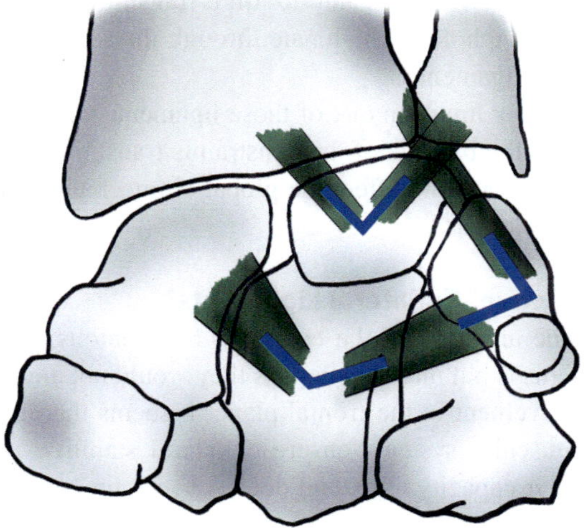

Fig. 1.37 "V" shape of the extrinsic volar ligamentous system

Oval-Ring Theory (Fig. 1.39)

The oval-ring theory helps us understand the way constraints are transmitted in the wrist. According to this concept, the wrist depends on four essential ligaments, whose role is to transmit the constraints from the second carpal row towards the first one (scapho-capital and triquetro-hamato-capital ligaments), and between the bones of the first row (scapholunate and lunotriquetral ligaments) (Garcia-Elias 2013).

In this theory, at the medial level, the triqeutro-hamato-capital ligament transmits constraints from the hamate to the triquetrum, which makes the triquetrum go in extension. This posterior tilt is transmitted from the triquetrum to the lunate through the lunotriquetral ligament.

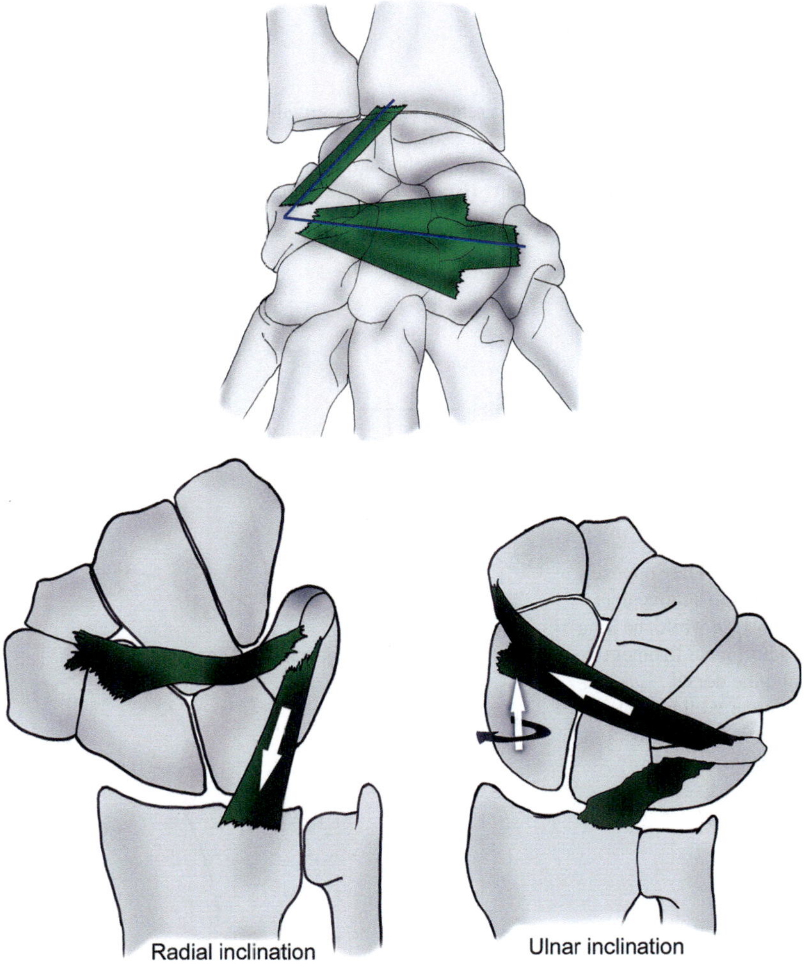

Fig. 1.38 "V" shape of the extrinsic dorsal ligamentous system, with a triquetral apex (1). In radial inclination, the dorsal radio-triquetral ligament is tense while the dorsal intercarpal ligament is relaxed. In ulnar inclination, the mechanism is reversed

At the radial level, the scapho-capitate ligament transmits the constraints from the bones of the second carpal row to the scaphoid, making it go in flexion. This anterior tilt is transmitted from the scaphoid to the lunate through the scapholunate ligament.

Any injury in one of those ligaments will disturb the balance of the constraints transmitted to the lunate and affect the global biomechanics of the carpus.

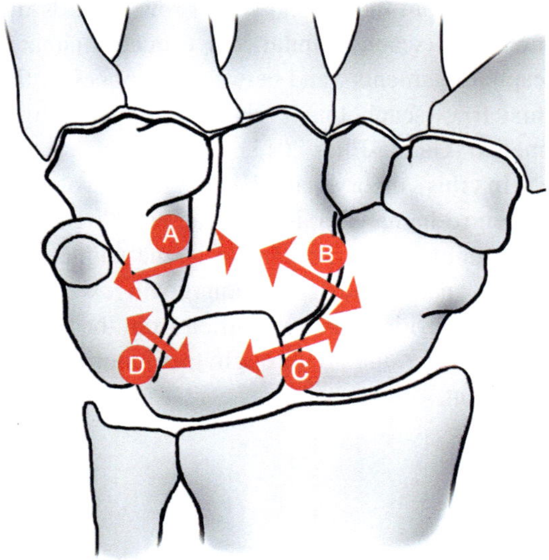

Fig. 1.39 The wrist kinematics is related to four essential ligaments. Their role is to transmit the stress from the second carpal row towards the first (triquetrohamatocapitate (**a**) and scapho-capitate ligaments (**b**)), and between the bones of the first carpal row (scapholunate (**c**) and lunotriquetral (**d**) ligaments))

"Active" Collateral Ligaments?

The anatomy of the collateral ligamentous systems is put into question, as they would not allow movement in the frontal plane. It seems that the muscular systems ensure collateral stability, as their capacity to extend does not restrain contralateral movements.

This active system is made of the extensor and flexor carpi ulnaris for the ulnar side, and the abductor pollicis longus, extensor pollicis brevis, extensor carpi radialis longus and flexor carpi radialis for the radial side.

Notion of Lunate "Mooring" (Fig. 1.40)

New mechanical models show the importance of extrinsic ligaments, that stabilize the lunate in the sagittal plane (Raja et al. 2022).

The dorsal radio-carpal (or dorsal radio-triquetral), triquetro-capital, and palmar scapho-

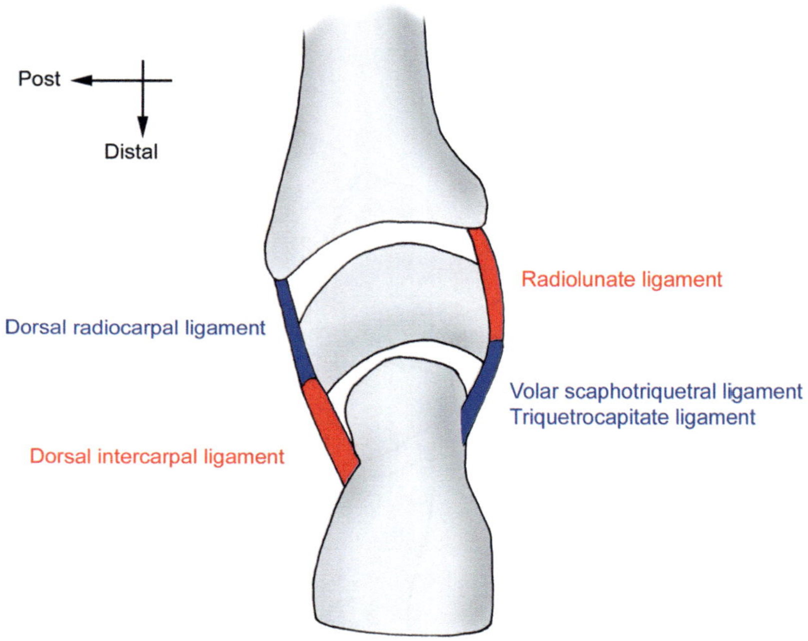

Fig. 1.40 "Mooring" concept for the lunate with the dorsal radio-carpal ligament (or dorsal radio-triquetral ligament), the volar scapho-triquetral ligament, and the triquetro-capitate ligament. They oppose the lunate's movement in flexion while the long radio-lunate ligament and the dorsal intercarpal ligament oppose its movement in extension

triquetral ligaments oppose the flexion of the lunate, while the long radioulnar and dorsal intercarpal ligaments oppose its extension.

Retinacular Ligaments

- *The flexors retinaculum*

It is the most powerful reflexion pulley in the human body. It optimizes the angle of the flexor system and protects the carpal tunnel. It is also the anchor for the thenar and hypothenar muscles.

- *The extensors retinaculum*

It is made of a transverse part and an oblique part. The transverse part plays the role of a reflexion pulley for the six synovial slides of the extensors of the long fingers, thumb, and wrist. The oblique part is oriented downwards and inwards and ties the ulnar side of the carpus and the extensor carpi ulnaris (with which it shares some fibres), before inserting on the pisiform.

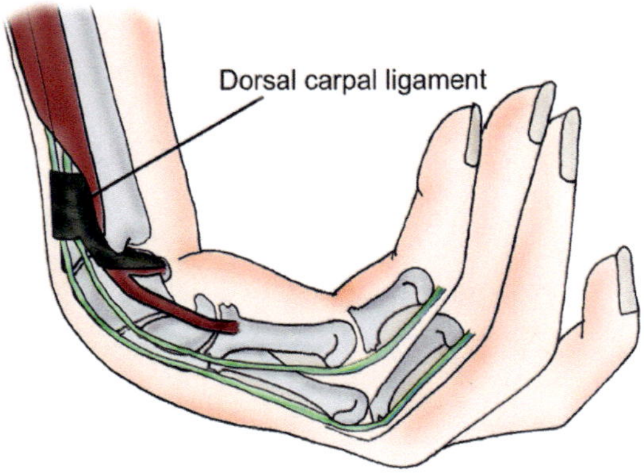

Fig. 1.41 The dorsal carpal ligament plays the role of a pulley for the extensor systems. Its oblique part ends on the pisiform and therefore participates in stabilizing the ulnar compartment of the carpus

This oblique portion participates in the formation of the triquetral anchor and therefore in the frontal carpal stabilization. It does not stabilize the ulnar head as it is more distal (Fig. 1.41).

Triangular Complex

Already described in the paragraph about the distal radioulnar joint, it is a fibrocartilage covered with cartilage helping to transmit the axial constraints from the carpus towards the forearm frame and participating in the stabilization of the distal radioulnar joint.

Proprioceptive Aspect

Proprioception is the ability to feel and perceive oneself. It is a key element in maintaining joint homeostasis, defined as a dynamic process in which the organism maintains and controls its environment despite external disturbances (Hagert 2010).

The ligamentous systems of the wrist are made of mechanoreceptors (Hagert 2010; Petrie et al. 1997) (Table 1.1) that send afferent information towards the posterior horn of the spinal cord in two ways:

- A monosynaptic way that relays information from the posterior horn to the anterior horn and allows a rapid reflex motor response.
- A polysynaptic way is destined to the somato-sensitivo-motor cortex and the cerebellum, where the information is treated to create a slower adapted motor response.

The distribution of mechanoreceptors is different in the dorsal ligaments (high density) and the palmar ligaments (lower density) (Hagert et al. 2005).

Table 1.1 Mechanoreceptors in the wrist ligaments

Name	Neurophysiological characteristics	Role in the joint's function
Ruffini	Slow adaption, low threshold	Joint position, modification of the speed/amplitude
Pacini	Fast adaptation, low threshold	Acceleration/deceleration
Golgi	Fast adaptation	High threshold, extreme amplitudes
Free nerve endings	Fast A ∂ fibres, slow C fibres	Pain, inflammation, harmful situation
Unclassifiable	Unknown	Unknown

Carpal Dynamics

Scapholunate Pair

The scapholunate pair is a key element in the carpal dynamics, as their permanent adaptation maintains the spatial alignment of the carpus by filling the "empty spaces".

To obtain this result, their "working distance" (distance between the radius and the second row) must adapt to the wrist positions.

In a straight position, the lunate's working distance is medium, and the scaphoid's is maximal.

In flexion, it is maximal for the lunate as its anterior horn (the biggest) interposes, and minimal for the scaphoid that is completely down.

In extension, it is minimal for the lunate that presents its posterior horn (the thinnest) and medium for the scaphoid that is upright, but the trapezium slides dorsally to reduce the working distance (Fig. 1.42).

Global Movements

During wrist movements, there is an adaptive carpal dynamics to maintain the joint cohesion. It is related to the conformation of the bones and the tension of the ligamentous systems.

According to I. A. Kapandji (2005), during flexion, the first carpal row performs a flexion/abduction/pronation while the second row performs a flexion/adduction/supination. The two flexions add up and the components of pronation/supination and abduction/adduction cancel each other out. This compensatory mechanism achieves a global simple flexion.

During extension, we observe the opposite movement of extension/adduction/supination

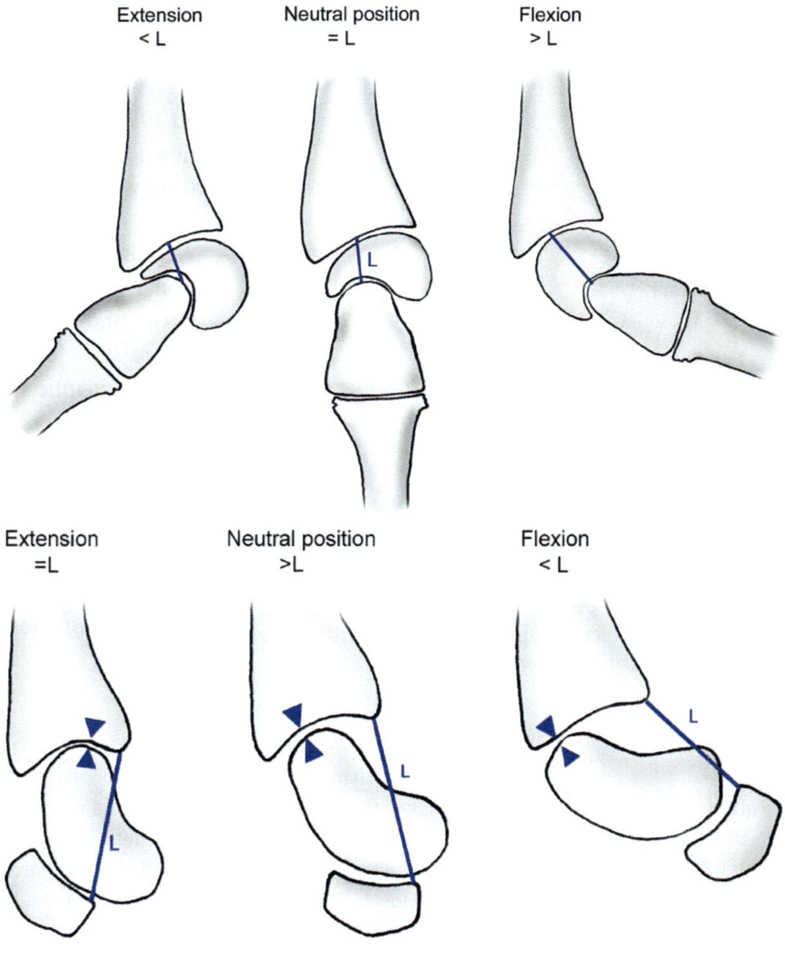

Fig. 1.42 The adaptability of the scapholunate pair allows modifying the space between the second carpal row and the radius, guaranteeing a good spatial consistency in the carpus

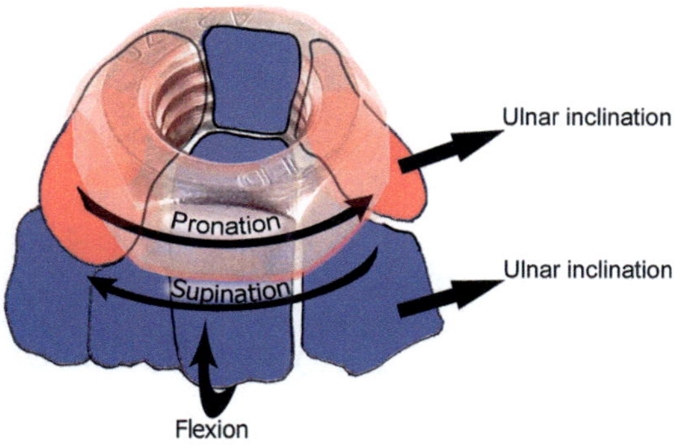

Fig. 1.43 In wrist flexion, both carpal rows go to flexion and ulnar inclination, but the scaphoid and the triquetrum go to pronation while the other carpal bones go to supination

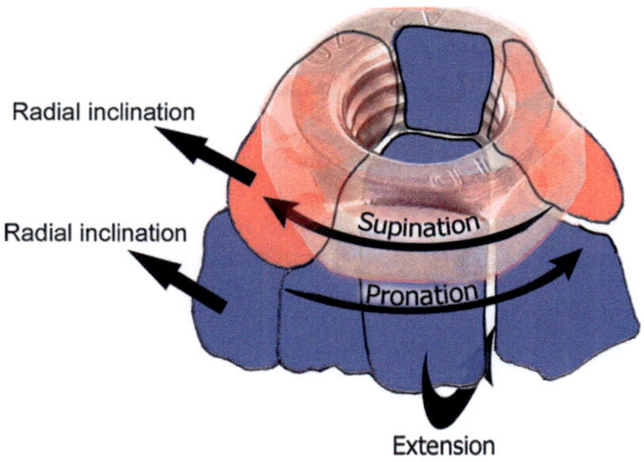

Fig. 1.44 In wrist extension both carpal rows go to extension and radial inclination, but the scaphoid and the triquetrum go to supination while the other carpal bones go to pronation

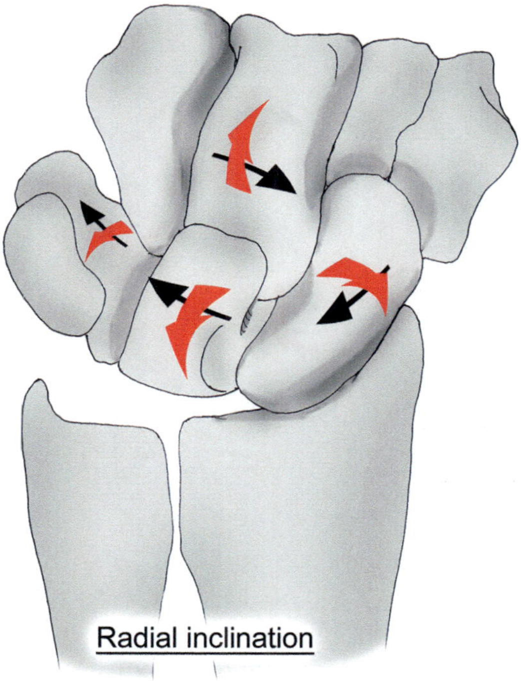

Fig. 1.45 In wrist radial inclination both carpal rows go to abduction, but the first row goes to flexion while the second row goes to extension. The resulting movement is a "simple" radial inclination

in the first row and extension/abduction/pronation in the second row. The two extensions add up and the components of pronation/supination and abduction/adduction cancel each other out.

According to other authors (Horii et al. 1991), in flexion the two rows perform a flexion and an ulnar inclination, but the scaphoid and the triquetrum perform a pronation while the other carpal bones perform a supination (Horii et al. 1991) (Fig. 1.43).

In extension, the opposite movements happen (Fig. 1.44).

In radial inclination, the trapezo-trapezoid joint moves upwards, thus reducing the radio-trapezo-trapezoid space, bringing the scaphoid to flexion. The triquetrum is maintained by the pyramidal "sling" and moves up the hamate slope towards the capitate, placing it in flexion. Therefore, the height of the radial column is reduced, and the height of the ulnar column is increased.

The scapholunate and lunotriquetral ligaments transmit this flexion component to the lunate, making the first row tilt in flexion. The lunate tilt brings the capitate frontwards, and then the rest of the second carpal row in extension (Fig. 1.45).

During an ulnar inclination, the triquetrum slides in an ulnar and palmar direction along the hamate, placing it in extension (Fig. 1.46). The height of the radial column increases and the height of the ulnar column decreases.

The scapholunate and lunotriquetral ligaments transmit this extension component to the lunate. The capitate performs a flexion and brings the second row with it.

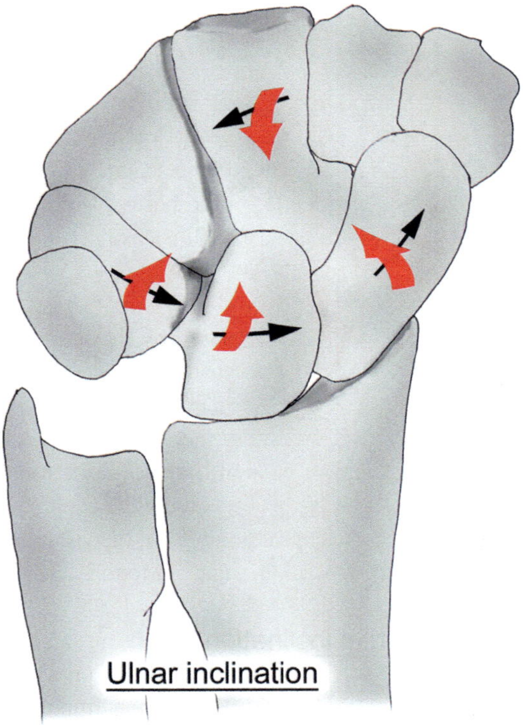

Fig. 1.46 In wrist ulnar inclination both carpal rows go to adduction, but the first row goes to extension while the second row goes to flexion. The resulting movement is a "simple" ulnar inclination

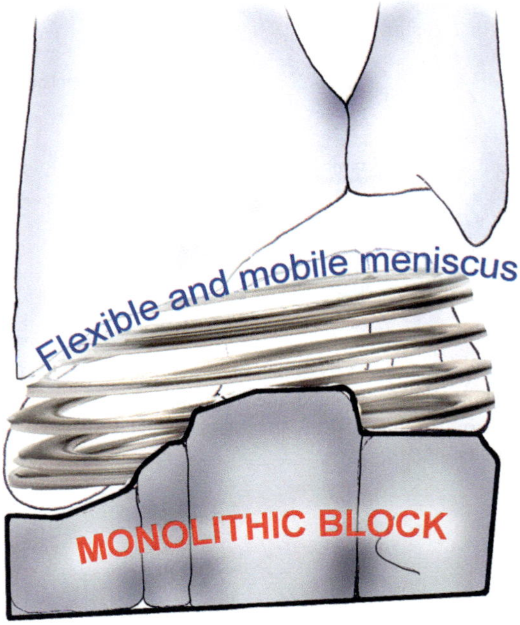

Fig. 1.47 The first carpal row is schematically identified as a flexible meniscus that adapts to the constraints imposed on it, while the second row is compared to a monolithic block with no adaptive capacity

"Variable Geometry" of the Carpus

The carpus is mostly under compressive constraints from the extrinsic muscles. Therefore, it requires great adaptative abilities to absorb part of these longitudinal constraints (Fig. 1.47).

These constraints are first transmitted to the second row, considered as a monolithic block, and then to the first row that can be compared to a flexible and mobile meniscus absorbing these longitudinal constraints.

Under these constraints, the scaphoid tends to perform a flexion and the triquetrum tends to go in extension (Fig. 1.48). However, according to some authors, in these conditions the flexion of the scaphoid is combined with a supination, and the extension of the triquetrum is combined with a pronation (Kobayashi et al. 1997). Other authors (Salva-Coll et al. 2011) describe a combination of flexion and pronation for the scaphoid, and of extension and supination for the triquetrum.

Dart Throwing Motion

The dart thrower's motion (DTM) is defined by the International Federation of Societies for Surgery of the Hand as the movement between radial extension and ulnar flexion. It is the most used movement in our daily activities (Crisco et al. 2005). It is in a movement plane of 45° between the sagittal and frontal planes. It is performed almost exclusively in the medio-carpal joint, without any participation of the radio-carpal joint.

Several studies have shown these dynamics without any ligamentous injury. However, in case of a total rupture of the scapholunate ligament, the DTM's dynamics are disturbed, and the scaphoid acts as a bone of the second carpal row: there is a decoaptation of the scapholunate joint in ulnar inclination (Garcia-Elias et al. 2014).

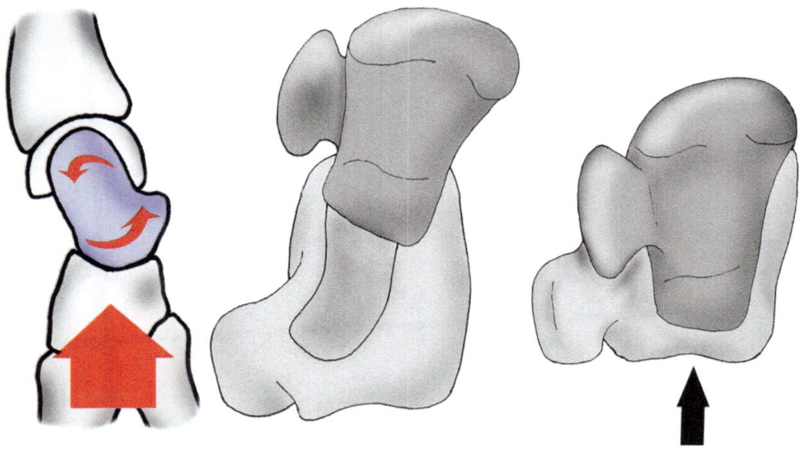

Fig. 1.48 Because of the axial stress transmitted to the first carpal row, the scaphoid moves towards flexion (1) and the triquetrum towards extension (2)

Muscular Anatomy and Physiology

The joints in the superior limb orient and stabilize the hand in the three planes. The wrist has a three-dimensional cinematics adapted to grasping and bearing.

The wrist muscles move the hand and stabilize it in gripping actions. They tend to co-contract and work in a static or dynamic way. There are six muscles:

- Three extensors on the dorsal side: the extensor carpi radialis longus (ECRL), the extensor carpi radialis brevis (ECRB), and the extensor carpi ulnaris (ECU).
- Three flexors on the palmar side: the flexor carpi radialis (FCR), the palmaris longus (PL), and the flexor carpi ulnaris (FCU).

These muscles pass like a bridge over the carpus and end with long tendons on the base of the metacarpal bones, where they have close contact with the hand's intrinsic muscles. Furthermore, their endings are off-centre relative to the rotation axis going through the head of the capitate.

In addition to the longitudinal compression, each wrist muscle has several actions on the joint (sagittal, frontal, and horizontal): for a "pure" movement, two muscles must be brought into play, as they are antagonist in one component but synergetic in another.

Overall, they are fusiform muscles that create an important active amplitude. Their fibres are set longitudinally with respect to their tendons. However, there also is the pronator quadratus: the only transversal, short, and mono-joint muscle, whose action is fully dedicated to the distal radioulnar joint.

The wrist can be divided into four quadrants around the joint centre.

In the front are the flexor muscles' tendons, while the extensor muscles' tendons are posterior. In the medial part are the tendons of the muscles performing ulnar inclination, and in the lateral part the ones performing radial inclination (Fig. 1.49).

Functional Anatomy of the Muscles in the Radioulnar Unity and the Wrist

Main Muscles of the Radioulnar Frame (Fig. 1.50)

Along with the biceps, they perform the rotation movements of the forearm thanks to the proximal and distal radioulnar joints.

There are pronator muscles (pronator teres and pronator quadratus) and supinator muscles (supinator and biceps), while the brachioradialis can be both a pronator and a supinator.

- *Pronator teres*

It is the most lateral superficial muscle of the forearm's anterior compartment. It has two heads, one from the medial humeral epicondyle (common epicondylar tendon) and the other from the

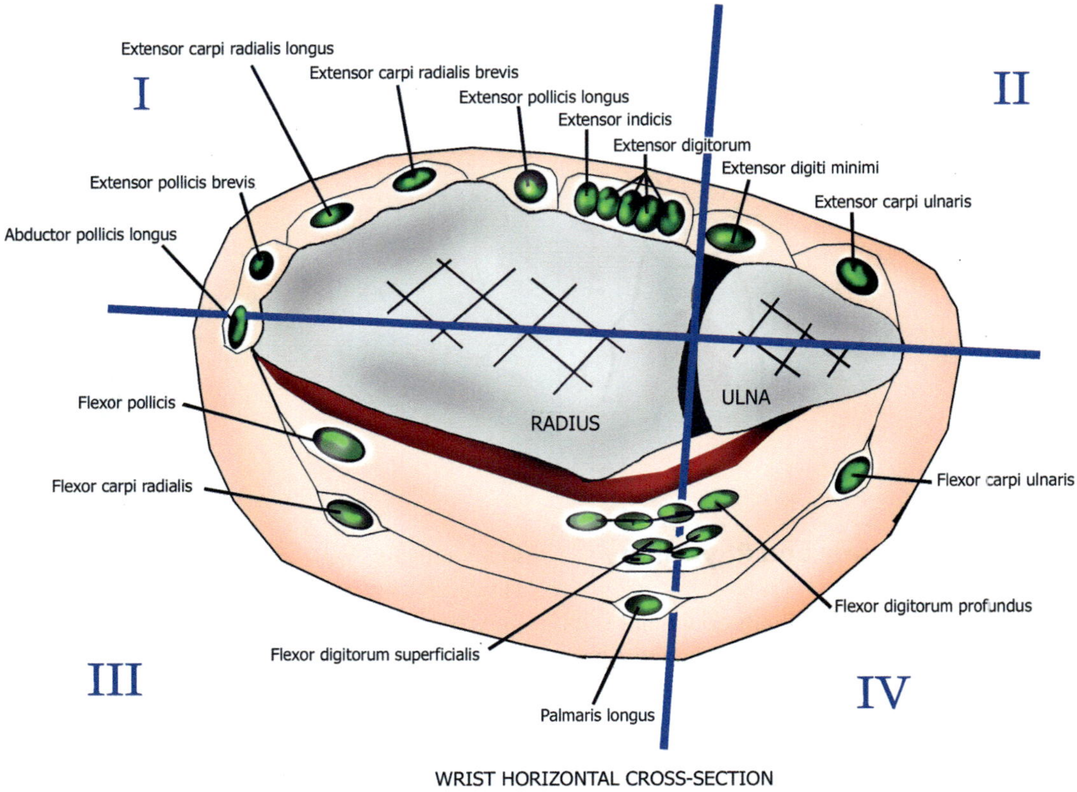

Fig. 1.49 Wrist cross-section

medial part of the coronoid process. The muscle ends on the middle third of the radius' lateral side.

- *Main action*: forearm pronation
- *Secondary action*: elbow flexion
- *Innervation*: median nerve (C6-C7)

- *Pronator quadratus* (Fig. 1.51)

It is the deepest muscle in the forearm's anterior compartment. It has a quadrilateral shape and is flat against the interosseous membrane, from the radius to the ulna in the inferior quarter, next to the distal radioulnar joint. It is a short, powerful muscle. It has its own aponeurosis and is composed of two bundles:

- A superficial bundle, made of transversal fibres and alike a flat muscle.
- A deep bundle made of fibres that are oblique downwards and outwards, twice as thick as the superficial bundle, and alike a pennate muscle (more stabilizing capacity).

The distal part of the muscle is larger than the proximal part and blends with the distal radioulnar joint capsule. Anatomically speaking, the architecture and location of the deep bundle allow it to efficiently stabilize this distal radioulnar joint.

- *Main action*: Forearm pronation and stabilization of the distal radioulnar joint.
- *Functional aspect*: The pronator quadratus acts automatically like a reflex, it is considered an "active ligament" (Mesplié 2007) of the distal radioulnar joint. It develops its maximum strength in an intermediary pronosupination position. Its maximal stabilizing action on the ulnar head is in pronation. Its action is facilitated by recruiting the abductor pollicis brevis.
- *Innervation*: Anterior interosseous nerve (C8-T1).

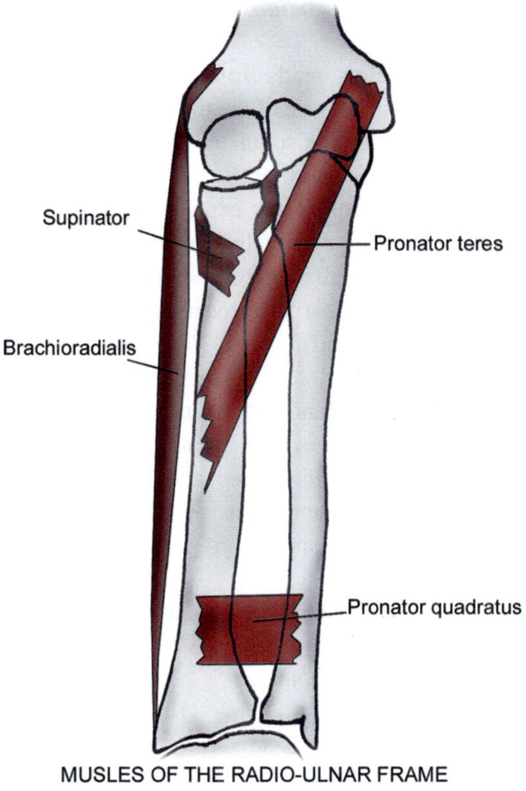

Fig. 1.50 Muscles of the radioulnar frame

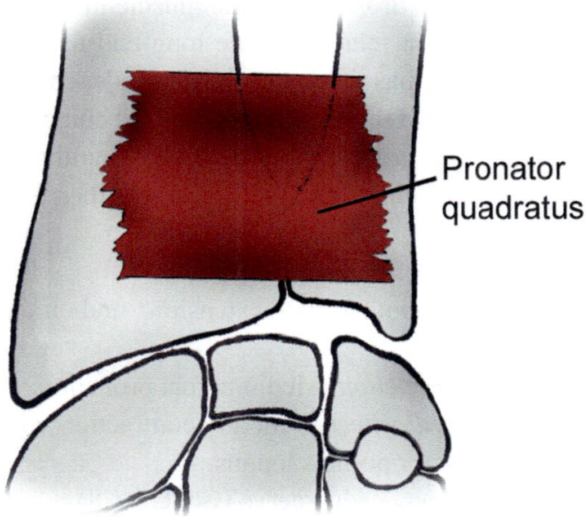

Fig. 1.51 Pronator quadratus

- *Brachioradialis*

It is a muscle bulging in the lateral side of the forearm in forced elbow flexion. It has no action on the wrist and is the only muscle in the body to start on the inferior extremity of one bone and end on the inferior extremity of another bone. It goes from the lateral supracondylar ridge of the humerus to the lateral side of the radial styloid process.

- *Main action*: Elbow flexion (weak action because of its parallelism with the radius and its proximal insertion close to the elbow joint).
- *Secondary action*: It is an accessory supinator in pronation and an accessory pronator in supination; it brings the forearm back into the intermediary position.
- *Innervation*: Radial nerve (C5-C6).

- *Supinator*

Short and flat, this muscle is wrapped around the radial head. Its origin is split into two bundles: a superficial bundle from the lateral humeral epicondyle and a deep bundle from the supinator crest of the ulna. It ends on the superior third of the lateral radial side, covering part of its anterior and posterior sides.

- *Main action*: Forearm supination in any elbow position.
- *Secondary action*: Coaptation of the lateral part of the elbow joint with its superficial head.
- *Innervation*: Radial nerve (C5-C6-C7).

Wrist Extensor Muscles (Fig. 1.52)

They are posterior muscles of the forearm, with tendons sliding in a synovial sheath at the level of the extensors' retinaculum. They end on the dorsal part of the base of the hand.

- *Extensor carpi radialis longus*

It spreads from the lateral inferior part of the humerus to the dorsal base of the second metacarpal. It is located outside the extensor carpi radialis brevis, under the brachioradialis. The muscle belly makes its way down the lateral part of the forearm and ends with a tendon in the middle third of the forearm. His tendon is right next to the extensor carpi radialis longus tendon,

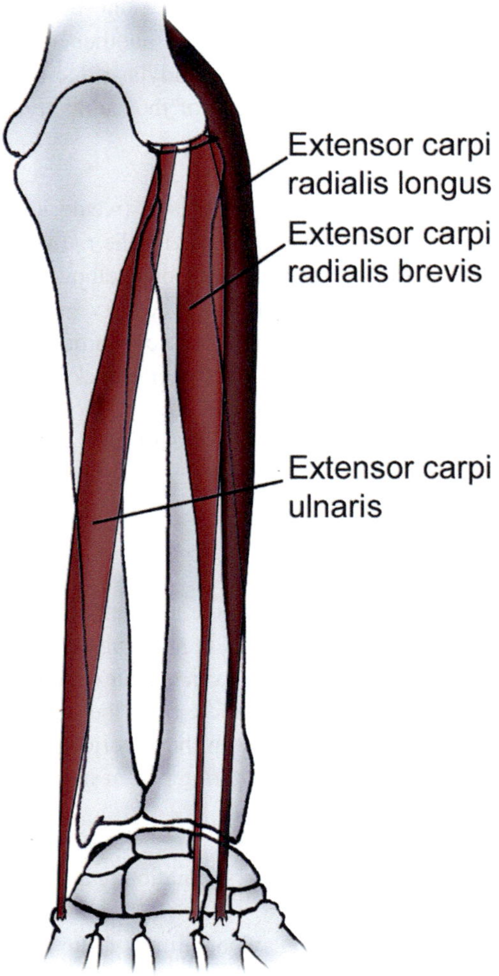

Fig. 1.52 Extensor muscles of the wrist

behind the brachioradialis. It then passes behind the radial styloid process, in the posterior groove on the lateral side of the inferior radial extremity.

- *Main action*: Wrist extension and radial inclination.
- *Secondary action*: Elbow flexion and medio-carpal supination.
- *Functional aspect*: It combines synergic-antagonist contractions with the flexor carpi radialis. It is the antagonist of the muscles realizing the ulnar inclination, and it stabilizes the radial side of the wrist.
- *Innervation*: Radial nerve (C6-C7).

- *Extensor carpi radialis brevis*

This muscle spreads from the lateral epicondyle to the dorsal base of the third metacarpal. Its origin is outside the supinator (common epicondylar tendon). The muscle belly is triangular, medial in relation to the extensor carpi radialis longus. Its tendon is right next to the extensor carpi radialis longus tendon and ends on the base of the third metacarpal (physically representing the axis of the hand).

- *Main action*: Hand extension.
- *Secondary action*: Medio-carpal supination.
- *Functional aspect*: It is synergic to the flexor digitorum profundus; its activity is reduced during the contraction of the fingers' extensors.
- *Innervation*: Radial nerve (C6–C8).

- *Extensor carpi ulnaris*

It is a fusiform muscle.

Its origin is on the epicondyle (common epicondylar tendon) and on the posterior part of the ulna (aponeurotic blade).

On its pathway, it is not in contact with the forearm aponeurosis a lot. The muscle fibres are longitudinal in relation to the long-end tendon. This tendon has its own sheath, independent from the dorsal retinaculum. It passes behind the ulnar styloid process in a resistant osteofibrous sheath and ends on the base of the fifth metacarpal.

- *Main action*: Wrist extension and ulnar inclination.
- *Secondary action*: Medio-carpal pronation.
- *Functional aspect*: Synergic contraction with the abductor pollicis longus.
- *Innervation*: Radial nerve (C6–C7–C8).

Wrist Flexor Muscles (Fig. 1.53)

They are anterior muscles of the forearm, from the medial epicondyle to the base of the hand. Their insertion on the medial epicondyle is a common tendon and is part of the superficial layer of the forearm (with the pronator teres).

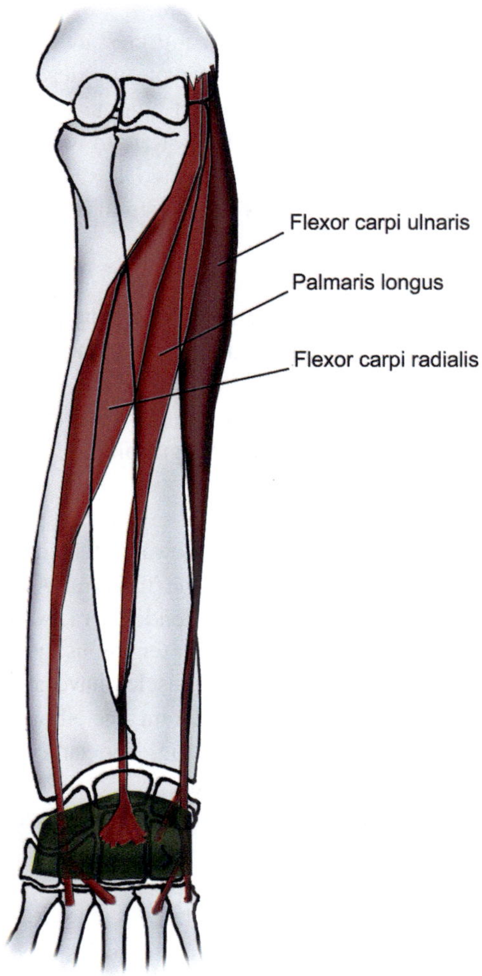

Fig. 1.53 Flexor muscles of the wrist

- *Flexor carpi radialis*

It belongs to the superficial plane of the anterior forearm compartment. Its origin is on the medial epicondyle. It is a fusiform muscle, flat in the front and in the back. Its fleshy muscle belly is followed by a long and voluminous tendon that goes down in front of the median nerve. The muscle belly is oblique downwards and a little outwards, placed in front of the flexor digitorum superficialis. It is followed by a tendon that appears in the middle of the forearm. This long tendon follows the gutter of the pulse.

At the level of the wrist, it crosses the carpus in its own osteofibrous groove, outside the carpal tunnel that contains the flexor tendons (limited in the back by the scaphoid and trapezium). The flexor carpi radialis tendon ends at the base of the second metacarpal and partly on the trapezium and the base of the third metacarpal.

- *Main action*: Wrist flexion, participates in the radial inclination.
- *Secondary action*: Elbow flexion, forearm pronation, and medio-carpal pronation.
- *Functional aspect*: It is synergic to the extensor digitorum when opening the hand. It performs the radial inclination of the wrist in co-contraction with the extensor carpi radialis longus.
- *Innervation*: Median nerve (C8–T1).

- *Palmaris longus*

This muscle belongs to the superficial plane of the anterior forearm compartment. Its origin is on the medial epicondyle. It is a fusiform muscle, thin, and not very powerful. Its muscle belly corresponds to the superior third and its tendon to the inferior two-thirds. The tendon goes down on the medial side of the flexor carpi radialis and ends up spreading on the flexors' retinaculum. The median fibres continue on the superficial palmar aponeurosis and the lateral fibres on the palmar aponeurosis of the thenar and hypothenar eminences.

- *Main action*: Wrist flexion, which puts tension in the superficial palmar aponeurosis.
- *Secondary action*: Small participation in elbow flexion and forearm pronation.
- *Particularity*: It is an inconstant muscle, absent in 13% of the cases and with multiple anatomical variations.
- *Innervation*: Median nerve (C8–T1).

- *Flexor carpi ulnaris.*

It is a bipennate muscle.

Its origin is epitrochlear (common epitrochlear tendon), with a tendinous blade on the internal part of the olecranon and on the superior two-thirds of the posterior ulnar part.

It sticks to the forearm aponeurosis. The insertion of the muscular fibres is oblique in relation to the tendon axis, and their end is purely tendinous, short, and inserted on the pisiform. It has expansions spreading towards the hamate, the flexors retinaculum, and the fourth and fifth metacarpals.

- *Action*: Wrist flexion and ulnar inclination.
- *Innervation*: ulnar nerve (C7, C8, T1).

Physiology of the Muscles in the Radioulnar Unity and the Wrist

Wrist motricity is ensured by agonist motor muscles assisted under certain circumstances by the fingers' muscles.

Wrist flexion is performed by the flexor carpi radialis, the palmaris longus, and the flexor carpi ulnaris. When the fingers are flexed, these muscles are assisted by the powerful flexor digitorum muscles.

Wrist extension is performed by the extensor carpi radialis longus, the extensor carpi radialis brevis, and the extensor carpi ulnaris. They are assisted by the extensor digitorum when the fist is closed.

Ulnar inclination is performed by the flexor carpi ulnaris and the extensor carpi ulnaris, assisted by the extensor digiti minimi, the flexor digiti minimi, and the short muscles of the fifth finger.

Radial inclination is performed by the flexor carpi radialis and the extensor carpi radialis, assisted by the abductor pollicis longus, extensor pollicis longus, and extensor pollicis brevis.

Pronosupination is the result of a rotation of the wrist and the elbow. It is performed by the pronator teres and the pronator quadratus assisted by the medial epicondylar muscles, and by the biceps and supinator assisted by the lateral epicondylar muscles.

> N.B.: The wrist extensor muscles are synergetic of the fingers' flexor muscles. A wrist extension triggers an automatic fingers flexion. The maximal strength for finger flexion is around 45° of wrist extension as the flexor muscles are pre-stretched.

Kapandji defines the wrist functional position at 40–45° of extension and 15° of ulnar inclination, for a maximal efficiency of the fingers' motor muscles. This way, the hand is placed in the position most adapted for gripping.

Tendon Gliding

The wrist is a passage area towards which converge tendons come from the forearm. As the wrist is widely mobile, the tendon's races confirm the necessity for the myo-tendinous units to lengthen. The wrist flexor muscles have a race close to the race of the wrist joint: the elbow has no influence on their stretching. The same goes for the wrist extensor muscles.

The wrist muscles' tendons have a race of approximately 3.5 cm.

> N.B.: The radial extensor muscles, the flexor carpi radialis, and the flexor carpi ulnaris develop their maximal race in flexion-extension. The extensor carpi radialis and the extensor carpi ulnaris develop their maximal race in radial-ulnar inclinations.

Active Stability of the Distal Radioulnar Joint

The stability of the radioulnar unity depends on several elements that avoid joint dislocation. The main elements are the pronator quadratus, the ulnar sling, the extensor indicis, and the oblique thumb muscles.

The two muscles of the ulnar sling associated with the extensor digiti minimi play a main role in active joint stability. However, their longitudinal orientation prevents them from opposing the transversal joint constraints on their own. This deficit is compensated by the pronator quadratus.

This "stabilizing quatuor" (flexor carpi ulnaris, extensor carpi ulnaris, extensor digiti minimi, and pronator quadratus) could therefore efficiently oppose the different mechanical constraints imposed on the joint.

We should also note the role of the oblique muscles (extensor indicis, extensor pollicis longus, extensor pollicis brevis, abductor pollicis longus): they are accessory stabilizers and complete the action of the main stabilizers of the distal radioulnar joint.

Carpal Stability: Intracapral Supinator and Pronator Muscles

The anatomical disposition of the forearm muscles makes them carpal pronators or supinators (Garcia-Elias 2011) (Fig. 1.54).

With normal proprioceptive abilities, they complete the action of anti-pronation and anti-supination ligaments (Fig. 1.55) to avoid an extra-physiological intracarpal rotation that could lead to ligament injuries.

The abductor pollicis longus, the extensor carpi radialis brevis and longus, and the flexor carpi ulnaris realize a midcarpal supination. Therefore, they protect the anti-pronation ligaments, especially the scapholunate ligament.

The contraction of the flexor carpi radialis and the extensor carpi ulnaris causes a midcarpal pronation: they protect the anti-supination ligaments, especially the lunotriquetral ligament (Esplugas et al. 2016; Salva Coll et al. 2012).

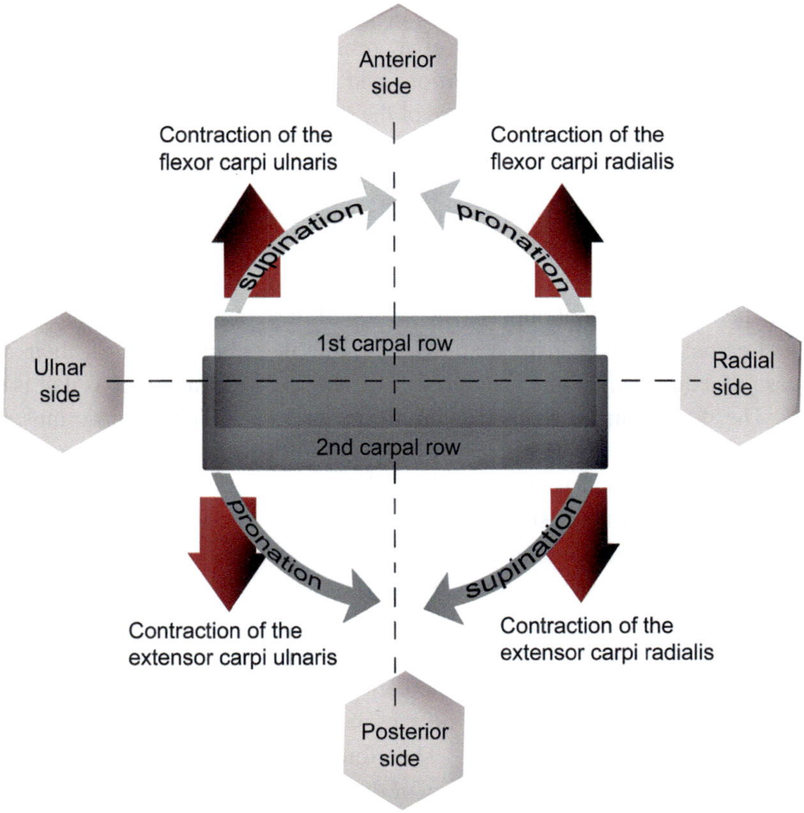

Fig. 1.54 Supination/pronation effects of the forearm muscles

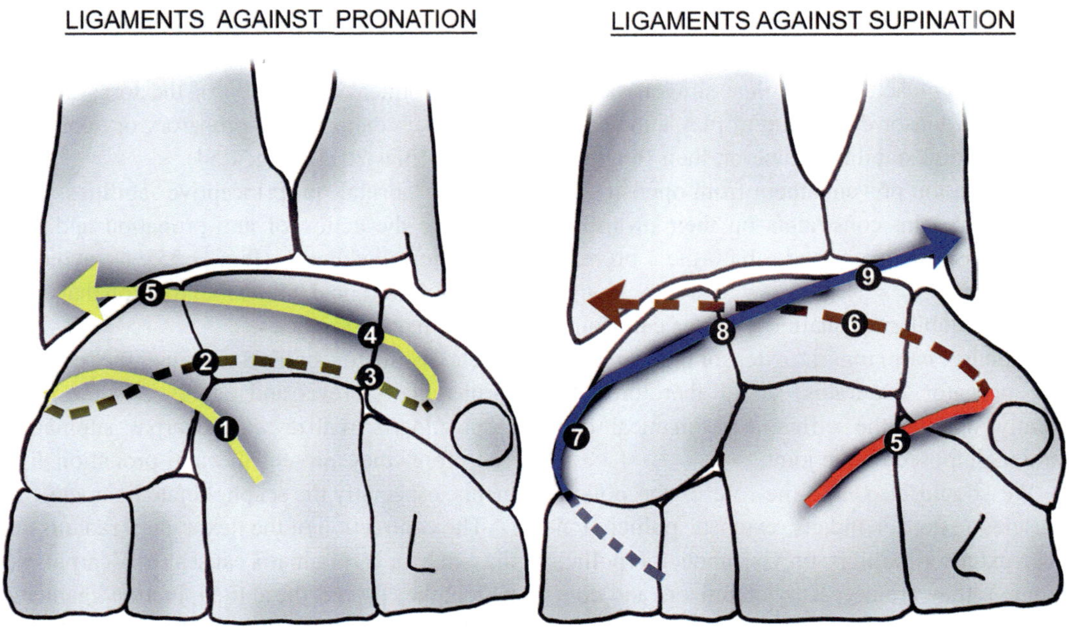

Fig. 1.55 Ligaments against intracarpal (or midcarpal) pronation (1) and against intracarpal (or midcarpal) supination (2) (according to Esplugas 2016 (Esplugas et al. 2016))

However, the flexor carpi radialis is special, as it is responsible for a midcarpal pronation because of its metacarpal insertion, and for a supination of the scaphoid because of the contact between its tendon and the tubercle of the scaphoid. It is the only muscle that is a pronator for the midcarpal joint and a supinator for the scaphoid (Fig. 1.56).

The extensor carpi ulnaris, midcarpal pronator, creates a force that opposes the flexion of the first carpal row. This gives it an essential role in case of palmar midcarpal instability.

The flexor carpi ulnaris, like the flexor carpi radialis, has two distinct roles: it supinates the midcarpal joint, and it applies a force from palmar to dorsal on the first carpal row through the pisiform. This last role has a stabilizing interest in palmar midcarpal instabilities (Fig. 1.57).

The isometric tensioning of the forearm muscles leads to a supination of the second carpal row, while the compression of the carpus from the third metacarpal bone with no muscle intervention leads to a pronation. Therefore, the "active" and "passive" compression of the carpus produce opposite effects (Esplugas et al. 2016; Salva Coll et al. 2012).

Strength of the Wrist Muscles

The study of forces allows to identify two types of activities: one in extension—radial inclination, and the other in flexion–ulnar inclination. It should be noted that the muscles doing the ulnar inclination develop a slightly superior force than the muscles doing the radial inclination. But above all, it is their torque with respect to the inclination axis that is significantly higher.

The extrinsic muscles of the fingers also participate in the wrist strength under certain conditions. Thus, the fingers' flexor muscles develop a strength that is four times higher than that of the direct wrist flexors, but they only become wrist flexors if the flexion of the fingers is blocked before the tendons come to the end of their race—for example in the flexion against resistance with a grip on a voluminous object. On the other hand, the fingers' extensor muscles become wrist extensors if the fist is closed, which means they are tensed by the flexion of the fingers.

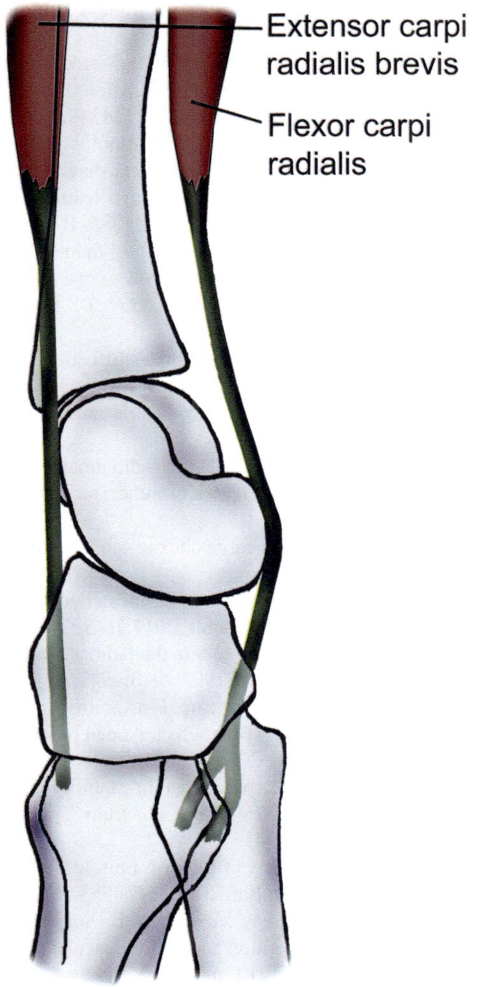

Fig. 1.56 Position of the flexor carpi radialis tendon giving it a role against the scaphoid pronation

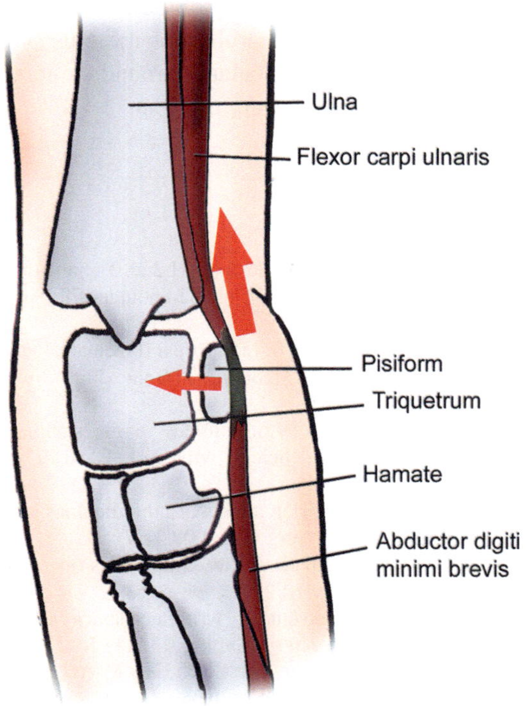

Fig. 1.57 The contraction in closed chain of the flexor carpi ulnaris creates a palmo-dorsal push on the triquetrum and therefore prevents the first row from moving towards flexion

Functional Aspects

The wrist muscles are motor muscles for the hand and participate in its orientation in space, in coordination with the rest of the superior limb's muscles. The wrist is the last element before the grip, so the muscles must always adapt their race depending on the context of the grip: the adaptation is constant. These fleshy and fusiform muscles have long tendons, so they have a great compliance and a high capacity to restore elastic energy during opposite movements. In a gripping situation, they have a high tendency to co-contraction and ensure the wrist stability regardless of its positions. The muscles have a protective role on the wrist to avoid its tendency to dislocation, due to external forces and compressive constraints imposed by the solicitation of the powerful flexor muscles of the fingers. The forces applied on the wrist are always compressive ones. Studying the functions faces us with a duality of mobility and stability, in the orientation of the palm, leaning on the hand, or the different types of prehension. The wrist muscles work in several ways: in open chain (free hand) the muscular recruitment is dynamic with isotonic contractions; in half-closed chain (mobile grips) it is dynamic or static with alternating contraction modes (concentric or eccentric isotonic, isometric); in closed chain (fixed grips) it is static with stabilizing isometric contractions.

The notions of force, endurance, and intermuscular coordination are integrated into the superior limb functionality, serving the displacement of the hand and the prehension.

The mobility and stability of the wrist require a three-dimensional control from the muscular system, a well-adjusted balance around the joint, and a coordination of every moment.

Bibliography

Arnold-peter C, Weiss AP, Hastings H 2nd. The anatomy of the proximal radioulnar joint. J Shoulder Elb Surg. 1992;1(4):193–9.

Crisco JJ, et al. In vivo radiocarpal kinematics and the Dart Thrower's motion. J Bone Joint Surg. 2005;87-A(12):2729.

Esplugas M, et al. Role of muscles in the stabilization of ligament-deficient wrists. J Hand Ther. 2016;29(2):166–74.

Fu E, et al. Elbow position affects distal radioulnar joint kinematics. J Hand Surg Am. 2009;34(7):1261–8.

Garcia-Elias M. Carpal instability. In: Green's operative hand surgery. Elsevier; 2011.

Garcia-Elias M. Understanding wrist mechanics: a long and winding road. J Wrist Surg. 2013;2(1):5–12.

Garcia-Elias M, Alomar Serrallach X, Monill Serra J. Dart-throwing motion in patients with scapholunate instability: a dynamic four-dimensional computed tomography study. J Hand Surg Eur Vol. 2014;39(4):346–52.

Gelberman RH, Menon J. The vascularity of the scaphoid bone. J Hand Surg. 1980;5A(5):508–13.

Hagert E. Proprioception of the wrist joint: a review of current concepts and possible implications on the rehabilitation of the wrist. J Hand Ther. 2010;23(1):2–16. quiz 17

Hagert E, Forsgren S, Ljung BO. Differences in the presence of mechanoreceptors and nerve structures between wrist ligaments may imply differential roles in wrist stabilization. J Orthop Res. 2005;23(4):757–63.

Hagert E, et al. Immunohistochemical analysis of wrist ligament innervation in relation to their structural composition. J Hand Surg Am. 2007;32(1):30–6.

Horii E, Garcia-Elias A, Han K. A kinematic study of luno-triquetral dissociations. J Hand Surg. 1991;16: 355–62.

Kapandji IA. Physiologie articulaire tome 1 - Membre supérieur. Maloine; 2005.

Kaufmann RA, et al. Kinematics of the midcarpal and radiocarpal joint in flexion and extension: an in vitro study. J Hand Surg Am. 2006;31(7):1142–8.

Kleinman WB. Stability of the distal radioulna joint: biomechanics, pathophysiology, physical diagnosis, and restoration of function what we have learned in 25 years. J Hand Surg Am. 2007;32(7):1086–106.

Kobayashi M, et al. Axial loading induces rotation of the proximal carpal row bones around unique screw-displacement axes. J Biomech. 1997;30(11–12):1165–7.

Markolf KL, Tejwani SG, Benhaim P. Effects of wafer resection and hemiresection from the distal ulna on load-sharing at the wrist: a cadaveric study. J Hand Surg Am. 2005;30(2):351–8.

Mesplié G. Stabilité de l'articulation radio ulnaire distale: quid du carré pronateur ? Kinésithérapie, la revue. 2007;68–69:58–62.

Mesplie G. Instabilités du carpe chez le sportif. Promanu; 2017.

Mesplie G, et al. Rehabilitation of distal radioulnar joint instability. Hand Surg Rehabil. 2017;36(5):314–21.

Petrie S, et al. Mechanoreceptors in the palmar wrist ligaments. J Bone Joint Surg. 1997;79-B:494–6.

Raja S, et al. New concepts in carpal instability. In: Wrist and elbow arthroscopy with selected open procedures; 2022. p. 173–85.

Salva Coll G, et al. Carpal dynamic stability mechanisms. Exp Study Rev Esp Cir Ortop Traumatol. 2012;2013(57):129–34.

Salva-Coll G, et al. Effects of forearm muscles on carpal stability. J Hand Surg Eur. 2011;36(7):553–9.

Salva-Coll G, Garcia-Elias M, Hagert E. Scapholunate instability: proprioception and neuromuscular control. J Wrist Surg. 2013;2(2):136–40.

Soubeyrand M, et al. Pathologie traumatique de la membrane interosseuse de l'avant-bras. Chir Main. 2007;26:255.

Soubeyrand M, et al. The middle radioulnar joint and triarticular forearm complex. J Hand Surg Eur. 2011;36(6):447–54.

Viegas S, et al. The dorsal ligaments of the wrist: anatomy, mechanical properties, and function. J Hand Surg. 1999;24:456–68.

2 Injuries of the Radioulnar Unity

Grégory Mesplié and Vincent Grelet

The radioulnar unity is a whole anatomical entity between the elbow and wrist. It is made of the two radioulnar joints, to which should be added the interosseous membrane and the two bones of the forearm (see Chap. 1).

A disturbance in one of these elements can lead to stiffness in pronosupination and an injury in two of them can lead to instability in the whole radioulnar frame.

Injuries of the radioulnar unity concern any damage of one of these elements.

Physiopathological Classification

M. Soubeyrand et al. classify the osteo-ligamentous injuries of the forearm depending on the number of damaged locks (Soubeyrand et al. 2007, 2011).

Stage 1: One Lock Damaged

It is a damage to the proximal lock (proximal radioulnar joint), middle lock (interosseous membrane), or distal lock (distal radioulnar joint).

If these injuries block the damaged lock, the global radioulnar mobility will be impaired.

If these injuries destabilize the damaged lock, the global radioulnar stability will be preserved thanks to the two other locks.

Taking the example of a door with three hinges helps in understanding this mechanism. If a hinge is rusted, the door cannot be moved. If a hinge is taken off or unscrewed, the door stays stable thanks to the two other hinges (Fig. 2.1).

Pathologies concerned by this stage are:

- Fractures of the radial head, resection of the radial head, radial head prosthesis, and injuries of the annular and quadrate ligaments for the proximal lock.
- Fractures of the ulnar or radial diaphyses, isolated injuries of the interosseous membrane (considered rare) for the middle lock.
- Fractures of the distal ulnar or radial extremities that damage the distal radioulnar joint, injuries of the triangular complex, and arthroplasty or resection of the ulnar head for the distal lock.

Stage 2: Two Locks Damaged

These damages concern the proximal and middle, middle and distal, or proximal and distal locks.

G. Mesplié (✉)
ISAMMS, Biarritz, France

V. Grelet
Institut Sud Aquitain de la Main et du Membre Supérieur, Biarritz, France

G. Mesplié (ed.), *Wrist Functional Anatomy and Therapy*,
https://doi.org/10.1007/978-3-031-42879-1_2

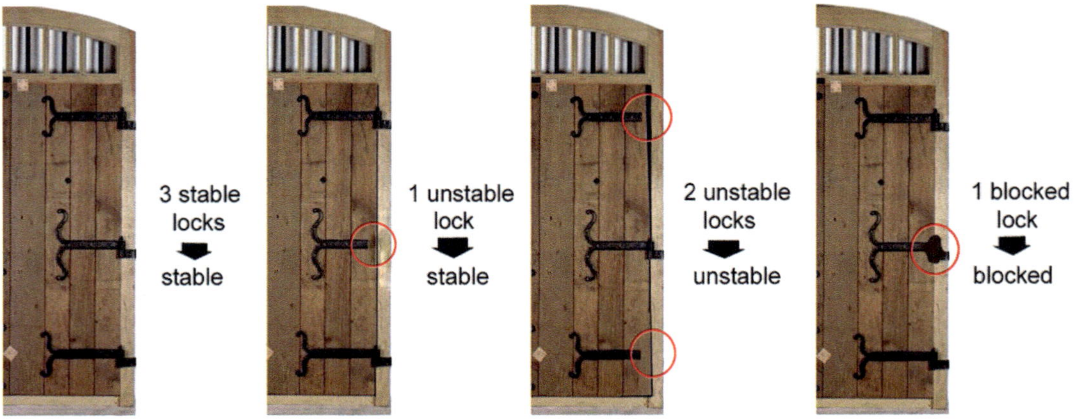

Fig. 2.1 The radioulnar unity acts like a door with three locks. If only one lock is blocked, the whole door is blocked. If two locks are taken away, the door is unstable

These injuries can block the radioulnar frame if one or two locks are blocked or destabilize it if both locks become unstable.

Pathologies concerned by this stage are:

- Monteggia fracture: An ulnar diaphyseal fracture combined with a dislocation of the proximal radioulnar joint. It is an injury of the middle (the fracture tears the interosseous membrane) and proximal locks (Fig. 2.2).
- Galeazzi fracture: A radial diaphyseal fracture combined with a dislocation of the distal radioulnar joint. It is an injury of the middle (the fracture tears the interosseous membrane) and distal locks (Fig. 2.3).
- Crisscross injuries: Fractures of the radial head combined with dorsal dislocations of the ulnar head. They are injuries of the distal and proximal locks. The injury mechanism is a pivot of the two bones around an axis made by the middle part of the interosseous membrane (Fig. 2.4).

Stage 3: Three Locks Damaged

These damages concern the three locks: it is an Essex–Lopresti syndrome combining a fracture of the radial head, a tear of the interosseous membrane, and a dislocation of the distal radioulnar joint (Fig. 2.5).

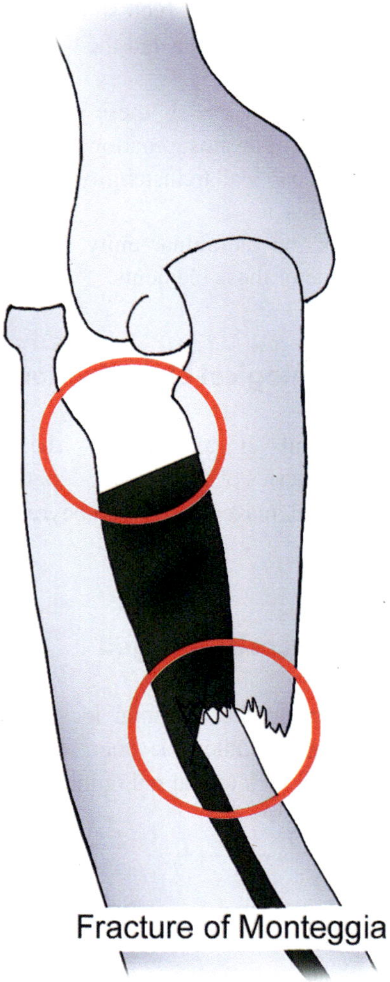

Fig. 2.2 Fracture of Monteggia combining an injury of the medium lock with one of the proximal locks

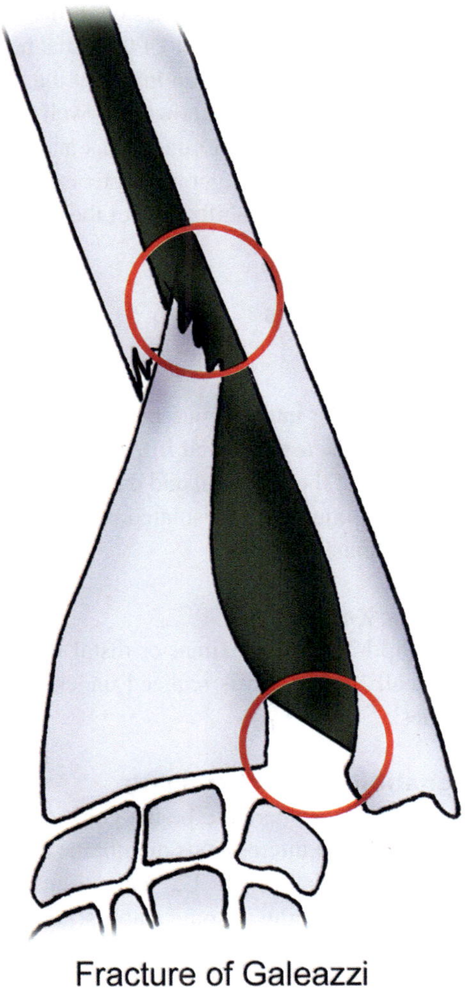

Fig. 2.3 Fracture of Galeazzi combining an injury of the distal lock with one of the medium locks

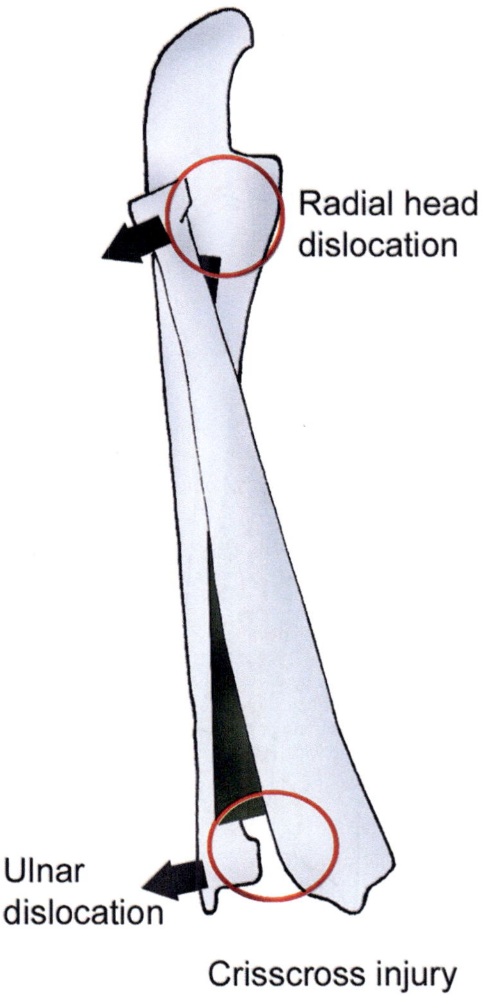

Fig. 2.4 Crisscross injury combining an injury of the distal lock with one of the proximal locks

Physiopathology

At the physiopathological level, injuries of the radioulnar unity correspond to a fall with the wrist in extension. The grade of pronosupination during the fall defines the anatomical damages observed:

- In total supination, fractures of the two forearm bones are frequent.
- In 45° of supination, simple fractures of the radial head are more frequent.
- In neutral position, Essex–Lopresti syndromes.
- In pronation, complex fractures of the radial head.

These are tendencies and must not be taken literally, as the exact position of the forearm during the traumatism can be uncertain. Moreover, other components like the violence of the traumatism have an important influence on the nature of the injuries.

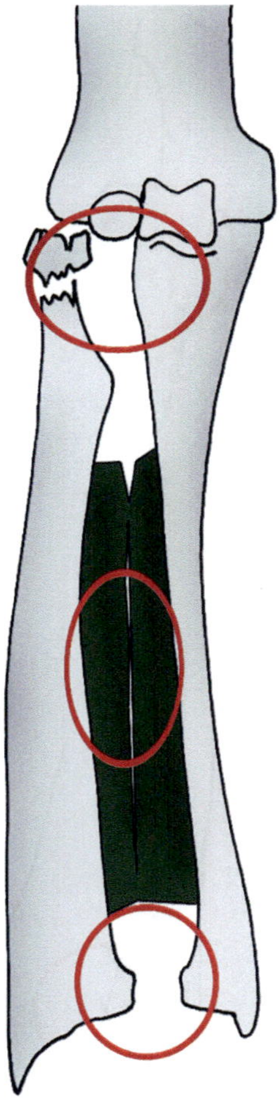

Fig. 2.5 Essex–Lopresti syndrome with injuries of the three locks

Clinical and Paraclinical Signs

Clinical Signs

It is important to differentiate between acute and old injuries. Chronic injuries are harder to treat, that is why it is important to make an early diagnosis. Symptoms vary depending on the number of damaged locks.

The limitation of mobility concerns pronosupination and the different amplitudes of the elbow and wrist, and it can evolve with time: formation of posttraumatic synostosis, or inversion of the distal radioulnar index after resection of the radial head.

The natural evolution of an injury of the interosseous membrane is unknown, as well as its healing mechanism. Ultrasound scans and MRIs have been made to try to get more precise indications for surgery and stabilization of the forearm.

Paraclinical Signs

Static X-rays

An injury of the interosseous membrane can be affirmed in the case of radial lift, combined with dislocations of the proximal and distal radioulnar joints. If the injury seems isolated, we must look for an associated injury.

Dynamic X-rays

They help highlight proximal or distal instabilities. Ideally, this exam is realized under general anesthesia.

Magnetic Resonance Imaging

This exam is considered to be the gold standard. We visualize the interosseous membrane directly with hyposignal T1 and T2, and a sensitivity above 87% according to some authors.

Ultrasounds

It is an exam easily realized in case of emergency, but it has the disadvantage of being operator dependent. However, several authors say it has excellent sensitivity and specificity, which can be potentiated by a dynamic study of the interosseous membrane (Soubeyrand et al. 2006a).

Therapeutic Process and Surgical Treatment

The treatment's results will be worse in old injuries, or in injuries that have not been treated well.

Osseous surgery: A radial or ulnar fracture requires perfect reduction and osteosynthesis with a plate to avoid any rotation or angulation

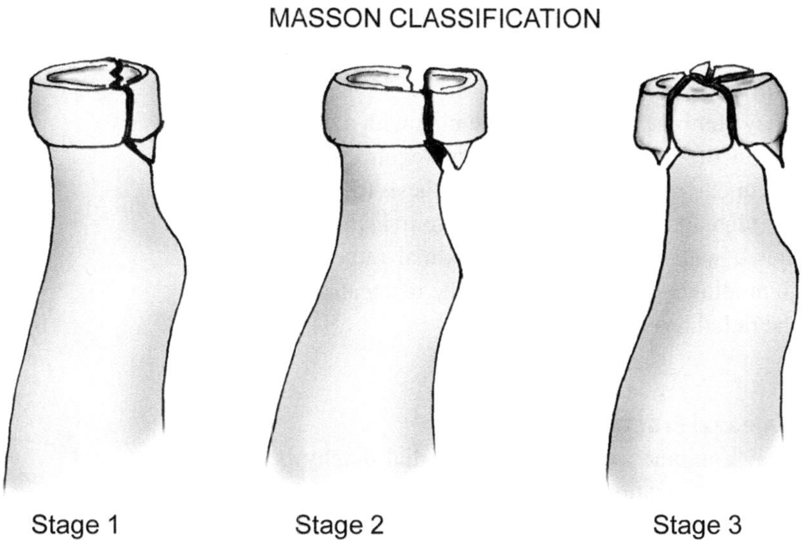

Fig. 2.6 Masson classification for radial head fractures

disorders that would have an immediate impact on pronosupination and joint stability. This perfect reduction will spontaneously produce a reduction of the dislocated joint.

Injury of the Proximal Radioulnar Joint

The most common injury is the radial head fracture. It happens after a fall on the palm of the hand with the elbow more or less flexed, or after a direct impact on the elbow.

Masson's classification (Fig. 2.6) orients the treatment:

Type 1

There is no displacement: the treatment will be functional with an analgesic immobilization for a few days, combined with an anti-inflammatory medical treatment and ice. The goal is to avoid stiffness as it is the main consequence of this type of fracture.

Type 2

There is a displacement, requiring an anatomical reduction with an osteosynthesis (screw or pin) and allowing early mobilization.

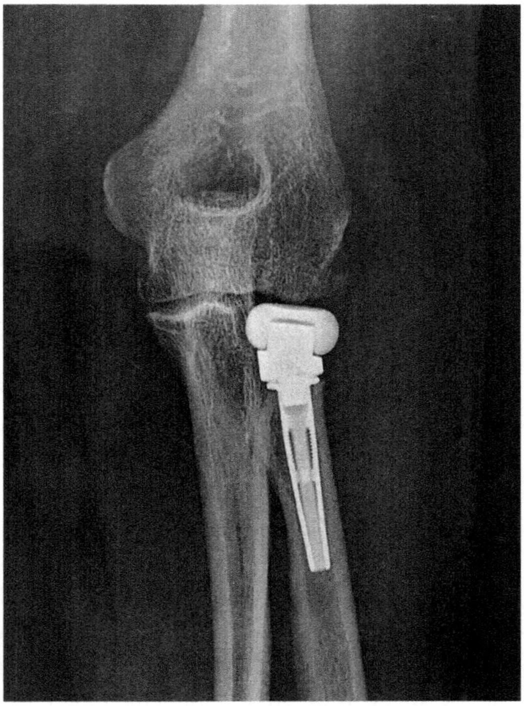

Fig. 2.7 Radial head prosthesis

Type 3

This comminuted fracture can only be treated with a radial head prosthesis (Fig. 2.7).

Injury of the Radioulnar Unity

Monteggia Fractures

They combine a fracture of the ulna with a dislocation of the radial head. They require urgent treatment: reduction and osteosynthesis (plate) of the ulna allowing the ulnar fracture to heal, associated with pinning of the proximal radioulnar joint allowing the reduction of the dislocation of the radial head.

Galeazzi Fractures

They combine a fracture of the radial diaphysis with a dislocation of the distal radioulnar joint. They also require urgent treatment: reduction and osteosynthesis (plate) of the radius giving the bone its length back. The distal radioulnar joint can also be temporarily pinned, to stabilize the joint.

Essex–Lopresti Syndrome

It was described in 1952. It is often treated when it has already become a chronic injury, therefore it is a true surgical challenge... with only 20% of good results. In most cases, a radial head prosthesis, a shortening ulnar osteotomy, and an interosseous membrane repair are necessary.

The initial diagnosis only happens in 25% of the cases, however, it is essential to implement the appropriate treatment for the interosseous membrane (IOM) and the triangular fibrocartilage complex (TFCC) to heal.

The key element is to restore the radial length with a stable osteosynthesis or a radial head prosthesis if we want the IOM to have a chance of healing. Moreover, it is necessary to pin the distal radioulnar joint and repair the TFCC.

The IOM itself is difficult to repair (Soubeyrand et al. 2006b), so some authors have suggested reinforcing it with the pronator teres or using an endo-button to improve global stability (Fig. 2.8).

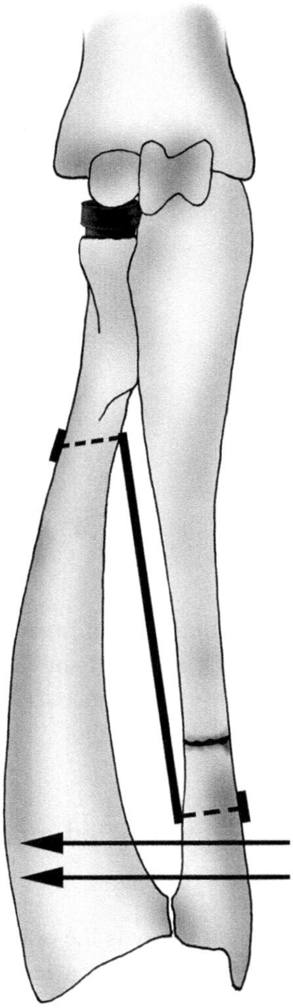

Fig. 2.8 Using an endo-button to repair the interosseous membrane (according to Soubeyrand 2006)

Injury of the Distal Radioulnar Joint

TFCC Injuries

The role and anatomy of the triangular ligament are better understood thanks to the work of Palmer and Nakamura (Palmer et al. 1984; Nakamura et al. 1999), and more recently the work of Atzei (Atzei and Luchetti 2011)—in fact, it is more of a fibrocartilage complex than a ligament. The TFCC plays a stabilizing role in the distal radioulnar joint and transmits constraints between the carpus and the ulna.

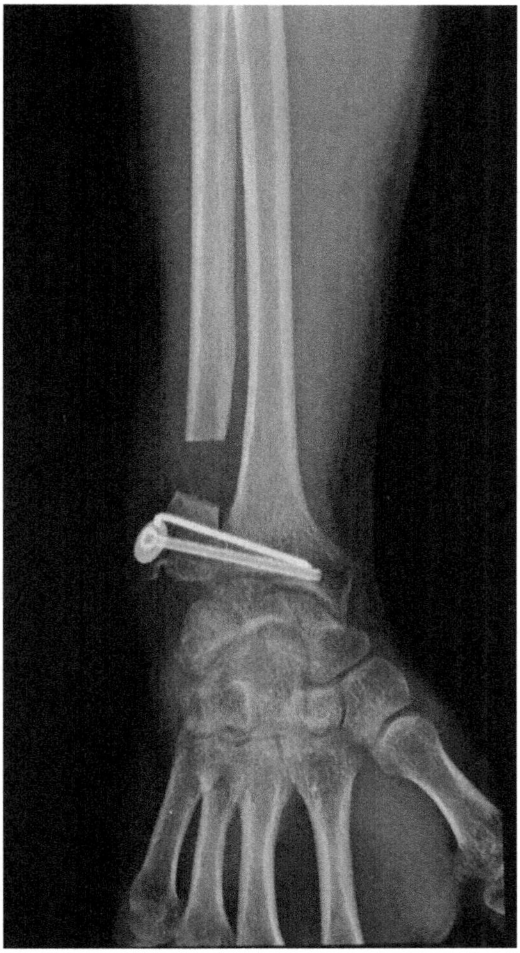

Fig. 2.9 Sauvé-Kapandji surgery

Wrist arthroscopies have helped us to discover new injuries, and to treat them accordingly to their location: peripheral injuries are reinserted while central injuries require a debridement. If the TFCC is disinserted from the ulna, it is repaired by an anchor system on the ulnar head.

The Sauvé–Kapandji Procedure

Fractures in the distal extremities of the radius and the ulna can create malunions with a loss of the distal radioulnar congruence, the pronosupination will then be limited.

The Sauvé–Kapandji procedure is an arthrodesis of the distal radioulnar joint combined with the creation of an intentional ulnar pseudarthrosis. It allows gaining pronosupination back (Fig. 2.9).

Rehabilitation and Orthotic Treatment

Given the variety and complexity of the possible injuries, we will not detail a precise rehabilitation protocol but rather elements to work with to regain good functionality of the radioulnar unity.

These elements concern the post-immobilization phase after the damaged elements are solid and the pain and trophic disorders have disappeared.

They are based on a global comprehension of the radioulnar unity, a "major" injury of one lock being possibly associated with a less important injury of another lock and "hidden" during the paraclinical exam.

Mobility of the Radioulnar Unity

As described in the Chap. 1, stiffness in one radioulnar lock blocks the whole radioulnar joint.

Therefore, it is essential to check the mobility of each radioulnar joint after any injury in the forearm.

Distal Radioulnar Joint

It is a trochoid joint with a cylindrical ulnar surface and a radial cavity.

It participates in the pronosupination movements: the radius and the ulna perform a rather circular movement around their respective rotation axis. The ulna only performs a rotation of 6° while the radius performs a more important rotation. Between the position of maximal supination and a 45° pronation, the radius performs a rotation of 140°. Between a 45° pronation and the position of maximal pronation, the radius stops rotating and performs a palmar translation. This translation seems to happen because of the morphology of the distal radioulnar joint and the contraction of the pronator quadratus (Nakamura et al. 1999). This specificity must be considered when passively mobilizing the distal radioulnar joint.

Between the position of maximal supination and a 45° pronation, the patient's elbow is placed

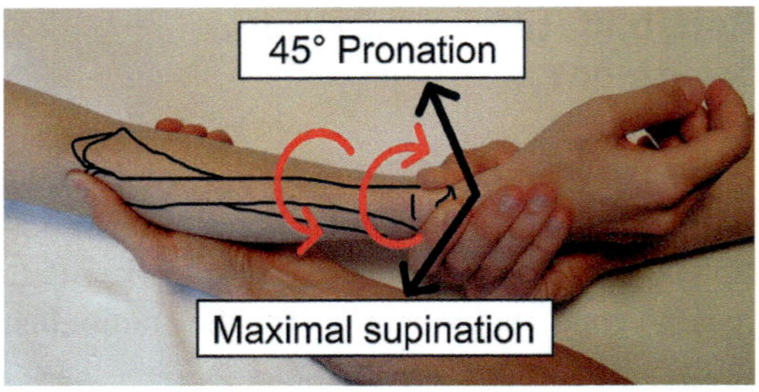

Fig. 2.10 Mobilization of the distal radioulnar joint from maximal supination to 45° of pronation. In this range of motion, the radius turns around the ulna

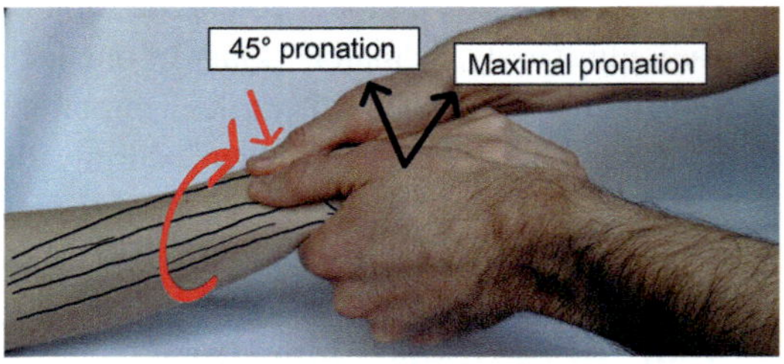

Fig. 2.11 Mobilization of the distal radioulnar joint after 45° of pronation. The radius performs an anterior translation relative to the ulna

at 90° of flexion and the therapist takes the distal and proximal radioulnar joints. The proximal hand is the fix point while the distal hand makes a pronosupination movement between maximal supination and 45° of pronation (Fig. 2.10).

Between a 45° pronation and the position of maximal pronation, the patient's elbow is placed at 90° of flexion and the therapist takes the distal extremity of the radius and the ulnar head. The ulnar hand is the fix point. The radial hand brings the forearm between 45° of pronation and the maximal pronation while performing an anterior gliding of the distal extremity of the radius (Fig. 2.11).

Interosseous Membrane

Fibrosis in the interosseous membrane can also produce stiffness in the radioulnar unity.

Several techniques are used but their efficiency on the interosseous membrane has yet to be demonstrated:

- *Deep massage*

These techniques do not have a direct effect on the membrane but can favor its mobilization by relaxing radioulnar muscles.

We use glided pressures, sanding, and palpating-rolling techniques that have been described in Volume 1—chapter "Scar massage and treatment."

- *Contraction-stretching of the muscles inserted on the interosseous membrane*

Alternating contractions and stretching improves the local microcirculation (pumping effect), favors the fiber remodeling during the healing phase, and improves mobility in the different gliding planes.

We progressively use static intermittent, concentric, and eccentric contractions. Resistance and speed are increased and adapted to the patient's evolution.

These techniques concern:

– *Flexor digitorum profundus*

Contractions are realized in all the pronosupination positions. The therapist places the resistance on the third phalanges of the long fingers.

Stretching is realized in the same position; the therapist applies a soft, progressive pain-free stretching (Fig. 2.12).

– *Flexor digitorum superficialis*

It is in relation with the interosseous membrane through the oblique cord.

The modalities are the same as those for the flexor digitorum profundus, but the resistance is placed on the second phalanges of the long fingers.

– *Flexor pollicis longus*

The modalities are the same as those described previously but the resistance is placed on the second phalanx of the thumb.

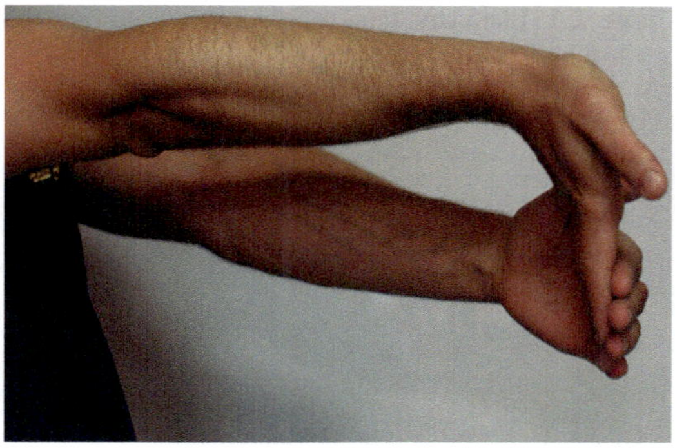

Fig. 2.12 Stretching of the fingers and wrist flexors. Resistance is placed at the level of the third phalanx. With a resistance on the second phalanx, we do not stretch the flexor digitorum profundus, and with a resistance on the palmar side of the metacarpals we do not stretch the flexor digitorum superficialis (only the wrist flexors)

– *Extensor pollicis longus*

Contractions are realized in all the pronosupination positions. The therapist places the resistance on the dorsal side of the second phalanx of the thumb.

Stretching is realized with the elbow extended and the forearm pronated; the therapist applies a radial inclination in the wrist, with his thumb against the palm.

– *Extensor pollicis brevis*

The modalities are the same as the ones for the extensor pollicis longus, but the resistance is placed on the dorsal side of the first phalanx.

The stretching is the same as the one for the extensor pollicis longus.

– *Abductor pollicis longus*

The modalities are the same as those described previously but the resistance is placed on the dorsal side of the first metacarpal.

The stretching is the same as the one for the extensor pollicis longus.

– *Extensor indicis*

Contractions are realized in all the pronosupination positions. The therapist places the resistance on the dorsal side of the first phalanx of the index.

Stretching is realized with the elbow extended and the forearm pronated; the therapist applies a flexion in the wrist and the metacarpophalangeal joint of the index.

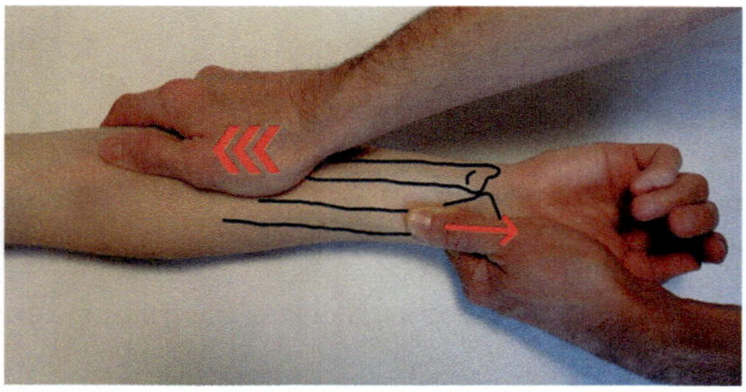

Fig. 2.13 Radius traction

- *Global mobilization of the radius in relation to the ulna*

Mobilization techniques for the IOM consist in moving the radius with respect to the ulna.

– *Mobilizations with longitudinal radial traction*

The therapist takes the inferior extremity of the radius and pulls it along the radial axis while the other hand stabilizes the anterior part of the forearm (Fig. 2.13).

– *Antero-posterior mobilizations*

The therapist takes the radius and glides it in an anteroposterior way while the other hand stabilizes the ulna. This mobilization should be realized in the different parts of the IOM (Fig. 2.14).

– *Mobilizations in pronosupination*

The therapist places the patient's elbow in flexion and takes the distal and proximal radioulnar joints. The mobilization is done by the therapist's distal hand in every pronosupination amplitude (Fig. 2.15).

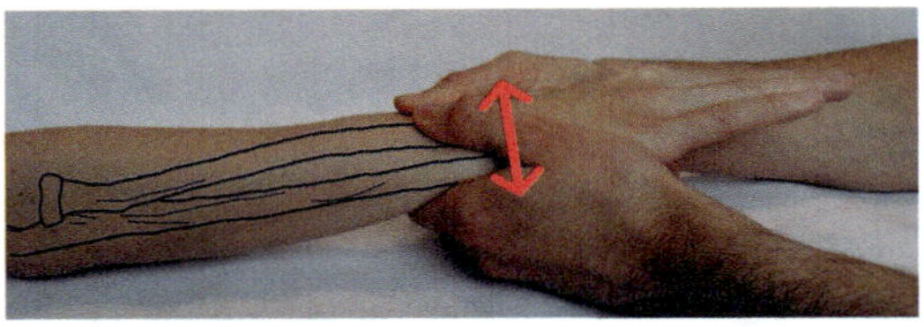

Fig. 2.14 Antero-posterior gliding of the radius relative to the ulna

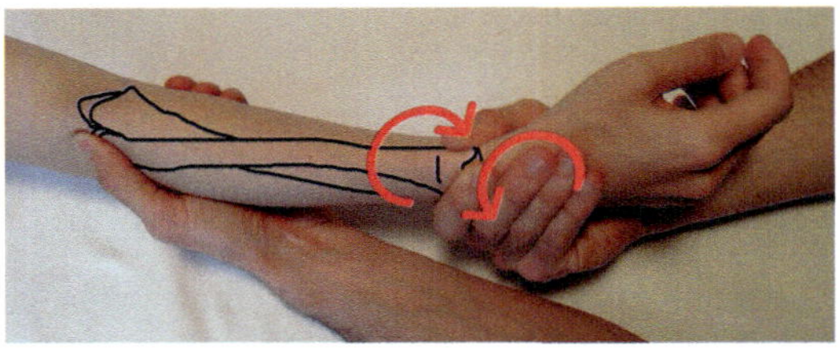

Fig. 2.15 Global mobilization in pronosupination

Proximal Radioulnar Joint

It is part of the elbow complex and shares its joint capsule with the humeroulnar and humeroradial joints. It is a trochoid joint, with the cylindrical radial head and the concordant radial notch of the ulna, stabilized by the annular ligament and the quadrate ligament (Weiss and Hastings 1992).

During pronosupination, the radial head does not only move in rotation: it also glides from anterior to posterior (Weiss and Hastings 1992). In pronation, the radial head performs a medial rotation and an anterior gliding. In supination, it performs a lateral rotation and a posterior translation (Ghossoub et al. 2009) (Table 2.1).

Regarding the anteroposterior glidings, some authors doubt that we can recreate those movements with mobilizations (Dufour et al. 2008), especially in a supination position.

Furthermore, there is little evidence regarding the impact of the position of flexion or extension of the elbow on the proximal radioulnar joint's mobility in pronosupination. Therefore, pronation mobilizations are performed with the elbow extended, and supination mobilizations with the elbow flexed—as it is easier for the therapist.

To mobilize the proximal radioulnar joint in pronation, the therapist takes the inferior third of the forearm, maintains the elbow extension, and mobilizes towards pronation. On the other hand, the therapist places the thumb on the dorsal side of the radial head and pushes it frontwards (Fig. 2.16).

Table 2.1 Summary table of the various movements while mobilizing the proximal radioulnar joint

	Mobilization in pronation	Mobilization in supination
Elbow position	Extension	Flexion
Radial head translation	Anterior	Posterior

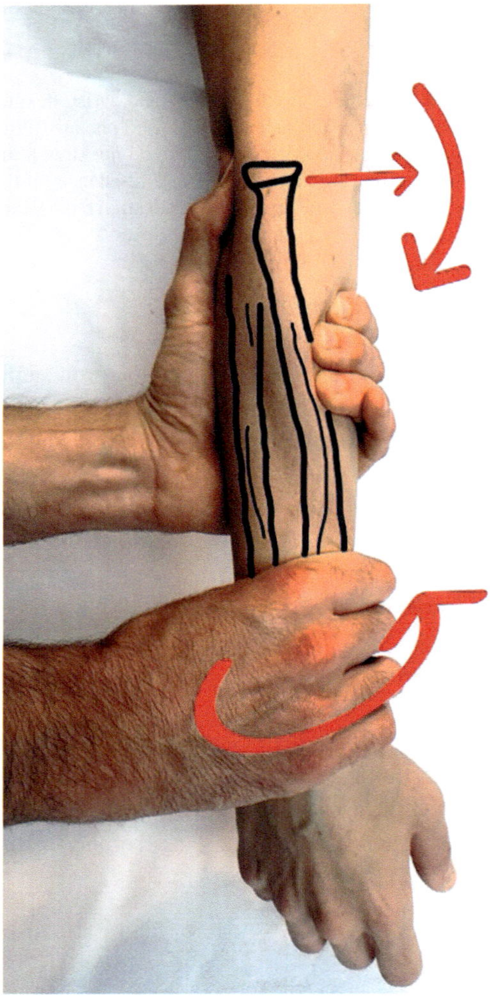

Fig. 2.16 Mobilization of the proximal radioulnar joint in pronation

The mobilization of the proximal radioulnar joint in supination is done in elbow flexion. The therapist takes the inferior third of the forearm and moves it toward elbow flexion and forearm supination. On the other hand, the therapist takes

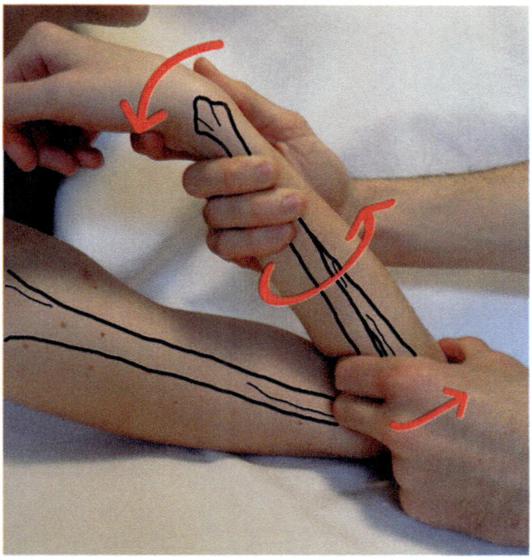

Fig. 2.17 Mobilization of the proximal radioulnar joint in supination

the proximal extremity of the radius and pushes it backward (Fig. 2.17).

Stability of the Radioulnar Unity

The instability or loss of one radioulnar lock can be compensated by the two other locks, but instability in two locks induces instability in the third lock.

However, important instability in one lock can be clinically observed even when there are no diagnosed injuries in the two other locks. This leads to three hypotheses:

- The associated injury is major but went unnoticed.
- The associated injury was minor after the traumatism but has evolved into a major injury destabilizing the radioulnar unit.
- The associated injury is minor but sufficient to destabilize the radioulnar unit.

In any case, it is important for the therapist to improve the neuromuscular capacities of the stabilizing muscles (Hagert 2010) after any injury in the forearm, with precise parameters as some of these muscles also have destabilizing components!

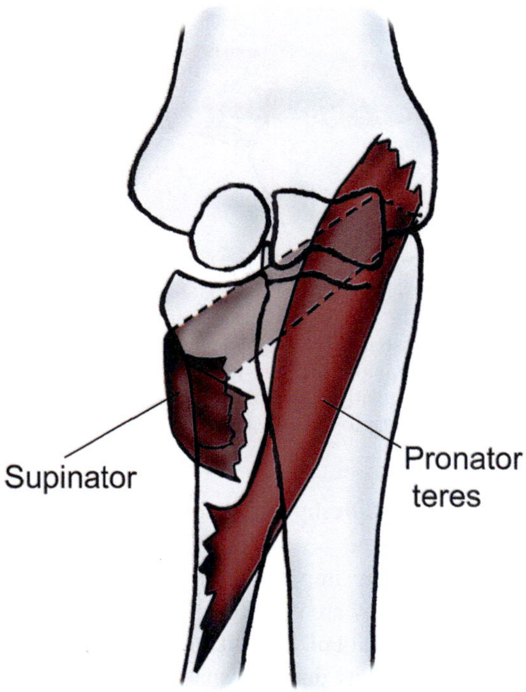

Fig. 2.18 The supinator and the pronator teres have a synergic action and work in parallel to stabilize the radial head

Like in any strengthening protocol, exercises inducing significant tissular constraints are prohibited during the period of fragility.

Key Muscles in Radioulnar Stability

- *Transverse muscles*

They play an essential role in coaptation.

They must be reinforced after any injury in the forearm as they do not destabilize the radioulnar unity.

The supinator and the pronator teres "surround" the superior extremity of the radius. They work in synergy to stabilize the radial head (Fig. 2.18). These three muscles are short "tonic" muscles, so the reinforcement protocol is based on static or stato-eccentric progressive exercises, proprioception, and rhythmic stabilization.

- *Pronator quadratus* (Mesplié 2007; Hagert and Hagert 2010)

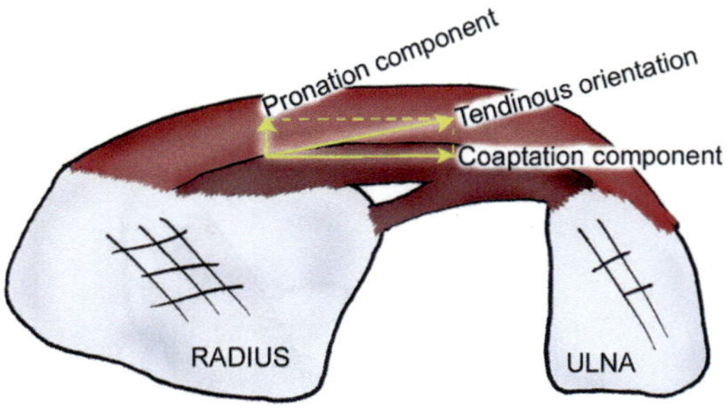

Fig. 2.19 The kinesiological study of the pronator quadratus demonstrates that its stabilizing action on the distal lock is more important than its pronation action. This action is particularly important for the deep fibers, which are perpendicular to the bony lever

It is a short, fleshy muscle against the interosseous membrane.

Its fibers are important for coaptation, especially since they are deep (Fig. 2.19).

Its superficial bundle is like a flat muscle, with an electric activity during pronation but not during supination. Its deep bundle is like a pennate muscle, with an electric activity during pronation and supination (Gordon et al. 2004). This makes it an "active ligament" of the distal radioulnar joint: this muscle has the anatomical situation of a ligament combined with the contractile capacity of a muscle.

Its action does not depend on the elbow's position.

– *Supinator* (Gordon et al. 2003)

Its action does not depend on the elbow's position. Therefore, it is important to reinforce it in all the elbow's positions.

However, we know the biceps has a supination action that changes depending on the elbow's position. It is most efficient at 90° of elbow flexion, but its contraction has a dislocation effect on the radial head! (Fig. 2.20).

Its action can be limited with a flexion of the glenohumeral joint.

In case of important instability of the proximal radioulnar lock, we recommend avoiding a 90° elbow flexion or working with the glenohumeral joint in flexion.

– *Pronator teres*

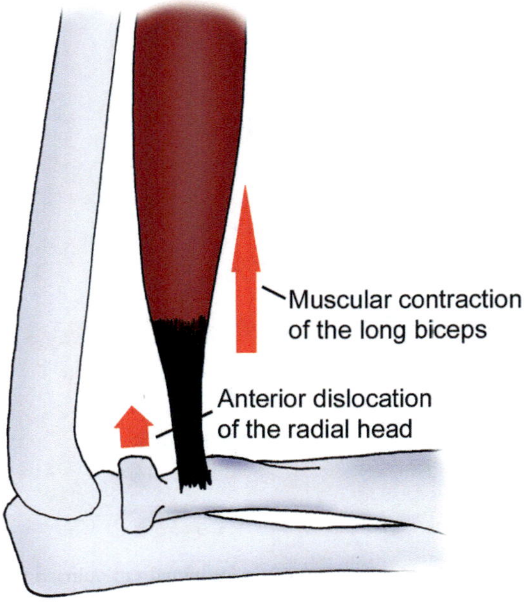

Fig. 2.20 With 90° of elbow flexion, the biceps has an anterior dislocation component of the radial head

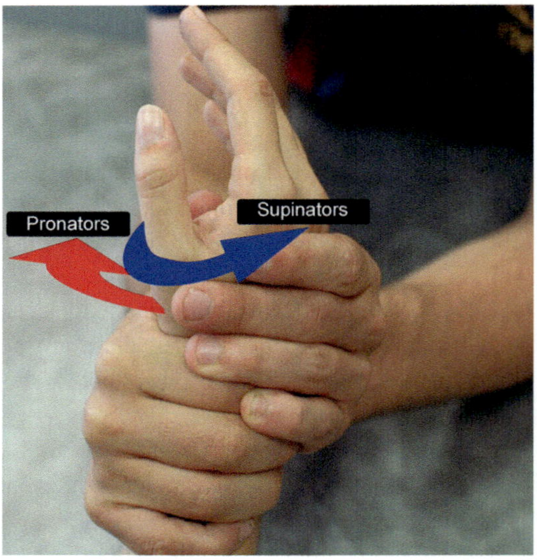

Fig. 2.21 Manual exercise with static and stato-eccentric contractions, and rhythmical stabilizations, adapted to the tonic muscles

Its action is favored with an elbow flexion, which is why this position is preferred for strengthening this muscle (even if we work in all the elbow amplitudes).

Strengthening exercises start with "manual" exercises: the therapist can control the applied resistance (Fig. 2.21). Static reinforcement with

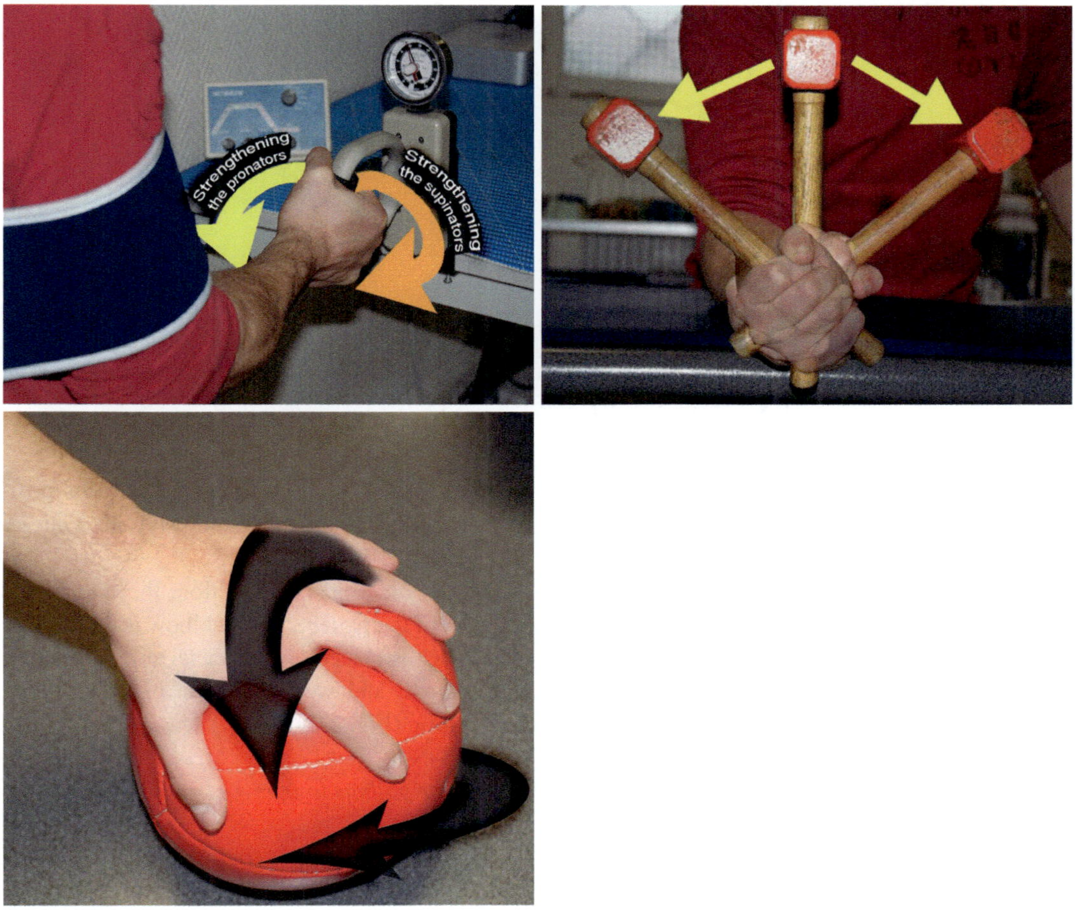

Fig. 2.22 Instrumental exercise with visual feedback and pronosupination dynamometer precisely focusing on the muscular work we want (1). This exercise can be proposed with a hammer (2) or a ball (3)

feedback, proprioception, and feedforward are added to optimize muscle strengthening and radioulnar stability (Fig. 2.22).

It should be noted that its orientation downward and outward makes it pull the radius upwards with respect to the ulna.

- *Longitudinal muscles*

Their role is more complex as they sometimes have destabilizing longitudinal effects. Like in transverse muscles, static exercises are preferred as it is the type of contraction corresponding to the "locking" of the radioulnar unity.

– *Flexor carpi radialis*

It is an epitrochlear muscle, oblique downward and outward. It ends on the bases of the second and third metacarpals.

This orientation gives it a stabilizing action in the frontal plane, but a longitudinal destabilizing action favoring the radial head going upward (Fig. 2.23). Therefore, it must be strengthened carefully, especially in cases of radial head fractures.

– *Radial extensors of the carpus*

They do not cross the radioulnar space and therefore do not have any stabilizing role in the frontal plane, but they forbid the radius from going backward with t-respect to the ulna.

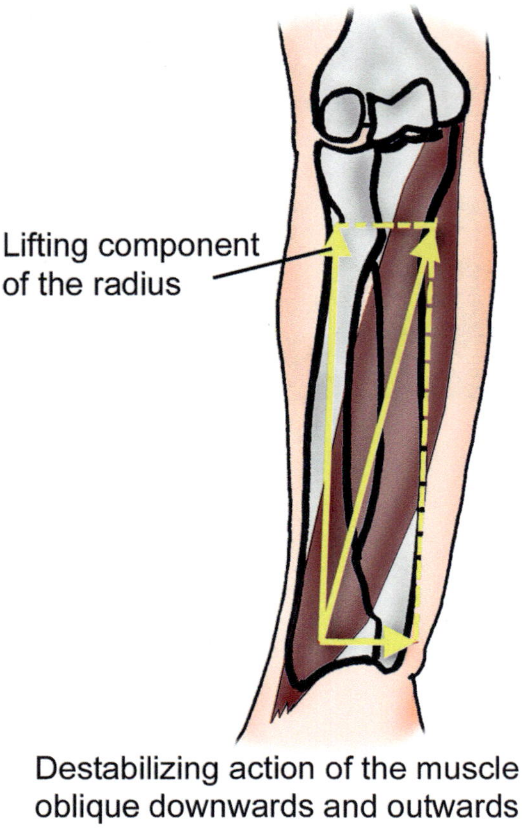

Fig. 2.23 The orientation downward and outward of the flexor carpi radialis gives it an important lifting component of the radius. Its reinforcement must therefore be realized very cautiously in case of fracture of the radial head for example

– *Abductor pollicis longus and extensor pollicis brevis*

They are oblique downward and outward, until the first extensor compartment, therefore, they stabilize the distal radioulnar joint in the frontal plane (Garcia-Elias et al. 2021) (Fig. 2.24). They also bring the radius upwards with respect to the ulna.

– *Extensor carpi ulnaris* (Salva-Coll et al. 2012; Pfirrmann et al. 2001)

It is an epicondylar muscle ending on the dorsal side of the fifth metacarpal's base. Its sheath is part of the TFCC. It helps stabilize the radioulnar joint, mostly in pronation where it

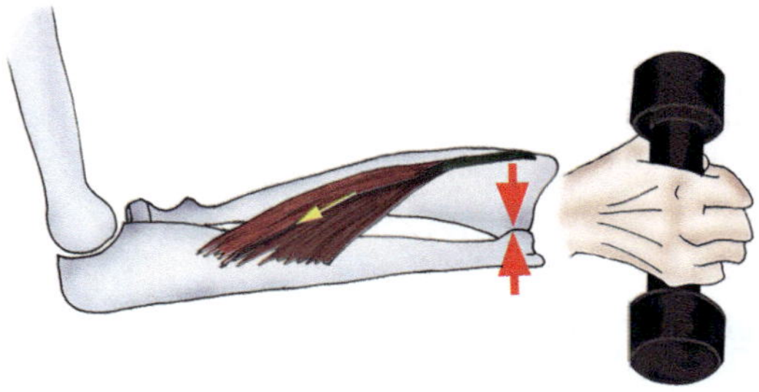

Fig. 2.24 The abductor pollicis longus and the extensor pollicis brevis coapt the proximal radiolunar joint in the frontal plane. These muscles also have an ascending component on the radius relative to the ulna

dynamically coapts the joint thanks to its position as opposed to the radial styloid (Garcia-Elias et al. 2021).

For an analytical contraction, the therapist is in front of the patient, whose elbow is flexed. The resistance is placed on the dorsal side of the fifth metacarpal, and we ask for an extension/ulnar inclination (Fig. 2.25).

– *Flexor pollicis longus*

It does not cross the radioulnar space, but it has notable longitudinal and anteroposterior components thanks to its radial insertion.

In closed chain, it prevents the inferior part of the radius from going frontward.

In fractures of the radial head, it is preferentially strengthened in the closed chain to increase the radioulnar space (Fig. 2.26).

The therapist is in front of the patient and puts a resistance at the level of the palmar side of the thumb's second phalanx. He/She asks for a contraction against a fix resistance if he/she wants to work in closed chain and against a mobile resistance if he/she wants to work in open chain. This exercise is realized in all the pronosupination amplitudes.

– *Flexor digitorum superficialis*

It does not cross the radioulnar space, but its double radioulnar insertion gives it a stabilizing role for the proximal part of the radioulnar frame, in all the planes.

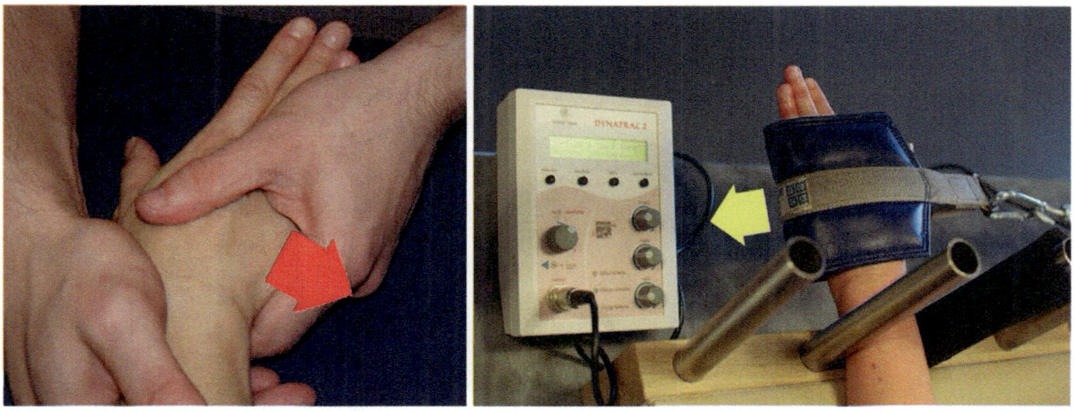

Fig. 2.25 Exercise for the ulnar stabilizers: manually (1) or with a dynamometer and visual feedback precisely focusing on the muscular work we want (2)

In closed chain, its contraction stabilizes the radioulnar frame as it brings its radial and ulnar insertions closer together (Fig. 2.27).

In open chain, it has a destabilizing effect on the distal radioulnar joint as it improves the longitudinal constraints imposed on it.

Therefore, it must be strengthened cautiously in injuries of the distal radioulnar joint, avoiding working in open chain.

The therapist is in front of the patient and puts resistance on the palmar side of the second phalanx of the long fingers. An exercise in closed chain is preferred.

– *Flexor digitorum profundus*

It has an ulnar insertion and does not cross the radioulnar space, which limits its direct stabilizing action. However, it has an indirect stabilizing effect due to its insertion on the interosseous membrane.

The therapist places manual or instrumental resistances on the palmar side of the third phalanges of the long fingers. This exercise is realized in closed chain, as it requires a displacement of the proximal muscle insertion.

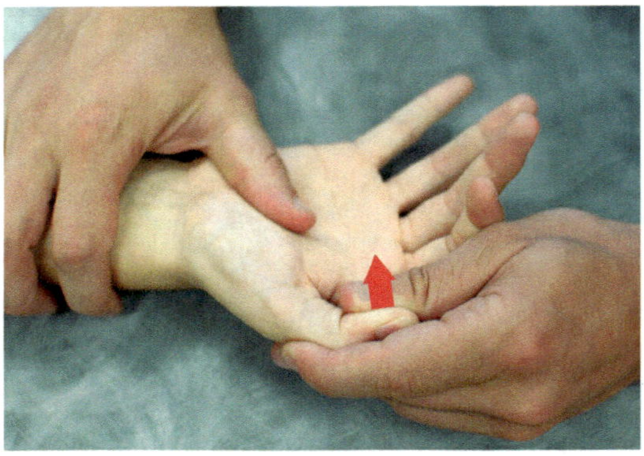

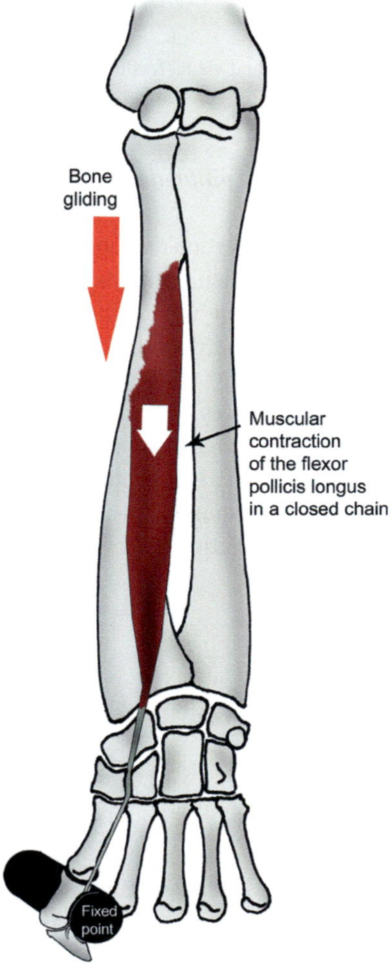

Fig. 2.26 Working in a closed chain with the flexor pollicis longus (resistance is stronger than contraction) (1) to decoapt the radio-humeral joint (2)

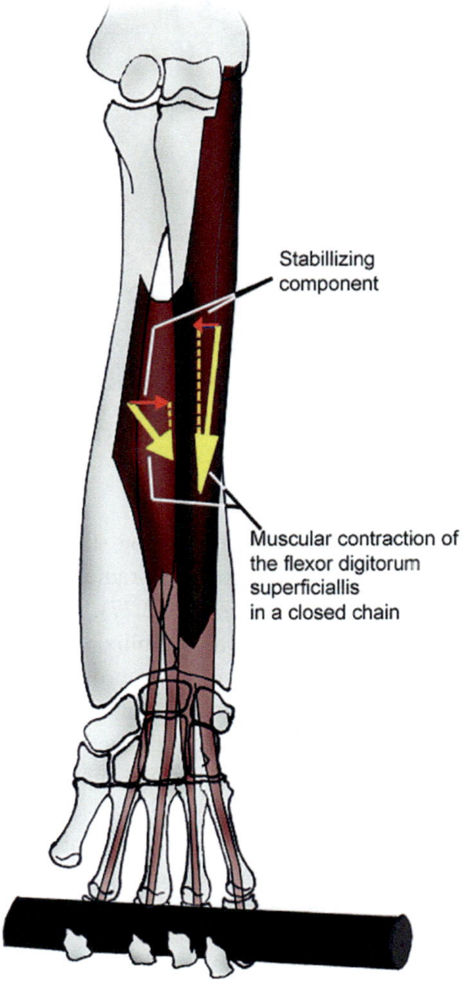

Fig. 2.27 In closed chain, the contraction of the digitorum superficialis induces a radioulnar coaptation

Bibliography

Atzei A, Luchetti R. Foveal TFCC tear classification and treatment. Hand Clin. 2011;27(3):263–72.

Dos Remedios C, et al. Pronator quadratus preservation for distal radius fractures with locking palmar plate osteosynthesis. Surg Tech Chir Main. 2009;28(4):224–9.

Dufour M, Neumayer M, P. M., Recherche de mobilités en glissements sagittaux dans l'articulation radio-ulnaire supérieure. Kinesitherapie Rev. 2008;5(37):35–40.

Garcia-Elias M, et al. Ligaments and muscles stabilizing the radio-ulno-carpal joint. J Hand Surg Eur Vol. 2021;47:17531934211042316.

Ghossoub P, et al. Mobilisations spécifiques. EMC - Kinésithérapie - Médecine physique – Réadaptation. 2009;5(2):1–20.

Gordon KD, et al. Influence of the pronator quadratus and supinator muscle load on DRUJ stability. J Hand Surg Am. 2003;28(6):943–50.

Gordon KD, et al. Electromyographic activity and strength during maximum isometric pronation and supination efforts in healthy adults. J Orthop Res. 2004;22(1):208–13.

Hagert E. Proprioception of the wrist joint: a review of current concepts and possible implications on the rehabilitation of the wrist. J Hand Ther. 2010;23(1):2–16. quiz 17

Hagert E, Hagert CG. Understanding stability of the distal radioulnar joint through an understanding of its anatomy. Hand Clin. 2010;26(4):459–66.

Kihara H, et al. Stabilizing mechanism of the distal radioulnar joint during pronation and supination. J Hand Surg Am. 1995;20A:930–6.

Mesplié G. Stabilité de l'articulation radio ulnaire distale : quid du carré pronateur ? Kinésithérapie, la revue. 2007;68–69:58–62.

Mesplie G, et al. Rehabilitation of distal radioulnar joint instability. Hand Surg Rehabil. 2017;36(5):314–21.

Nakamura T, et al. In vivo motion analysis of forearm rotation utilizing magnetic resonance imaging. Clin Biomech (Bristol, Avon). 1999;14(5):315–20.

Palmer AK, Glisson RR, Werner FW. Relationship between ulnar variance and triangular fibrocartilage complex thickness. J Hand Surg Am. 1984;9(5):681–3.

Pfirrmann CW, et al. What happens to the triangular fibrocartilage complex during pronation and supination of the forearm? Analysis of its morphology and diagnostic assessment with MR arthrography. Skelet Radiol. 2001;30(12):677–85.

Salva-Coll G, et al. Role of the extensor carpi ulnaris and its sheath on dynamic carpal stability. J Hand Surg Eur. 2012;37(6):544–8.

Soubeyrand M, et al. The "muscular hernia sign": an original ultrasonographic sign to detect lesions of the forearm's interosseous membrane. Surg Radiol Anat. 2006a;28(3):372–8.

Soubeyrand M, et al. Ligamentoplasty of the forearm interosseous membrane using the semitendinosus tendon. Anatomical study and surgical procédure. Surg Radiol Anat. 2006b;28(3):300–7.

Soubeyrand M, et al. Pathologie traumatique de la membrane interosseuse de l'avant-bras. Chir Main. 2007;26:255.

Soubeyrand M, et al. The middle radioulnar joint and triarticular forearm complex. J Hand Surg Eur. 2011;36(6):447–54.

Weiss AP, Hastings H. The anatomy of the proximal radioulnar joint. J Shoulder Elb Surg. 1992;1(4):193–9.

3 Recent Fractures of the Inferior Extremity of the Radius

Grégory Mesplié, Nicolas Christiaens,
and Amélie Faraud

Physiopathology

The fractures of the distal extremity of the radius represent up to 18% of all the fractures in adults, and 1.5% of the reasons for consultations in the emergency services (Nellans et al. 2012).

The carpus is the element making the radius vulnerable: during a fall with the wrist in hyperextension, the position of the proximal carpal row will cause anterior, central, or posterior fractures. The strength of the traumatism can then complicate the fracture, from a simple transversal metaphyseal fracture to a complex metaphyso-epiphyseal one.

With a traumatism in hyperextension, there is a dorsal displacement. The joint surface becomes horizontal in both planes (there can even be a dorsal orientation in the sagittal plane), combined with a supination of the joint surface.

With a traumatism in hyperflexion, there is an anterior tilt, with a pronation of the joint surface. These injuries are rare (less than 10%) and are more unstable than the ones with a posterior tilt. There often is an epiphyseal component: in up to 70–80% of the cases (Turner et al. 2010; McKay et al. 2001; Castaing 1964; Laulan et al. 2016). The postero-medial fragment, called "die punch," is the most important one to reduce. It is present in 14–70% of joint fractures and is one of the therapeutic issues in joint reduction, as it is difficult to reduce. Several authors say they failed to reduce it with external maneuvers (Knirk and Jupiter 1986; Porter and Tillman 1992; Beck et al. 2014).

The "die punch" fragment is often separated from the lateral side by a sagittal fracture line, and from the antero-medial side by a frontal fracture line. The "die punch" fragment and the antero-medial side form a medial complex described by Melone (Melone 1984; Laulan and Obert 2009) (Fig. 3.1).

We use Laulan's MEU classification (Laulan et al. 2016), which separates the Metaphyseal, Epiphyseal, and Ulnar components (Table 3.1).

Moreover, there are frequent associated ligamentous injuries (20–30%) (Fontes et al. 1992) that can lead to degenerative injuries in the wrist if they are not well treated (Geissler et al. 1996a; Geissler et al. 1996b). There are in fact 30% of scapholunate injuries and 30% of TFCC injuries diagnosed with arthroscopy (Christiaens et al. 2017).

In practice, fractures in elderly patients and patients with osteoporosis are mostly metaphyseal fractures without associated injuries, while

G. Mesplié (✉)
ISAMMS, Biarritz, France

N. Christiaens · A. Faraud
Institut Sud Aquitain de la Main et du Membre Supérieur, Biarritz, France

G. Mesplié (ed.), *Wrist Functional Anatomy and Therapy*,
https://doi.org/10.1007/978-3-031-42879-1_3

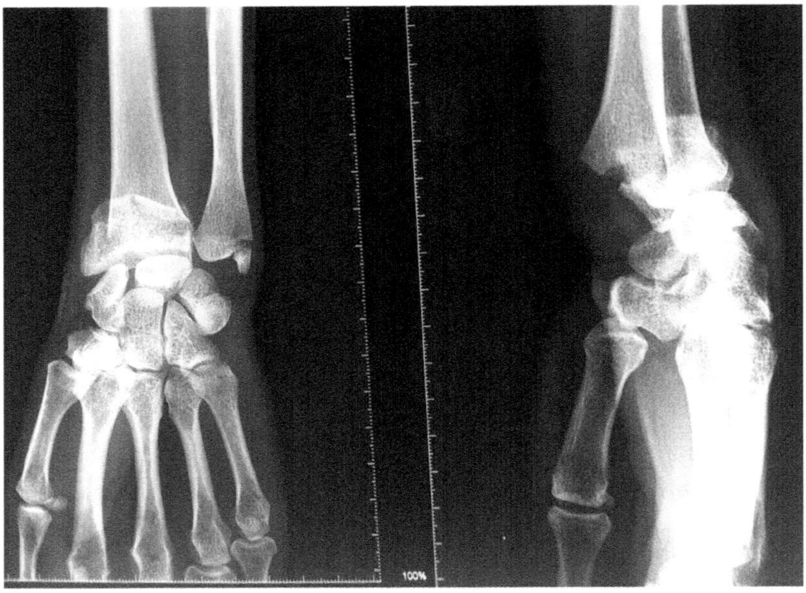

Fig. 3.1 Example of fracture with "die punch" fragment

fractures in younger patients caused by more violent traumatisms will often be complex with associated injuries.

This type of fracture can modify the radioulnar index with an injury of the triangular complex and/or another radioulnar lock, disturbing the dynamics and/or stability of the radioulnar frame (see chapter *"Injuries of the radioulnar unity"*).

In this chapter, we will only see the injuries of the inferior extremity of the radius that do not lead to these complications.

Table 3.1 Laulan's MEU classification

Components of the distal radius fractures	Classification criteria	Injury ranks 0	1	2	3	4
M (metaphyseal)	Metaphyseal fracture line: cortical comminution	No metaphyseal fracture	No comminution of the metaphyseal line	Localized comminution (<½ circumference)	Wide comminution (>½ circumference)	Circumferential comminution
M' (metaphyseal)	Metaphyseal line ending in the distal radioulnar joint					
E (epiphyseal)	Articular fracture line(s): presence and displacement, type (shear or depression), area	No articular fracture	Articular fracture with no displacement	Fracture with displacement because of shearing	Localized articular recess. There still are simple reduction criteria	Wide recess (epiphyseal fragmentation, >3 articular fragments)
U (ulnar)	Ulnar fracture line: presence and displacement, location	No ulnar fracture	Ulnar fracture with no displacement	Displaced fracture of the ulnar head (>2 mm)	Displaced metaphyso-diaphyseal fracture (±styloid)	Displaced metaphyso-diaphyseal fracture (±styloid)

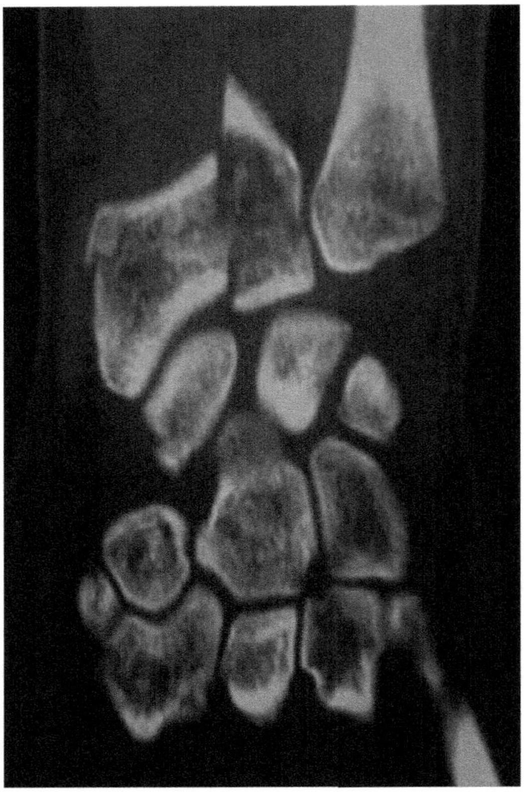

Fig. 3.2 Wrist scanner

Clinical and Paraclinical Signs

A radiological assessment must be done after any injury causing pain or wrist deformity. It must be complemented by a wrist scan if it is not sufficient (Fig. 3.2).

We always check the radial pulse and the absence of injury of the median nerve. This verification can require a quick reduction of the fracture, or even emergency surgery.

Therapeutic Process and Surgical Treatment

The orthopedic treatment is used in stable and non-displaced fractures of the distal radius.

On the other hand, surgery is used in displaced fractures of the metaphysis or joint surface, and that are unstable after reduction. The therapeutic indications depend on the injury and on the M and E parameters of J. Laulan's classification (Laulan et al. 2016) (Table 3.2).

The surgery's aims are:

- To obtain an anatomical restitution of the joint surface, the relative length of the radius with respect to the ulna (radioulnar index), and the orientation of the joint surface (radial slope in the frontal and sagittal planes).
- To obtain the joint reduction closest to the original anatomy to prevent the risk of radiocarpal and midcarpal arthrosis.
- To diagnose and treat the associated injuries (ligamentous injuries or carpal bone fractures).

This guarantees a quality functional recovery.

Reduction

It is always performed with an external maneuver at first, with the help of an image intensifier. We also take shots in traction to analyze better the fracture lines.

In joint fractures, arthroscopy can be interesting to check the quality of the joint reduction and diagnose possible associated ligamentous injuries.

In children, the periosteum is thick and of good quality: displaced fractures of the radial metaphysis are usually stable once reduced and do not require complementary surgical fixation.

Generally, in adults, fractures are unstable once reduced and require osteosynthesis in most cases.

Osteosynthesis

The goal is to obtain a stable fixation allowing consolidation with no secondary displace-

Table 3.2 Schematical therapeutical indications depending on the injuries of the M and E parameters, and their combinations

	M0	M1	M2	M3	M4
E0		Ortho	Pin or plate[a]	Pin or plate with locked screws	Pin + external fixator[b] or plate with locked screws
E1	Ortho	Ortho	Pin or plate	Pin or plate with locked screws	Pin + external fixator[b] or plate with locked screws
E2	Pin or plate	Pin or plate	Pin or plate	Pin or plate with locked screws	Pin + external fixator or plate with locked screws
E3	Pin or plate with locked screws	Pin or plate with locked screws	Pin or plate with locked screws	Plate with locked screws (or external fixator + pin) ± graft	Plate with locked screws (or pin + external fixator) ±
E4	Pin + external fixator or plate with locked screws ± external fixator	Pins + external fixator or plate with locked screws ± external fixator	Pin + external fixator or plate with locked screws ± external fixator	External fixator + pin (or external fixator + plate with locked screws) ± graft	±

[a] The choice between pins and screwed plate depends on the direction of displacement or the location of a reduction default: dorsal (pins) or palmar (plate), as well as the bone quality (degree of osteoporosis)
[b] In these cases, the external fixator can only be radio-radial (and not radio-carpal)

ment, ideally with an early mobilization of the wrist.

There are three ways to perform the osteosynthesis:

Pins

They are generally put percutaneously and can only be dorsal or lateral as there is a major risk of injury for the noble palmar elements (radial artery and median nerve). Pins can only be put in extra-articular fractures with a dorsal tilt, and with little to no posterior comminution.

Screwed Plates

They are more stable than pins, and this stability is even more important since the screws can have angular stability inside the plate (locked screws). This osteosynthesis can be used in fractures with an anterior or a dorsal tilt, fractures with several fragments, and joint fractures.

It has many advantages, regarding radiological, functional, and clinical criteria. It is also more stable (Geissler et al. 1996a) and allows earlier wrist mobilization.

External Fixator

This last resort technique is used in complex fractures in which the other osteosynthesis techniques are not enough. The principle is to use the ligamentotaxis induced by the wrist distraction. The problems of this technique are the high number of complex regional pain syndromes related to distraction and the inaccessibility of the postero-medial fragment of the radius on which no ligament is inserted.

To prevent these complications, it is recommended to realize the smallest distraction possible, and to place at least one postero-medial pin combined with the external fixator.

Rehabilitation and Orthotic Treatment

Rehabilitation Protocol (Fig. 3.3)

This protocol can follow the surgery or orthopedic treatment and can be modified depending on the healing evolution. It must be started as early

FRACTURES OF THE INFERIOR EXTREMITY OF THE RADIUS	Post-surgery / trauma (A)	Relative fragility (B)	Solidity (C)
REHABILITATION	**Goals:** 1 – To reduce trophic disorders 2 – To reduce pain 3 – To prevent the risk of stiffness in the free joints 4 – To maintain the proprioceptive abilities **Techniques:** 1 – Draining massages and compressive bandage, vacuum therapy for draining, low-frequency electrical currents 2 – Cryotherapy, TENS, TVS (100Hz) 3 – Mobilization of the free joints in passive and active (fingers +++) 4 – TVS (70-80Hz) and varied sensitive stimulation without constraints **Risks:** Bad healing (pseudarthrosis, vicious callus) in case of non-observance, type 1 CRPS (favored by maladapted immobilization), EPL rupture (pins), adherences of the FDP and FPL (anterior plate)	**Goals:** 1 – Same as in phase A with intensified techniques if necessary 2 – To recover joint mobility (except flexion if capsulodesis) 3 – To gradually recover the protective muscles' proprioceptive abilities **Techniques:** 1 – Pressotherapy for draining, vacuum therapy on the scar, defibrosing massage if the scar is not inflammatory and closed (A1), manipulation of light objects (A4) 2 – Soft mobilizations (instrumental and manual), work in ulnar decoaptation if the RUI is positive 3 – Gradual conscious proprioceptive work, then global conscious neuromuscular rehabilitation, NO BALL CLENCHING and no exercise in pronation if there is a long ulna **Risks:** Same as phase A + type 1 CRPS	**Goals:** 1 – Same as in phases A and B with intensified techniques if necessary 2 – Total functional recovery **Techniques:** 1 – Intensification of the mobilizations with specific joint mobilizations, postures, and electrostimulation (B2) 2 – Unconscious neuromuscular rehabilitation and recovery of normal muscular ratios (B3) 3 – Functional activities adapted to the patient's professional and sports needs **Risks:** Same as in phases A and B
ORTHOSES	2 options: - Strict immobilization (limiting the rehabilitation options) - Removable orthosis	Gradual removal	Functional orthosis for resumption of activity
	D3 to D21/45	D21/45 to D90	After D90

Fig. 3.3 Rehabilitation protocol (2) and progression pyramid (2)

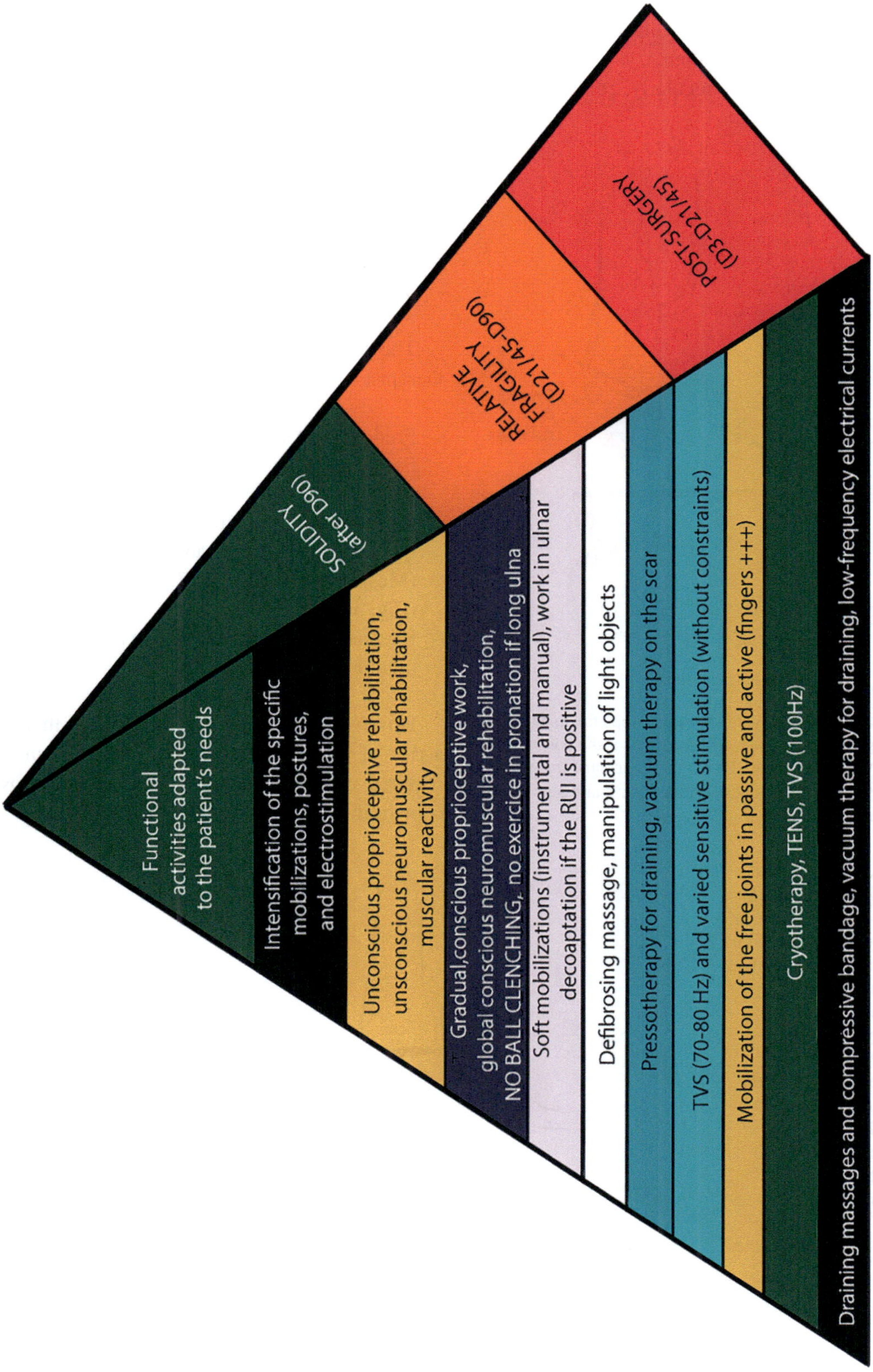

Fig. 3.3 (continued)

as possible to limit the risk of complications (Thomas and Zanin 2016; Gillespie et al. 2016), and adapted to bone healing.

This evolution is regularly controlled with X-rays.

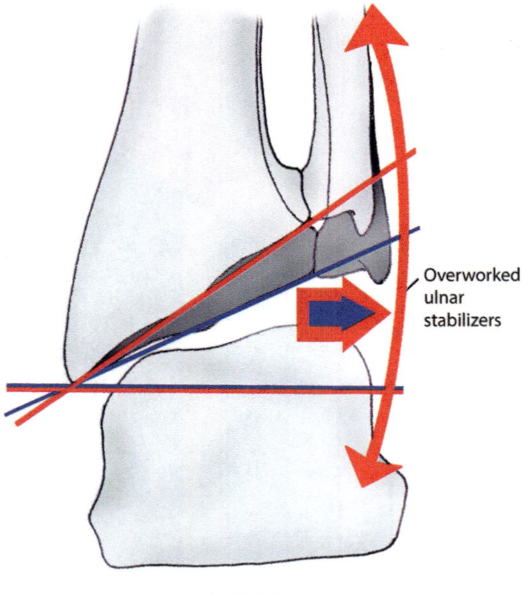

Fig. 3.4 The increase of the radial slope favors the carpal gliding toward the ulna, which increases the constraints at this level. In this case, the rehabilitator must intensify the strengthening techniques for the ulnar stabilizers to fight this phenomenon

From a symptomatic point of view, the patients often describe pain on the ulnar side of the wrist that can have various causes (Kramer et al. 2013):

- Increase of the radial slope leading to overwork of the ulnar stabilizers.
- Associated injury of the distal radioulnar ligaments.
- Changes in the radioulnar index with a "long" ulna increases the ulnocarpal constraints.

The consequences of these unbalances for the therapist are:

- Predominant strengthening of the ulnar stabilizers in case of increased radial slope (Fig. 3.4).
- Predominant strengthening of the pronator quadratus in distal radioulnar instabilities (Mesplie et al. 2017; Mesplié 2007) (Fig. 3.5).
- Exercises in ulnar decoaptation in case of long ulna (Fig. 3.6).

However, if the symptoms persist or if there is a risk of arthrosis, a corrective surgery can be required (Wafer procedure, osteotomy, arthroscopy of the TFCC).

Fig. 3.5 A combined injury of the triangular complex can cause pain, or even instability if it is associated with an injury of one of the two other radioulnar locks (1). Strengthening the pronator quadratus (active ligament for the distal radioulnar joint) helps limit pain and instability (combined with the other "key" radioulnar muscles—see Chap. 2) (2)

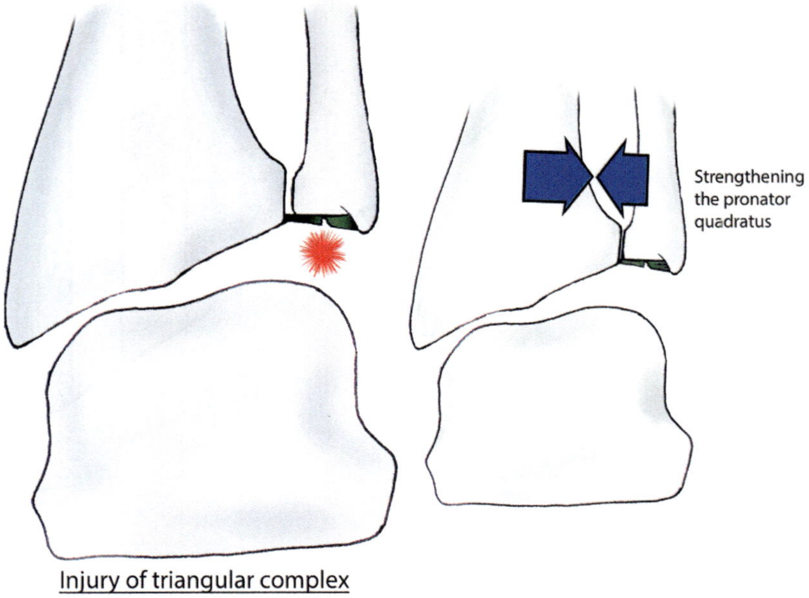

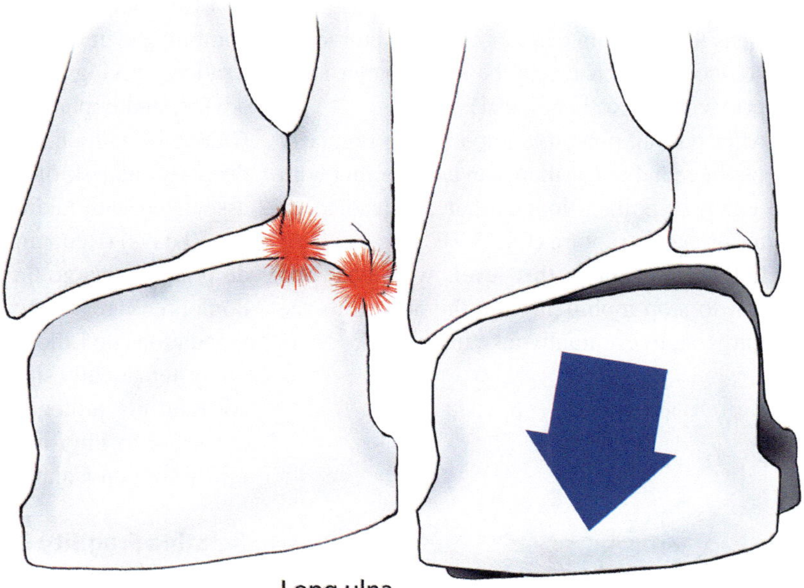

Fig. 3.6 A long ulna increases ulnocarpal constraints (1). Decompressive maneuvers are preferred as they limit this phenomenon, as well as exercises in supination where the radioulnar index decreases (2)

Post-surgical or Post-traumatic Phase (D0 to D21/45)

The duration of immobilization after surgery depends on the initial fracture, the type of surgery, and the evolution of the bone healing.

The treatment is based on the PRICE protocol to fight against trophic disorders and pain:

- P for protection of the fracture site during the whole phase, realized immobilizing the wrist and informing the patient about the tissue fragility in this phase.
- R for rest of the damaged area that must not be solicited during the immobilization phase, aside from self-rehabilitation exercises explained by the therapist.
- I for ice, put cold packs several times a day on the fracture zone. If there is a cast it is impossible, but if there is no wound and we immobilize the patient with a thermoformed orthosis the patient can do a cold bath against edema.
- C for compression that can be performed in the fingers if they are swollen.
- E for elevation of the wrist to avoid edema.

Finger stiffness is frequent, and an adapted early mobilization protocol is essential to optimize recovery (Smith et al. 2004).

During this whole phase, rehabilitation is mostly simple active self-mobilization in the healthy joints, especially the metacarpophalangeal joints that can easily get stiff.

The patient should do a short series of exercises (10–15 repetitions), several times a day (3 times in the morning and 3 times in the afternoon). These exercises must be stopped in case of pain.

The use of transcutaneous vibratory stimulations (TVS) with a frequency of 70–80 Hz is interesting at the level of the myotendinous junctions, as they stimulate motor and premotor areas and reduce disturbances in the motor pattern and proprioception (Roll et al. 2012).

After putting pins, it is important to regularly check the radial pin as there can be a conflict with the extensor pollicis longus that can lead to an injury or even a rupture (Fig. 3.7).

If there is pain at this level, we advise the patient to stop mobilizing the thumb and to see his surgeon, to eventually take the pin off.

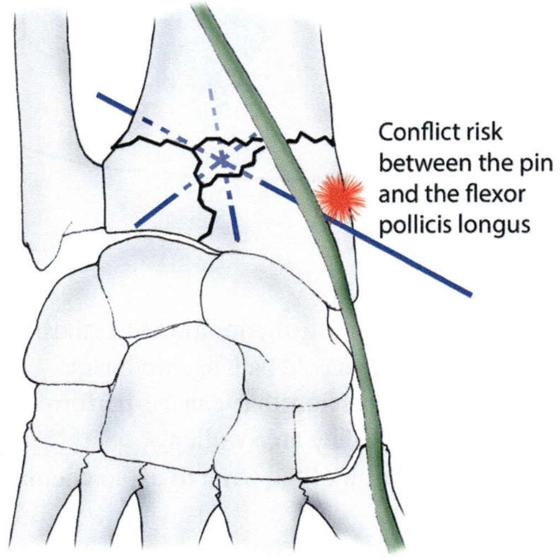

Fig. 3.7 After putting a pin, it is very important to check if there are not any conflicts between the pin and the extensor pollicis longus. This conflict could lead to a rupture of the tendon

Liverpool's guidelines (Gillespie et al. 2016) combine the importance of checking the immobilization, giving the patient self-mobilization advice, and explaining the patient his pathology (Mathews and Chung 2015). They considerably decrease the risk of CRPS (Fig. 3.8) and can be associated with taking vitamin C (500 mg a day for 50 days) (Recommandations diagnostiques et de prise en charge thérapeutique des syndromes douloureux régionaux complexes : les recommandations de Lille 2019; Shah et al. 2009).

Systematically starting a mirror therapy protocol (and not motor imagery) in this phase does not seem to improve the results in this type of injury (Bayon-Calatayud et al. 2016).

Relative Fragility Phase (D21/45 to D90)

In this phase, we start putting load on the fracture site and the patient progressively goes back to his daily activities. We fight against pain and trophic disorders if they are still present, try to regain functional amplitudes and start working on conscious and unconscious proprioceptive abilities. This work must allow the patient to regain functionality in his daily activities.

- *Fight against trophic disorders and pain*

It is essential as it sets the possibilities for other exercises. Therefore, it is the key element of this phase. We can use:

Fig. 3.8 The Liverpool advice to significantly reduce the risks of CRPS

1 – Do not immobilize with excess or without reason, a distal radial fracture.
2 – Make sure the casts are well adjusted and comfortable, avoiding excessive flexion and sharp edges, and making sure the phalanges can move freely.
3 – Encourage contraction/release exercise every hour, with the hand higher than the elbow, to control the edema.
4 – Control the immobilized limb.
5 – Every verbal information must come with an information brochure for the patient.
6 – Every advice given must be written down on a paper for the patient.
7 – Always change a cast if the patient signals that it is too tight and/or uncomfortable.
8 – Propose a consultation with a specialized orthopedist, if the patient frequently asks for the cast to be changed or signals a claustrophobia in the cast.

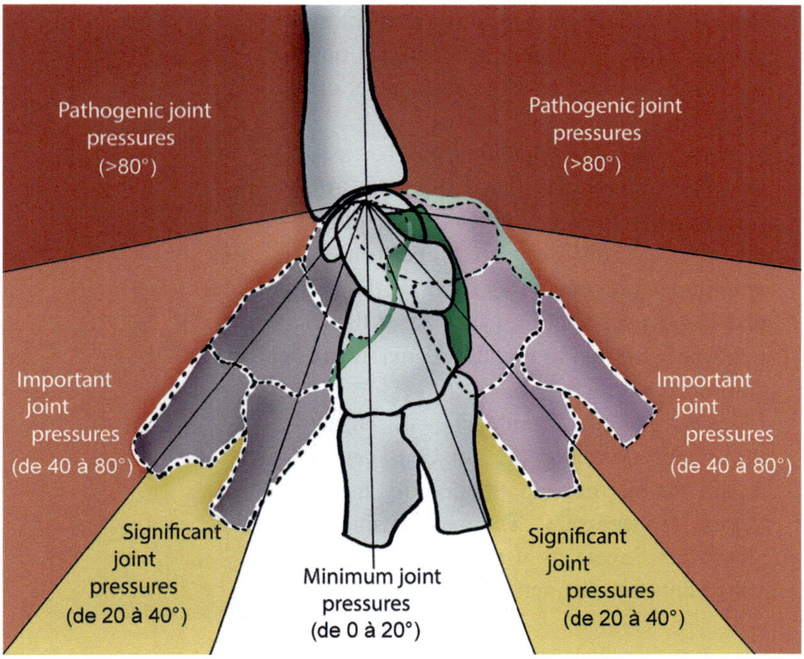

Fig. 3.9 Joint pressures depending on the wrist amplitudes

- In case of surgery, scar massages can be done if the recoloring time is over 2 s in the diascopy test. Decontracting massages for the forearm can also be done if we observe hypertonia in the extrinsic musculature, which is frequent.
- Analgesic electrotherapy can be used with the parameters described in Volume 1—Chapter "Physical agents."
- Pressotherapy from distal to proximal helps drain the wrist (cf. Volume 1—Chapter "Physical agents"). In this phase, this technique can be badly tolerated by the patient; we will then delay its use.
- Transcutaneous vibratory stimulations and infrasound are used for their analgesic and vasomotor effect (cf. Volume 1—Chapter "Physical agents"). Vibrations with more than 1 mm amplitude are realized far from the fracture site in order not to disturb the healing process.

• *Regaining functional amplitudes*

Mobilizations must not harm the healing process of the fracture site: if the cartilaginous callus bears hypoxia well, the osseous callus does not. An excess of constraints on the fracture site during this phase can cause hypoxia and prevent the osseous callus from developing, leading to pseudoarthrosis.

Therefore, it is important to know the relation between joint amplitudes and supported pressures (Fig. 3.9).

All these elements allow for defining "risky" areas in which the exercises to regain amplitude will have to be realized very cautiously, without any force.

These areas are after 20° in flexion/extension and ulnar inclination and from 5° in radial inclination (Kapandji 2005).

Trying to regain total amplitudes at all costs is, in this phase, useless and dangerous.

We use the same techniques as for scaphoid fractures, but being more careful with pronosupination movements as they often cause problems:

- Fluidotherapy to relax the muscles and tissues. We use it at the beginning of the session to warm-up the wrist.
- Passive manual mobilizations are basic exercises to regain joint amplitude. They are soft, pain free, and can be realized increasing the joint spaces a little.

- Active mobilizations are performed after the passive ones, in various finger positions to improve tendinous glidings at the level of the wrist.
- Active-assisted mobilizations can be assisted by an arthromotor. We ask the patient to participate actively in the movements applied by the device. This exercise is performed in amplitudes previously regained by the therapist in passive. It has an interest at the joint level, but also in draining the edema. It can be combined with icing.
- Electrostimulation, combined with an active movement (winding the fingers), can help regain the last degrees of mobility in finger flexion if necessary. The patient must not clutch his fingers as it would put important constraints on the fracture site.

The dart thrower's motion (DTM) is defined by the International Federation of Societies for Surgery of the Hand as the movement between radial extension and ulnar flexion. It is the most used movement in our daily activities (Crisco et al. 2005). It is in a movement plane of 45° between the sagittal and frontal planes. It is performed almost exclusively in the medio-carpal joint, without any participation of the radio-carpal joint.

Mobilizations following the DTM plane help us maintain functional mobility in the wrist while reducing radio-carpal movements and movements within the first carpal row. Therefore, it is a particularly interesting exercise right after taking the immobilization off.

In this phase, specific radio-carpal and radio-ulnar mobilizations are forbidden as they can be dangerous for the fracture site.

- *Proprioceptive abilities of the wrist*

It is important to propose a coherent evolution for the exercises depending on the healing phase, in order not to disturb the consolidation process. The recovery stage of the proprioceptive abilities must also be considered so that the patient does not develop compensative pathologies such as tendinopathies or reflex contractures.

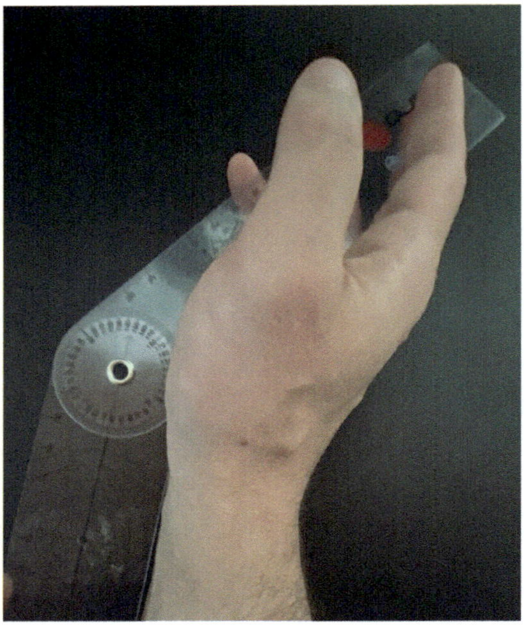

Fig. 3.10 Assessment of the joint position perception (statesthesia or position sense)

- *Perception of joint position (Hagert's stage 3)*

It is defined as the ability to precisely reproduce a given joint angulation (Hagert 2010).

The rehabilitation of this perception is done in three steps. In the first step, the therapist places the patient's wrist in a defined joint position and controls the joint amplitude with a goniometer.

In the second step, the wrist is placed in another position, indifferently. In the third step, the patient must place his forearm in the first position (Hagert 2010; Karagiannopoulos et al. 2016) (Fig. 3.10).

The exercise is realized with the patient's eyes closed to avoid any visual afference. An error margin of 4° is considered normal in adults (at the level of the wrists).

This test is highly correlated with the wrist's sensorimotor abilities (Karagiannopoulos et al. 2016) and must therefore be done before any evolution of the rehabilitation protocol—especially before Hager's stage 5.

- *Kinesthesia (Hagert's stage 4)*

It is defined as the ability to detect a passive movement. The therapist realizes the movement

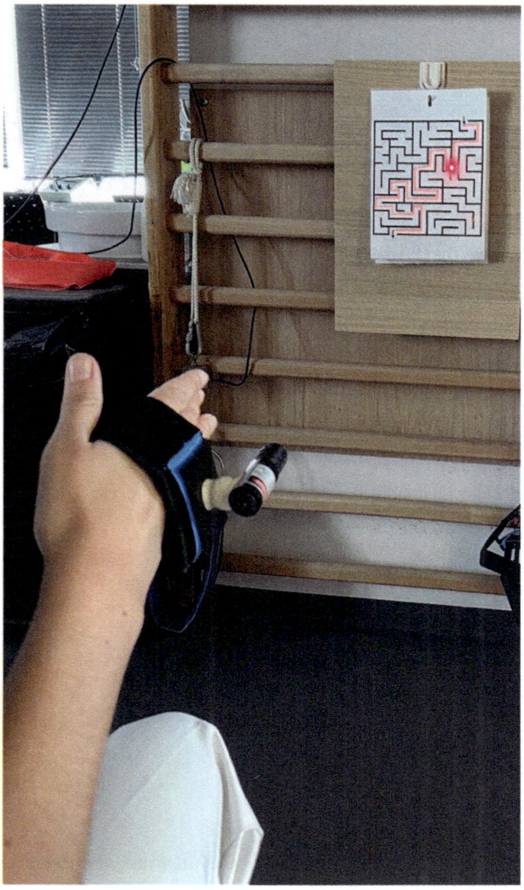

Fig. 3.11 Using a laser to improve conscious proprioceptive abilities

while the patient keeps his eyes closed and tells him when he perceives the movement.

This exercise is easy to realize at the physiotherapy office or at home but does not allow a precise analysis regarding the patient's perception threshold.

Using an arthromotor device allows for analyzing more precisely the movement speed and the studied angular sector.

A laser can also be a very helpful tool to improve conscious proprioceptive abilities. The patient must follow trajectories becoming increasingly complex, going faster and faster (Fig. 3.11).

– *Conscious neuromuscular rehabilitation (Hagert's stage 5)*

Several strengthening modes have been described to improve neuromuscular capacities. They help increase the basic muscle tone and therefore the joint's dynamic stability (Riemann and Lephart 2002a).

At this stage, we use muscular awakening techniques and static contractions in four directions, favoring the contraction of the ulnar stabilizers that have an essential stabilizing role, especially when the radial slope is increased.

These exercises can be manual, analytical, or global (Fig. 3.12).

Throughout the sessions, the joint position evolves from a stability position to a more unstable position, always respecting the tissue's healing phases and the "no pain" rule.

If the radioulnar index is modified with a (relative) long ulna, these exercises are performed with the forearm in a supination or neutral position, to decrease the stress on the TFCC's meniscus that is higher in pronation.

This protocol is completed by the muscular awakening of the pronator quadratus using the abductor pollicis longus as a "trigger" muscle (Fig. 3.13), and its strengthening using controlled manual and instrumental techniques (Fig. 3.14). This is especially true in case of a combined injury of the TFCC as the pronator quadratus is a powerful distal radioulnar stabilizer.

As in any wrist injury, strengthening the finger flexors is forbidden at this stage, especially clamping a ball as it produces important compressive constraints on the carpus and the two forearm bones (Fig. 3.15).

– *Unconscious neuromuscular rehabilitation or reflex muscle activation (Hager's sixth stage)*

Conscious neuromuscular rehabilitation intentionally targets the requested muscles. On the contrary, unconscious neuromuscular rehabilitation uses the reflexes that actively lock the joints, which can partially compensate a passive instability.

In this phase, the exercises are of a moderate intensity in order not to disturb the healing process.

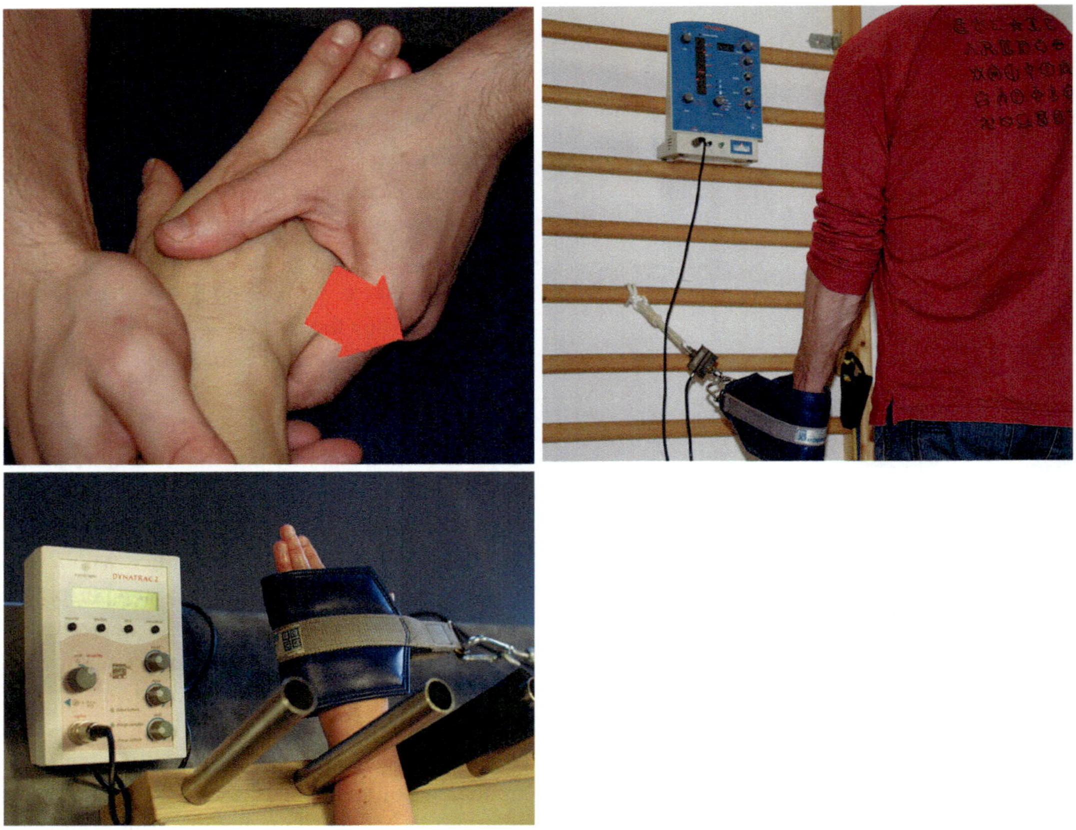

Fig. 3.12 Manual exercise for the ulnar stabilizers (1). Analytical instrumental exercise for the ulnar stabilizers with load cell and visual feedback for better control of the contraction parameters (2). Global instrumental exercise with a similar device (3)

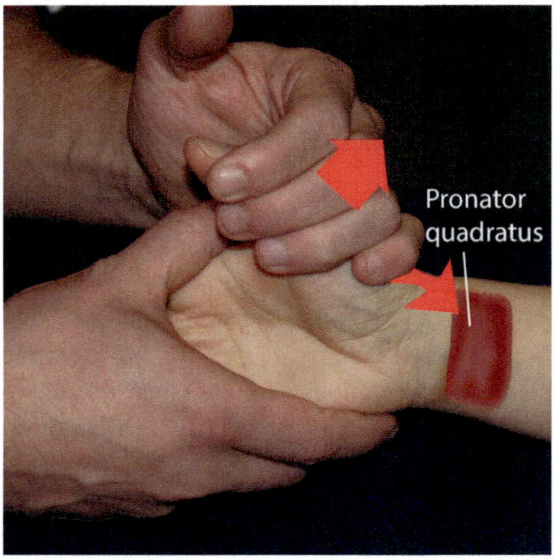

Fig. 3.13 Exercise for the pronator quadratus in irradiation from the abductor pollicis brevis

- *Table Tennis Racket*

  We ask the patient to maintain the ball on the racket, which implies a good sensorial analysis and a contraction adapted to the received information.

  Progressively, we ask the patient to throw the ball and receive it "softly" on the racket.
- *Exercise with a Plastic Ball*

  We use a light plastic ball and ask the patient to pass it from one hand to the other, to throw and catch it.

- *Coordination and dexterity*

We work on prehensions to improve coordination and dexterity and therefore improve functional capacities in daily activities.

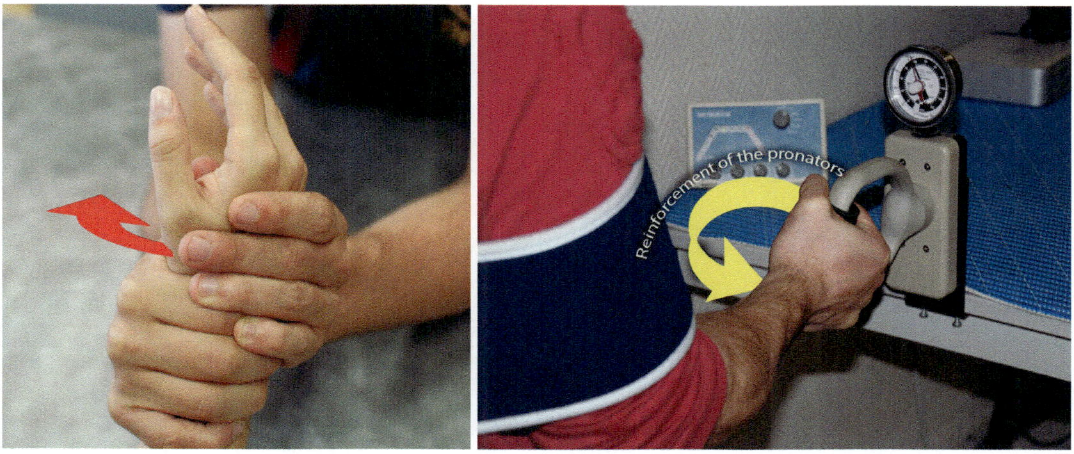

Fig. 3.14 Manual exercise for the pronator quadratus with direct resistance (1), and instrumental exercise with visual feedback for a precise control of the contraction's intensity (2)

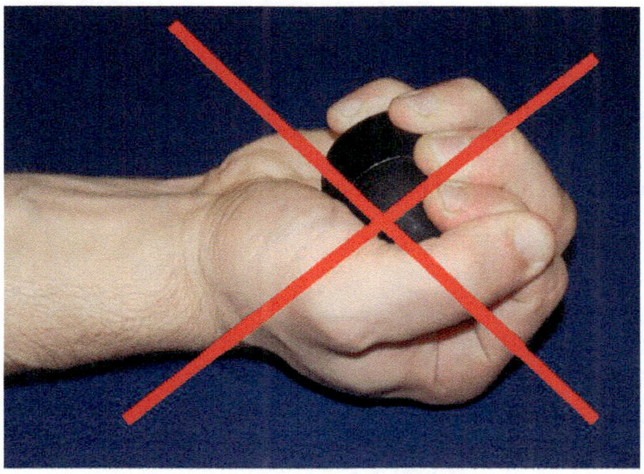

Fig. 3.15 Clamping a ball is forbidden during the healing phase as it puts important constraints on the wrist

These exercises are performed without clamping or putting excessive constraints on the callus.

Manipulating two golf balls or a small ball improves coordination and dexterity without excessive risks for bone healing (Fig. 3.16).

Consolidation Phase (after D90)

When the callus is solid, we can start more intensive techniques—but not aggressive ones.

In this phase, we try to reach a total recovery of strength and amplitude in the wrist. Rebalancing the strength ratios between the different muscular groups limits the risks of secondary tendinopathies.

Prehension and proprioception exercises meet the functional requirements related to the patient's professional and leisure activities.

- *Regaining amplitudes in the wrist*

We keep using the techniques from the previous phase, intensifying them if needed (always without pain) to recover the total wrist amplitudes.

In this phase, specific mobilizations are authorized and help with the carpal and radio-carpal dynamics.

– *Stretching*

  Stretching the forearm muscles helps fight against muscular stiffness by stretching the wrist flexors (stiffness in extension) or extensors (stiffness in flexion) (Fig. 3.17).

  Hypo-extensibility and adherences around the muscles and tendons are frequent in the wrist and finger flexors after putting an anterior plate, so these stretching techniques are especially adapted after this type of surgery.

– *Specific mobilizations*

  They require a good knowledge of the morpho-palpatory anatomy and the radio-carpal and intracarpal biomechanics. Tractions and glidings are realized between the radius and the first carpal row, between the first and second carpal row, and between the carpal bones if necessary.

- *Mobilization First Row/Carpus*

To perform the radio-carpal mobilizations, the therapist holds the first carpal row with one hand,

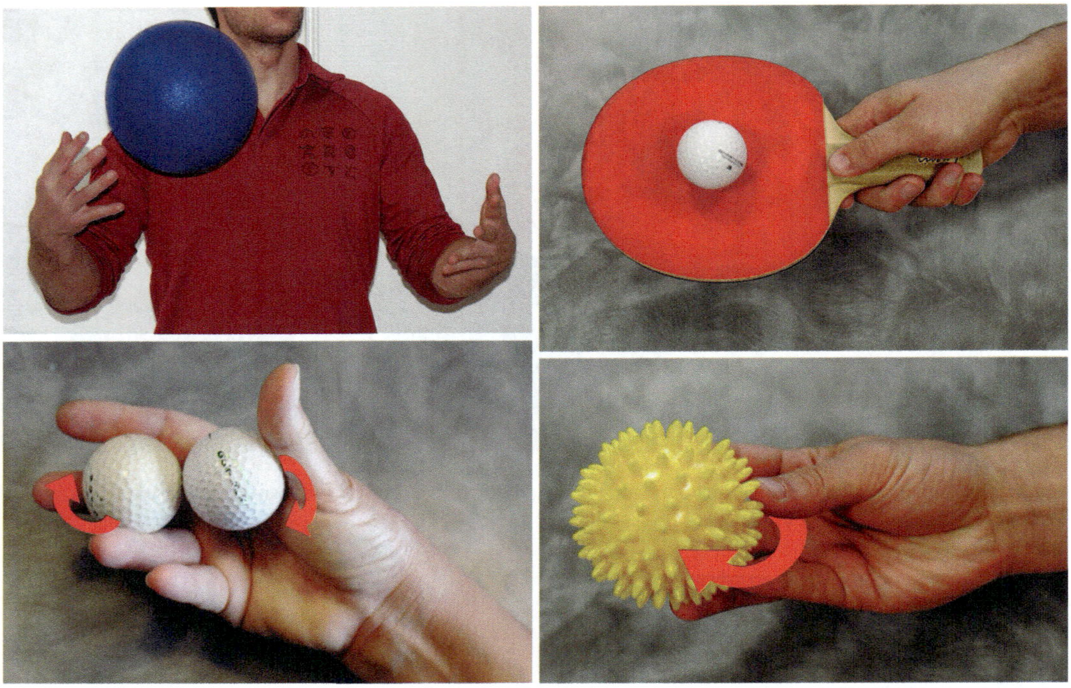

Fig. 3.16 Examples of exercises for unconscious neuromuscular rehabilitation (1–2) and coordination/manual dexterity (3–4)

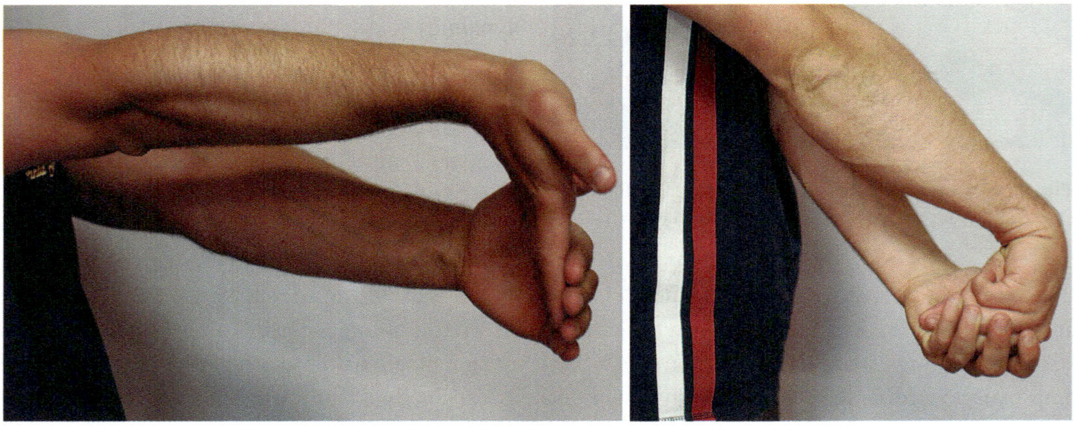

Fig. 3.17 Stretching of the wrist and finger flexors. It is even more important after putting and anterior plate (adherences or hypo-extensibility of the flexors) (1). Stretching of the extensors (2)

while the other hand immobilizes the inferior extremity of the radius, always respecting the radial slope (oblique downward and outward in the frontal plane) (Fig. 3.18).

The distal grip performs the mobilizations and the accessory movements. In practice, the manual realization of these mobilizations can be simplified and better controlled if we work with associated movements according to the combinations described in Tables 3.3 and 3.4. It is also interesting to vary the combinations (Figs. 3.19, 3.20, and 3.21). For example, when looking for wrist extension, we should use the associated movements (radial inclination and pronosupination) and the accessory movements (anterior and radial glidings). Therefore, the

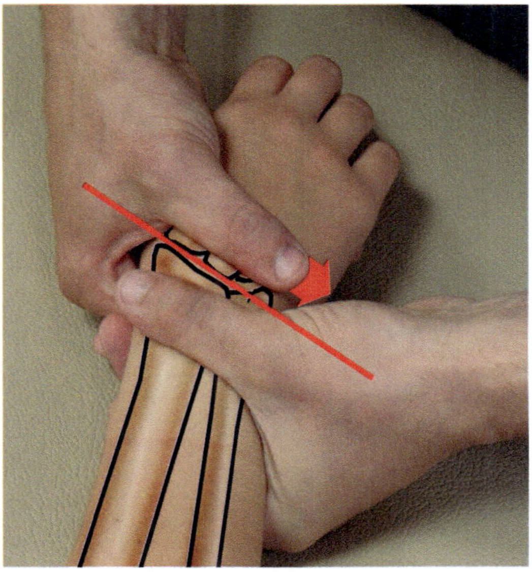

Fig. 3.18 Specific mobilization of the first carpal row with respect to the two bones of the forearm, respecting the axes of movement (the radial slope is oblique downwards and outwards in the frontal plane and downward and backward in the sagittal plane)

Table 3.3 Summary table of the combinations of radio-carpal movements in the different planes depending on the wrist movements

	Sagittal plane	Frontal plane	Transversal plane
Wrist flexion	Flexion	Slight ulnar inclination	Scaphoid and triquetrum: very slight pronation Lunate: very slight supination
Wrist extension	Extension	Very slight radial inclination	Scaphoid and triquetrum: very slight supination Lunate: very slight pronation
Wrist ulnar inclination	Extension	Ulnar inclination	Scaphoid and lunate: slight pronation Triquetrum: very slight supination
Wrist radial inclination	Flexion	Radial inclination	Slight supination

mobilizations for extension in the radio-carpal joint can be broken down into four distinct mobilizations: extension and radial inclination, extension and pronosupination, extension and anterior gliding, and extension and radial gliding.

In practice, the accessory gliding movements must respect the anatomy of the inferior extremity of the radius: the radial and ulnar glidings must follow the frontal obliquity of the radial slope (downward and outward), while the anterior and posterior glidings must follow the sagittal slope (oblique downward and backward).

Among the radio-carpal complex, the radio-scaphoid joint is particularly requested in wrist flexion and extension. Specific mobilizations with scaphoid glidings in relation to the radius can be performed when these movements are limited.

With one hand, the therapist immobilizes the inferior extremity of the radius. With the other, he holds the scaphoid through its tubercle and its dorsal side between the thumb and the index. The therapist then applies antero-posterior glidings with his distal hand (Fig. 3.22).

Traction can be added to lower the stress on the joint surfaces when performing glidings. Using a finger grasping device also helps maintain this traction during the mobilization. Depending on the situation, it can be useful to decoapt the radial or the ulnar compartment. In the first case, the finger grasping device is placed on the index and the third fingers. In the second case, it is placed on the fourth and fifth fingers (Luchetti and Atzei 2017).

- *Mobilization Second Row/First Row*

According to the same principle, the proximal grip is on the second carpal row and the distal grip is on the first carpal row at the level of the pisiform and the scaphoid's tubercle. We apply antero-posterior glidings and perform mobilizations in flexion/extension and pronation/supination:

Table 3.4 Summary table of the accessory movements depending on the mobilization of the radiocarpal joint

	Mobilization in flexion	Mobilization in extension	Mobilization in ulnar inclination	Mobilization in radial inclination
Antero-posterior glidings	Posterior	Anterior	–	–
Radioulnar glidings	Insignificant	Radial	Radial	Ulnar

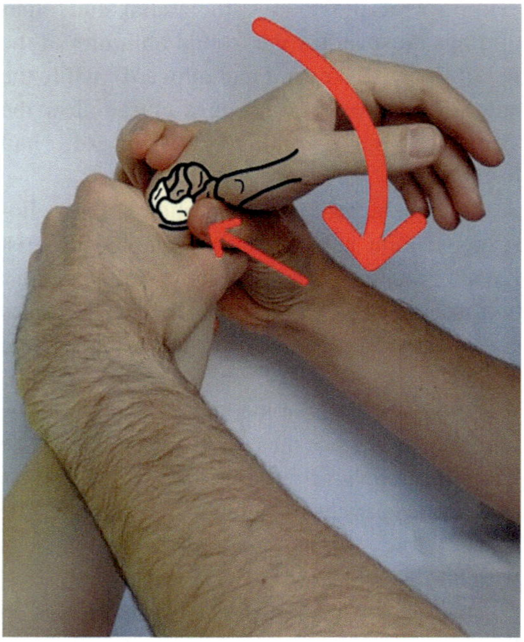

Fig. 3.19 Mobilization of the radiocarpal joint in flexion and posterior gliding

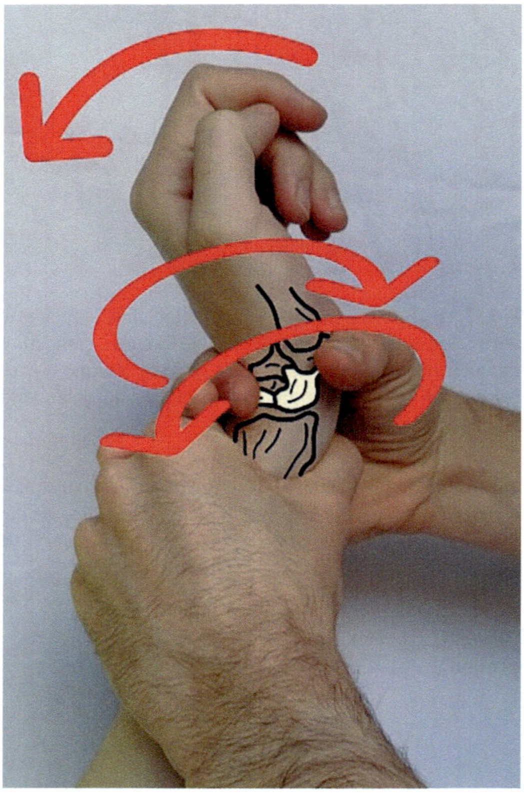

Fig. 3.20 Mobilization of the radiocarpal joint in extension and pronosupination

– For antero-posterior glidings, the therapist is in the same position as before. The distal hand mobilizes the second carpal row while performing anteroposterior tractions (Fig. 3.23).
– For mobilizations in flexion/extension, the therapist places the patient's wrist in a neutral position and immobilizes the first carpal row with one hand. His other hand holds the second carpal row. The distal hand mobilizes the second carpal row and performs flexions and extensions (Fig. 3.24).
– For mobilizations in pronation/supination, the techniques will replicate the rotation movements of the second carpal row in relation to the first one. The therapist places his hands the same way as to perform intracarpal flexions and extensions. The proximal hand is the fixed point while the distal hand makes rotation movements in the transversal plane. The mobilization in medial rotation brings the second carpal row in pronation, and the mobilization in lateral rotation brings it in supination (Fig. 3.25).
– *Intracarpal Mobilization*

These techniques are described in the chapter *"Fractures of the carpal bones."*

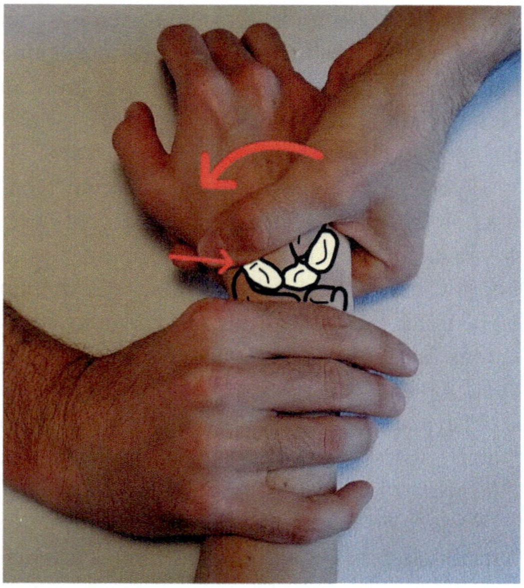

Fig. 3.21 Mobilization of the radiocarpal joint in radial inclination and ulnar gliding

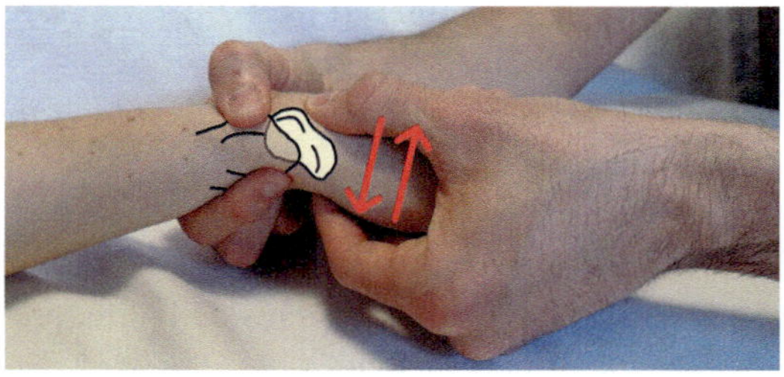

Fig. 3.22 Antero-posterior glidings of the radio-scaphoid joint

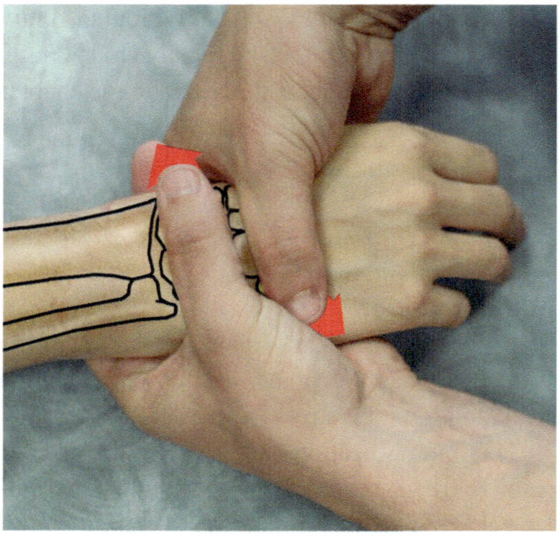

Fig. 3.23 Antero-posterior glidings of the second carpal row relative to the first carpal row

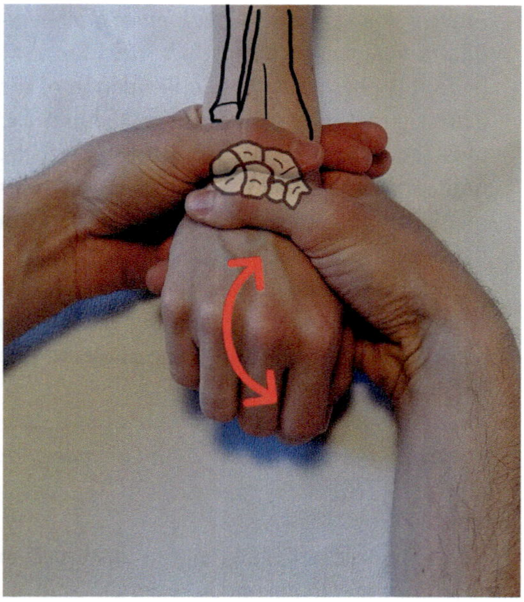

Fig. 3.24 Mobilization of the midcarpal joint in the sagittal plane

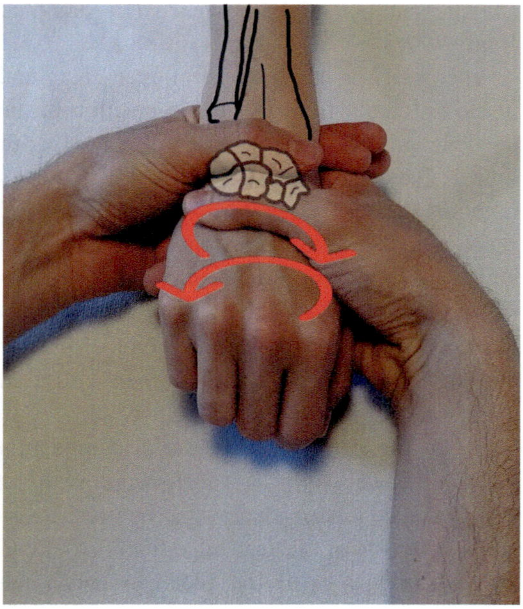

Fig. 3.25 Mobilization of the midcarpal joint in pronation and intracarpal supination

- *Recovering proprioceptive capacities*

The osseous callus is solid; therefore, we can perform more intensive reinforcement techniques.

- *Intensifying conscious neuromuscular rehabilitation techniques (Hagert's stage 5)*

  In this phase, there often is a deficit of the extrinsic muscles with respect to the intrinsic muscles. This unbalance is likely related to the limitations imposed during the previous phases to protect the scaphoid (exercises with the fingers in extension).

  We use the same reinforcement techniques with force sensors as in scaphoid fractures to recover muscular ratios comparable to the healthy side.
- *Intensifying unconscious neuromuscular rehabilitation techniques, or reflex muscular activation (Hagert's stage 6)*

Reflex muscle activation can be disturbed in any joint with ligamentous injuries and its adapted rehabilitation helps get back protective neuromuscular reflexes that exist in all normal joints (Karagiannopoulos and Michlovitz 2016) and prevent potential recurrence (Lephart and Henry 1996).

The exercises can be done in open chain and in closed chain, from the stable position to the unstable position to get closer to the superior limb's global function, targeting the patient's functional needs.

To work on reflex neuromuscular control in a closed chain, the exercise can be, for example, using a medicine ball with the patient's hands on it (two hands then one hand), and the therapist destabilizing the ball in different directions.

When the patient knows the destabilization modalities, we work on feedforward with an anticipated contraction happening before the sensorial detection of the destabilization.

We can also work on feedback when the patient has his eyes closed and does not know what the destabilization modalities are going to be. This corresponds to a corrective contraction after the sensorial detection of the destabilization (Riemann and Lephart 2002b).

A similar exercise in semi-closed chain can be realized with a plastic tube half-full of water. The patient holds it in the palm of his hand and controls the oscillations in pronation and supination.

Other reflex muscle activation exercises can be done using a ball on a racket or an oscillating bar. Other more specific and complex devices can be interesting too, such as the "inimove" © and the "powerball" © (Fig. 3.26).

Plyometric exercises refer to an eccentric contraction immediately followed by a concentric contraction. They have shown their interest in improving the global stability of the inferior limb by bettering muscle activation and creating adaptations in the sensorimotor system (Chimera et al. 2004).

They can be realized by asking the patient to "jump" against a wall or against the floor first, then against a Swiss ball (Fig. 3.27).

Respecting the progression in proprioceptive rehabilitation is key for an optimized functional recovery, and to limit the risks of recurrence. A settled proprioceptive disorder can decrease neuromuscular control, creating a ligamentous overwork leading to recurrence (Lephart and Henry 1996; Lephart et al. 1997) (Fig. 3.28).

- *Functional recovery (professional and leisure activities)*

We realize exercises with grips similar to those needed by the patient in his daily life, professional, and sports activities.

Important Note

There are frequent associated injuries of one other or two other locks of the radioulnar unity (Sammer and Chung 2012; Soubeyrand et al. 2007). Their treatment is described in the chapter *"Injuries of the radioulnar unity."*

Orthotic Treatment

Immobilization

The wrist is placed in a neutral position in the frontal and sagittal plane, as this is a position with the least joint stress (Kapandji 2005).

The immobilization can be a cast or made of resin, but we prefer using perforated thermoformable plastic (2,4 mm thick) to make a nonremovable orthosis (Fig. 3.29).

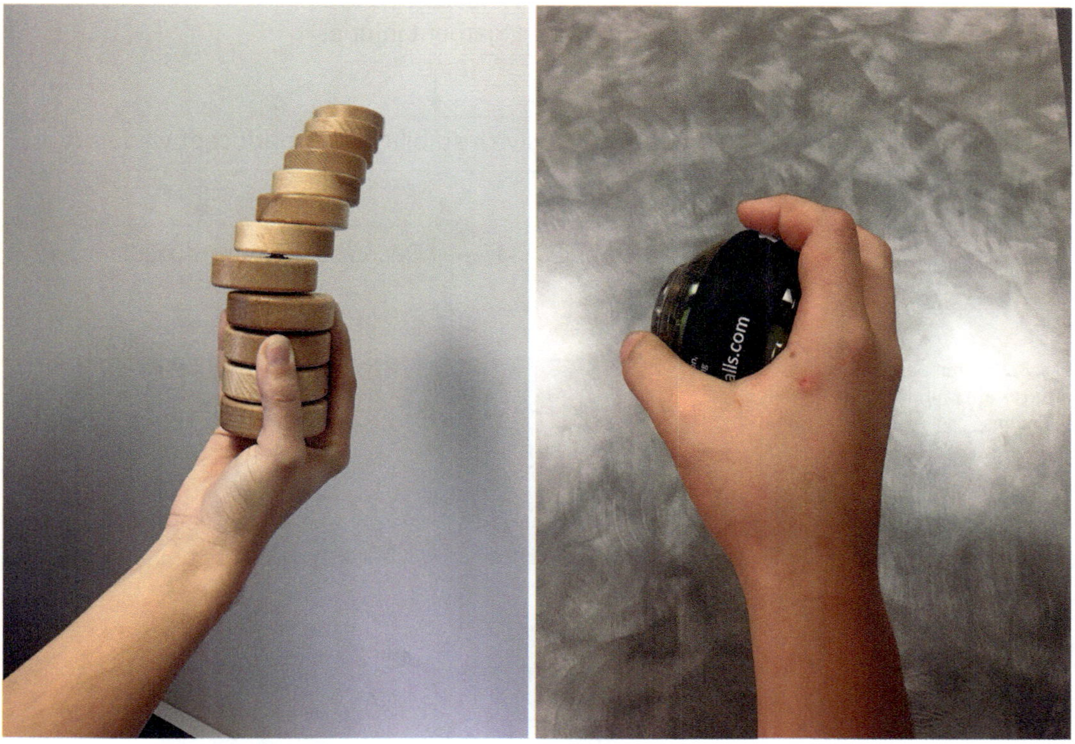

Fig. 3.26 Intensification of the unconscious neuromuscular rehabilitation techniques with Inimove © (1) or Powerball © (2)

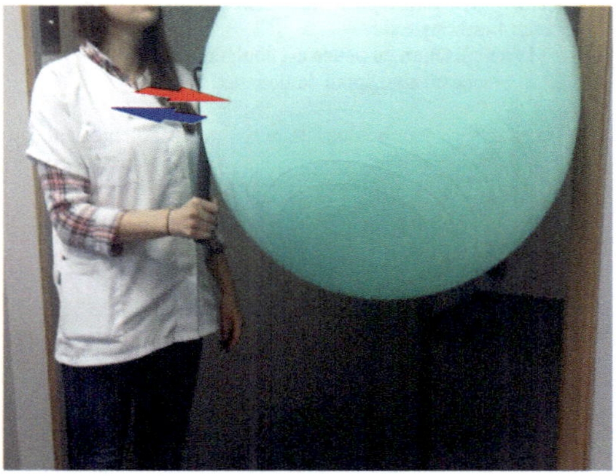

Fig. 3.27 Example of plyometric exercise with Swiss ball

With this technique, we achieve a precise immobilization that is eight times lighter than a resin. It can go in water (if the patient has no wound), is radiolucent, and has perforations allowing the skin to "breathe."

"Advice sheets" are always given to the patients. They are about the terms of use and maintenance of the orthosis, and self-rehabilitation exercises the patient must realize during the immobilization phase (Fig. 3.30).

New 3D technologies can also create quality orthoses that help optimize the patients' functional recovery (Fig. 3.31).

Relative Fragility

It is not realized all the time, but a resting orthosis can be useful in case of nocturnal pain or in daily activities.

However, we make sure the patient gets rid of the orthosis so that it does not impede his functional evolution.

The orthosis maintains the wrist in a neutral position. The plastic is perforated, and its thickness depends on the patient's morphology (Fig. 3.32).

Consolidation

A neoprene orthosis can be realized by going back to professional and sports activities.

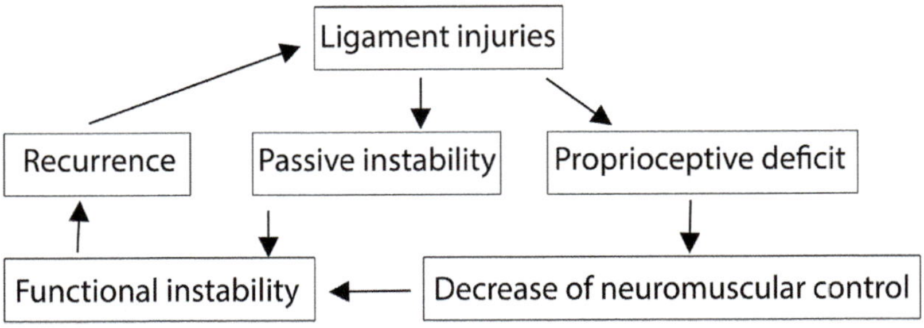

Fig. 3.28 Interest in proprioceptive rehabilitation to prevent recurrence by improving neuromuscular control

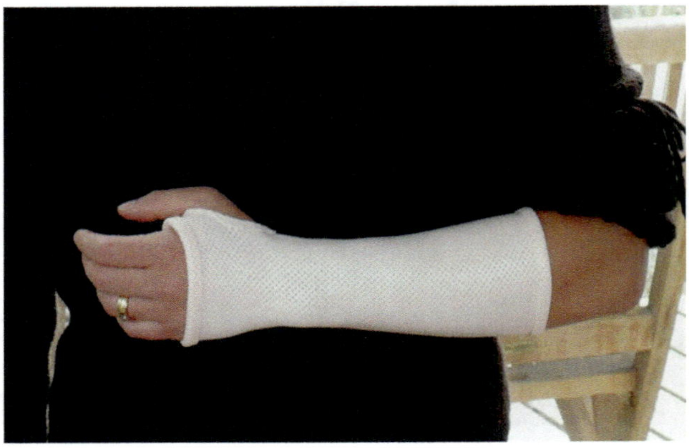

Fig. 3.29 Immobilization orthosis after a fracture of the radius

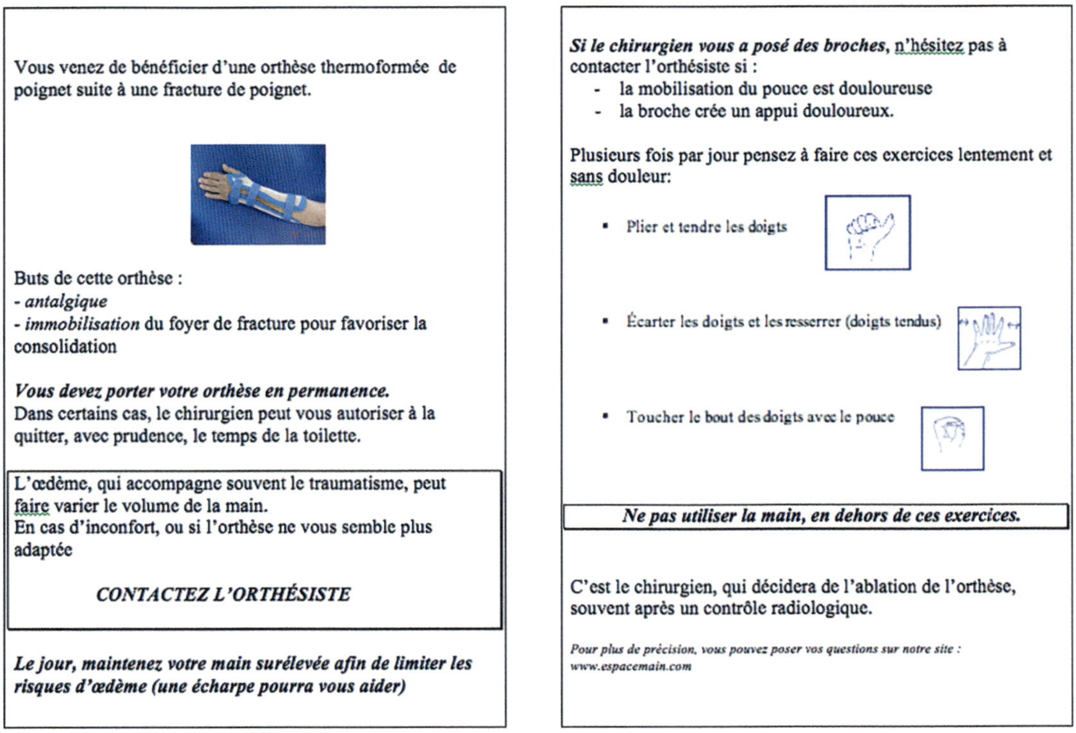

Vous venez de bénéficier d'une orthèse thermoformée de poignet suite à une fracture de poignet.

Buts de cette orthèse :
- *antalgique*
- *immobilisation* du foyer de fracture pour favoriser la consolidation

Vous devez porter votre orthèse en permanence.
Dans certains cas, le chirurgien peut vous autoriser à la quitter, avec prudence, le temps de la toilette.

L'œdème, qui accompagne souvent le traumatisme, peut faire varier le volume de la main.
En cas d'inconfort, ou si l'orthèse ne vous semble plus adaptée

CONTACTEZ L'ORTHÉSISTE

Le jour, maintenez votre main surélevée afin de limiter les risques d'œdème (une écharpe pourra vous aider)

Si le chirurgien vous a posé des broches, n'hésitez pas à contacter l'orthésiste si :
- la mobilisation du pouce est douloureuse
- la broche crée un appui douloureux.

Plusieurs fois par jour pensez à faire ces exercices lentement et sans douleur:

- Plier et tendre les doigts
- Écarter les doigts et les resserrer (doigts tendus)
- Toucher le bout des doigts avec le pouce

Ne pas utiliser la main, en dehors de ces exercices.

C'est le chirurgien, qui décidera de l'ablation de l'orthèse, souvent après un contrôle radiologique.

Pour plus de précision, vous pouvez poser vos questions sur notre site : www.espacemain.com

Fig. 3.30 Advice sheet given to the patient after giving him an orthosis

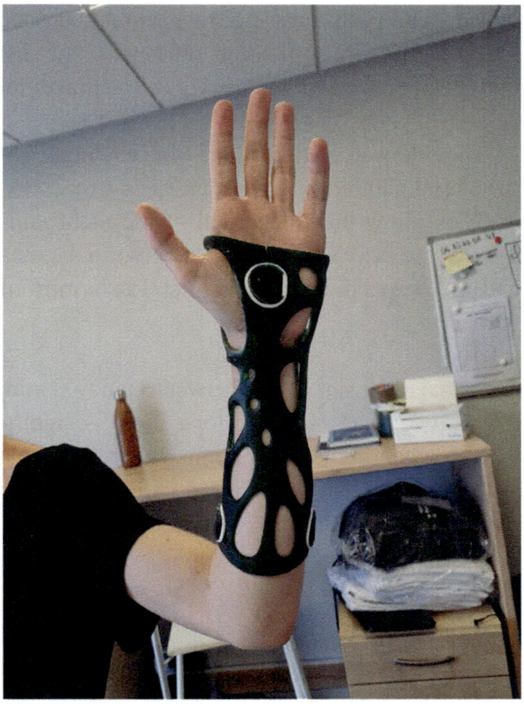

Fig. 3.31 Orthosis made with a 3D-printer and the Xkelet © technology

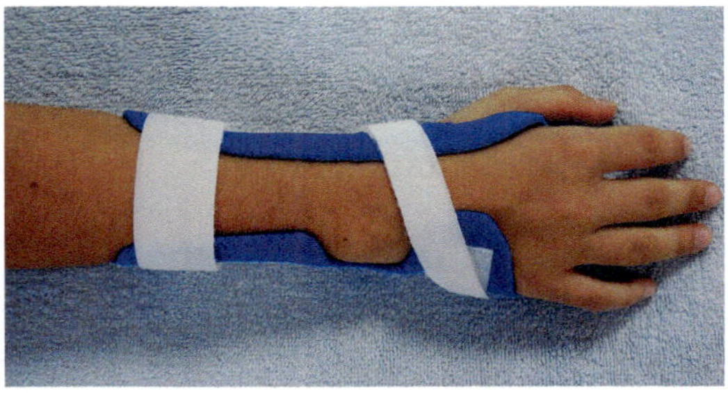

Fig. 3.32 Resting orthosis, not realized in every case but that can be useful in case of pain, especially during the night

It protects the wrist from shocks, and has an interesting contention effect, useful at a proprioceptive level and in the patient's apprehension.

Thermoformed plastic reinforcements can be added depending on the indications.

Complications

Common Complications (Except Ulnocarpal Conflict)

The Complex Regional Pain Syndrome (CRPS) is particularly frequent (Erhard 2016) in wrist injuries (25% of the fractures of the radius, regardless of the treatment (Roh et al. 2014; Atkins and Duckworth 1990)). Preventing this complication must be key for all the health care team to limit its impact (Gillespie et al. 2016).

Other complications in these types of fractures are frequent (Turner et al. 2010; McKay et al. 2001), with almost systematic extrinsic ligamentous injuries (Table 3.5) that must be considered in the rehabilitation protocol.

Table 3.5 Incidence of complications in distal radius fractures

Complications	Incidence
Motricity loss (significant deformation, mobility loss, joint fibrosis, Volkmann ischemic contracture, finger stiffness)	0%–31%
Delayed healing, pseudarthrosis	0,7%–4%
Nerve compression, neuritis	0%–17%
Painful syndromes (CRPS, shoulder-hand syndrome, persistent pain)	0,3%–8%
Complications related to the surgical materials	1,4%–2,6%
Osteomyelitis	4%–9%
Vicious callus	5%
Tendon injuries (rupture, lag, trigger, tenosynovitis)	0%–5%
Scar (keloid)	3%
Ligament injuries	98%
Radioulnar injuries (synostosis, perturbation)	0%–1,3%
Hematoma in a bone graft	1%
Dupuytren (nodes, palmar fascia strips)	2%–9%
Arthritis/arthrosis	7%–65%
Other pathology, unrecognized	2%

Ulnocarpal Conflict

This syndrome is characterized by pain on the wrist ulnar side caused by excessive pressure on the ulnar extremity—the ulna being too long compared to the radius.

This stress and length inequality produce friction that may result in ligamentous injuries (TFCC, lunotriquetral ligament) and arthrosis.

Biomechanically speaking, a positive ulnar variance increases the stress and shearing on the ulna (normally, 20% of the force is transmitted to the wrist by the ulna, and 80% by the radius (Palmer et al. 1982)).

Causes

The ulnocarpal conflict can be congenital, but in most cases, it is a sequel to a fracture of the distal extremity of the radius. The compaction of the radius induces an inversion of the distal radioulnar index with a positive ulnar variance (long ulna): there is a conflict between the ulnar head and the lunate's proximal part.

Other causes can result in this conflict: radial head resection, Madelung's disease, and Essex–Lopresti syndrome.

Clinical and Paraclinical Signs

- *Clinical signs*

There is usually pain on the ulnar side of the wrist, especially in wrist extension and ulnar inclination.

The patient describes strength loss, functional impotence, and sometimes painful snaps at the level of the wrist.

Nakamura's test (ulnocarpal stress test) is positive if we reproduce the patient's pain with an axial compression combined with a movement from neutral position to ulnar inclination.

There also is a strength loss measured with a JAMAR and compared with the contralateral side, especially in pronation.

- *Paraclinical signs*
  - *X-rays*

Face and profile wrist X-rays should be done in pronation, in supination, and with the fist closed, and must be compared to the contralateral side.

They show a relatively long ulna and highlight the causal pathology in most cases.

They allow the calculation of the ulnar variance on the face X-ray (distance between the ulna and the perpendicular to the distal extremity of the radius):

A normal ulnar variance is between 0 and −2 mm.
A positive ulnar variance (long ulna) is significant when higher than 2 mm. It is related to a higher frequency of TFCC injury and ulnar impaction syndrome.

- *MRI and arthro-TDM*

These exams can show the causes of conflict: degenerative central injury of the TFCC and injury of the lunotriquetral ligament. Focal chondromalacia at the beginning, and even sclerosis, cysts, and subchondral geodes in the later stages can be found on the lunate, the triquetrum, or the ulna.

Treatment Orientations

- *Conservative*

At first, the wrist should be put at rest, avoiding or modifying the patient's activities. To this end, pronations of more than 45° and ulnar inclinations should be limited.

An orthosis can help, made in a supination position and with a slight radial inclination. It is mostly worn during the night. The patient should also learn the movements that are stressful for his wrist, to limit them in his daily activities.

Proprioceptive rehabilitation is essential and targets the flexor and the extensor carpi ulnaris that stabilize the ulnar compartment and limit the ulnar gliding of the first carpal row (Mesplié and Lemoine 2015) (Fig. 3.33).

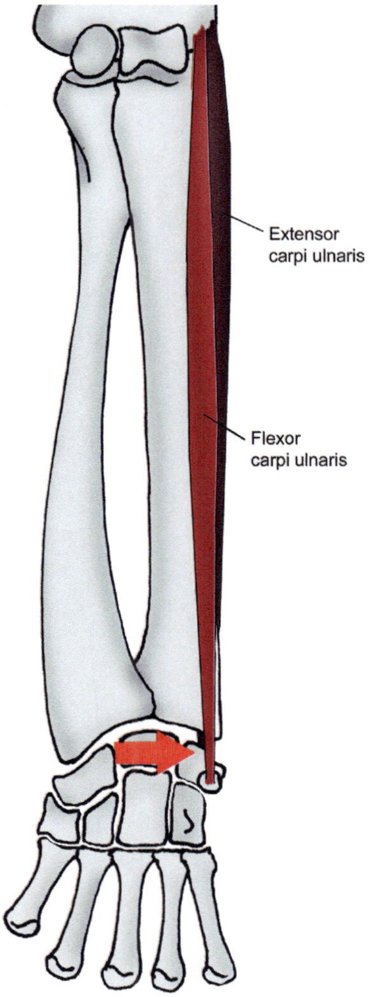

Fig. 3.33 Specific exercises for the flexor carpi ulnaris and the extensor carpi ulnaris, opposing the ulnar gliding of the first carpal row along the radial slope

A corticoid infiltration under ultrasound guidance can also be tried, as well as an anti-inflammatory drug treatment.

- *Surgery*

The surgery should target the cause of the pathology and must consider the injuries induced by the conflict (TFCC injuries, arthrosis of the lunate and/or ulna) that can be contraindications for some surgeries.

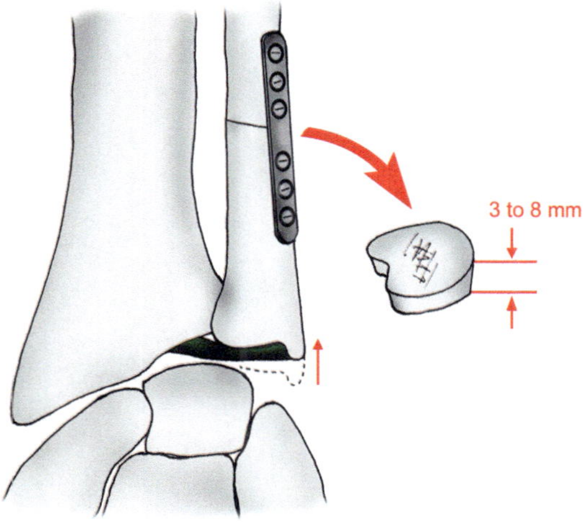

Fig. 3.34 Shortening of the ulna according to Milch, with diaphyseal osteotomy

- Correction of a radial vicious callus with bone graft.
- Ulna shortening according to Milch with diaphyseal osteotomy (Fig. 3.34).
- Hemisection of the ulnar head according to Bowers: oblique resection of the distal ulna, respecting the styloid with tendinous interposition (Fig. 3.35).
- Darrach's surgery: Total resection of the ulnar head with stabilization of the distal ulna (Fig. 3.36).
- Sauvé-Kapandji's surgery: Osteotomy of the ulnar neck with distal radioulnar arthrodesis (Fig. 3.37).
- Arthroscopic resection of the ulnar head, Wafer procedure (Fig. 3.38).

The surgical indications for these interventions depend on the cause of the conflict, the presence of secondary injuries, the patient's age, and his functional needs.

They must be assessed considering the advantages and disadvantages of each and every one of them, especially the mobility and strength loss, and the length of surgical follow-ups.

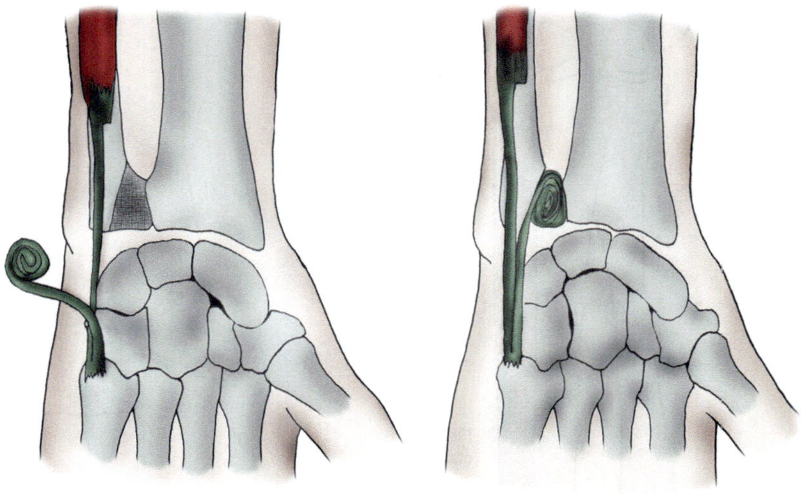

Fig. 3.35 Hemisection of the ulnar head according to Bowers

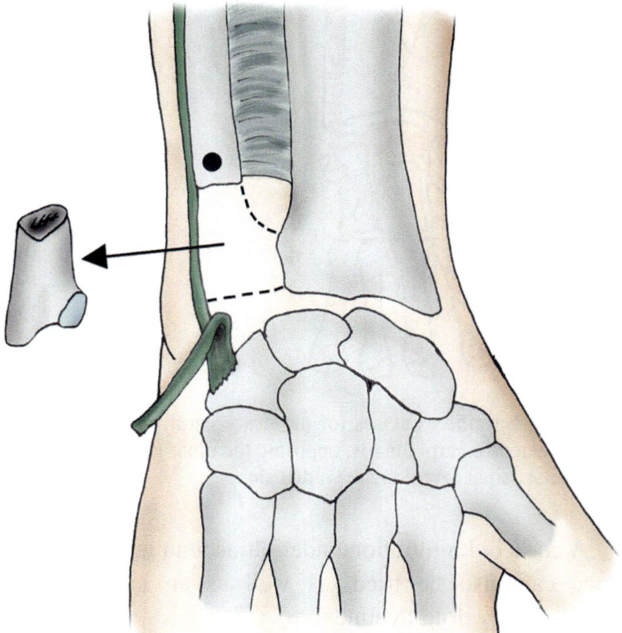

Fig. 3.36 Darrach procedure

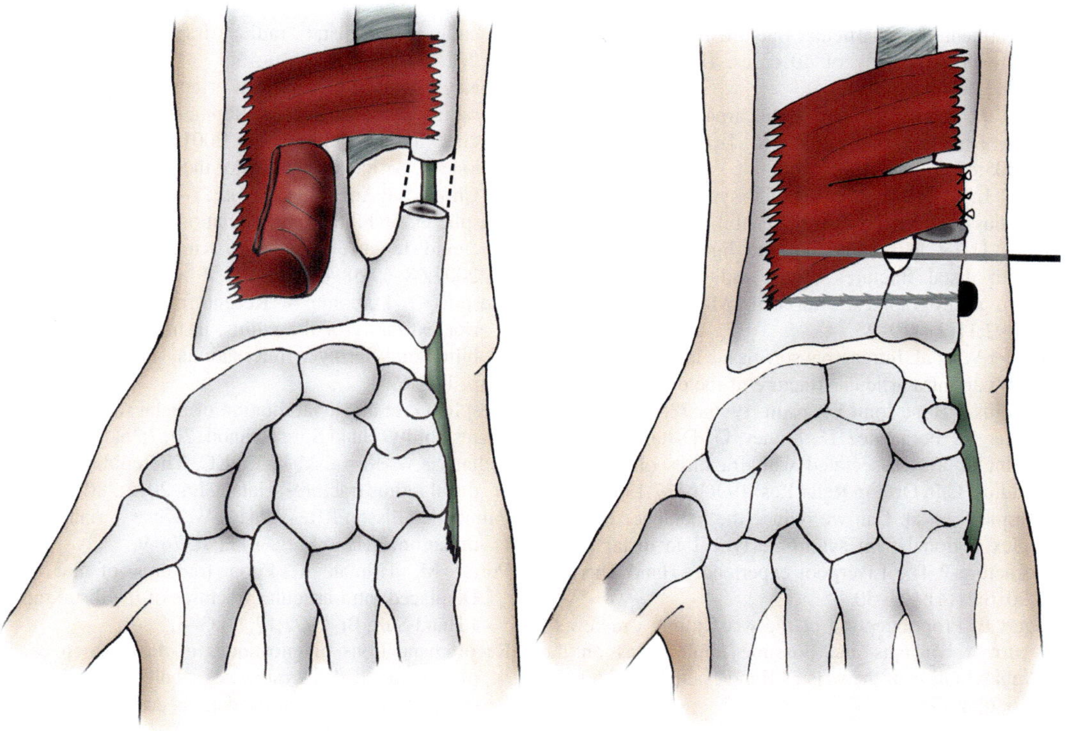

Fig. 3.37 Sauvé-Kapandji procedure with ulnar osteotomy (1), then distal radioulnar arthrodesis (2)

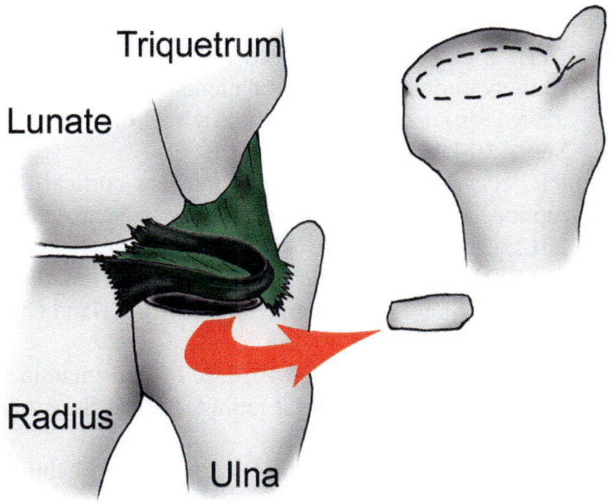

Fig. 3.38 Wafer procedure with arthroscopy, to decrease the ulna's length (<3 mm)

Bibliography

Atkins RM, Duckworth T, JA K. Features of algodystrophy after Colles' fracture. J Bone Joint Surg. 1990;72B:105–10.

Bayon-Calatayud M, Benavente- Valdepenas AM, Del Prado Vazquez-Munoz M. Mirror therapy for distal radial fractures: a pilot randomized controlled study. J Rehabil Med. 2016;48(9):829–32.

Beck J, Harness N, Spencer H. Volar plate fixation failure for volar shearing distal radius fractures with small lunate facet fragments. J Hand Surg Am. 2014;39(4):670–8.

Castaing J. Recent fractures of the lower extremity of the radius in adults. Rev Chir Orthop Reparatrice Appar Mot. 1964;50:581–696.

Chimera NJ, et al. Effects of plyometric training on muscle-activation strategies and performance in female athletes. J Athl Train. 2004;39(1):24–31.

Christiaens N, et al. Contribution of arthroscopy to the treatment of intraarticular fracture of the distal radius: retrospective study of 40 cases. Hand Surg Rehab. 2017;36(4):268–74.

Crisco JJ, et al. In vivo radiocarpal kinematics and the Dart Thrower's motion. J Bone Joint Surg. 2005;87-A(12):2729.

Erhard L. Complex pain regional syndrome after distal radius fractures. Hand Surg Rehabil. 2016;35S:S144–9.

Fontes D, et al. Lesions of the ligaments associated with distal fractures of the radius. 58 intraoperative arthrographies. Ann Chir Main Memb Super. 1992;11(2):119–25.

Geissler W, et al. Intracarpal soft-tissue lesions associated with an intra-articular fracture of the distal end of the radius. J Bone Joint Surg Am. 1996a;78(3):357–65.

Geissler W, Fernandez D, Lamey D. Distal radioulnar joint injuries associated with fractures of the distal radius. Clin Orthop Relat Res. 1996b;327:135–46.

Gillespie S, et al. Can we reduce the incidence of complex regional pain syndrome type I in distal radius fractures? The Liverpool experience. Hand Therapy. 2016;21(4):123–30.

Hagert E. Proprioception of the wrist joint: a review of current concepts and possible implications on the rehabilitation of the wrist. J Hand Ther. 2010;23(1):2–16. quiz 17

Kapandji IA. Physiologie articulaire tome 1 - Membre supérieur. Maloine; 2005.

Karagiannopoulos C, Michlovitz S. Rehabilitation strategies for wrist sensorimotor control impairment: from theory to practice. J Hand Ther. 2016;29(2):154–65.

Karagiannopoulos C, et al. Responsiveness of the active wrist joint position sense test after distal radius fracture intervention. J Hand Ther. 2016;29(4):474–82.

Knirk J, Jupiter J. Intra-articular fractures of the distal end of the radius in young adults. J Bone Joint Surg Am. 1986;68(5):647–59.

Kramer S, et al. The incidence of ulnocarpal complaints after distal radial fracture in relation to the fracture of the ulnar styloid. J Hand Surg Eur. 2013;38(7):710–7.

Laulan J, Obert L. Fractures de l'extrémité distale des deux os de l'avant-bras chez l'adulte. EMC - Appareil locomoteur. 2009;4(4):1–16.

Laulan J, Marteau E, Bacle G. The MEU classification system for distal radius fractures: prognostic and therapeutic value of an independent assessment of various fracture parameters. Hand Surg Rehabil. 2016;35S:S28–33.

Lephart S, Henry T. The physiological basis for open and closed kinetic chain rehabilitation for the upper extremity. J Sport Rehab. 1996;5:71–87.

Lephart S, et al. The role of proprioception in the management and rehabilitation of athletic injuries. Am J Sports Med. 1997;25:130–7.

Luchetti R, Atzei A. Arthroscopic assisted tendon reconstruction for triangular fibrocartilage complex irreparable tears. J Hand Surg Eur. 2017;42(4):346–51.

Mathews AL, Chung KC. Management of complications of distal radius fractures. Hand Clin. 2015;31(2):205–15.

McKay SD, et al. Assessment of complications of distal radius fractures and development of a complication checklist. J Hand Surg Am. 2001;26(5):916–22.

Melone C. Articular fractures of the distal radius. Orthop Clin North Am. 1984;15(2):217–36.

Mesplié G. Stabilité de l'articulation radio ulnaire distale : quid du carré pronateur ? Kinésithérapie, la revue. 2007;68–69:58–62.

Mesplié G, Lemoine S. Recent fractures of the inferior extremity of the radius, in hand and wrist rehabilitation. Springer International Publishing; 2015. p. 147–69.

Mesplie G, et al. Rehabilitation of distal radioulnar joint instability. Hand Surg Rehabil. 2017;36(5):314–21.

Nellans KW, Kowalski E, C. KC. The epidemiology of distal radius fractures. Hand Clin. 2012;28(2):113–25.

Palmer A, Glisson RR, Werner FW. Ulnar variance determination. J Hand Surg. 1982;7:376–9.

Porter M, Tillman R. Pilon fractures of the wrist. Displaced intra-articular fractures of the distal radius. J Hand Surg Br. 1992;17(1):63–8.

Recommandations diagnostiques et de prise en charge thérapeutique des syndromes douloureux régionaux complexes : les recommandations de Lille. Douleur et Analgésie. 2019;32(3):155–64.

Riemann B, Lephart S. The sensorimotor system, part 1: the physiologic basis of functional joint stability. J Athl Train. 2002a;37(1):71–9.

Riemann B, Lephart S. The sensorimotor system, part 2: the role of prprioception in motor and functional joint stability. J Athl Train. 2002b;37(1):80–4.

Roh YH, et al. Factors associated with complex regional pain syndrome type I in patients with surgically treated distal radius fracture. Arch Orthop Trauma Surg. 2014;134(12):1775–81.

Roll R, et al. Illusory movements prevent cortical disruption caused by immobilization. NeuroImage. 2012;62(1):510–9.

Sammer DM, Chung KC. Management of the distal radioulnar joint and ulnar styloid fracture. Hand Clin. 2012;28(2):199–206.

Shah AS, Verma MK, Jebson PJ. Use of oral vitamin C after fractures of the distal radius. J Hand Surg Am. 2009;34(9):1736–8.

Smith DW, Brou KE, Henry MH. Early active rehabilitation for operatively stabilized distal radius fractures. J Hand Ther. 2004;17(1):43–9.

Soubeyrand M, et al. Pathologie traumatique de la membrane interosseuse de l'avant-bras. Chir Main. 2007;26:255.

Thomas D, Zanin D. Hand rehabilitation after distal radius fracture. Hand Surg Rehabil. 2016;35S:S156–61.

Turner RG, Faber KJ, Athwal GS. Complications of distal radius fractures. Hand Clin. 2010;26(1):85–96.

Fractures of the Carpal Bones

4

Grégory Mesplié, Vincent Grelet, and Olivier Léger

Fractures of the carpal bones are injuries whose frequency depends on the injured bone, and whose functional consequences are important. They may go unnoticed and require specialized surgical care and rehabilitation for an optimal recovery.

Recent Fractures of the Scaphoid Bone

Fractures of the scaphoid are frequent, especially in young men, and represent 65% of the traumas of the carpus (Garcia-Elias 2001; Auffray 1970; Snodgrass 1937).

Their consolidation is difficult because of the important stress imposed on the scaphoid and the precarious vascularization of its proximal part (Gelberman and Menon 1980).

The efficiency of the treatment depends on an early diagnosis, which allows for avoiding evolutions toward a Scaphoid Nonunion Advanced Collapse (SNAC) wrist (Marcuzzi et al. 2014).

G. Mesplié (✉)
ISAMMS, Biarritz, France

V. Grelet · O. Léger
Institut Sud Aquitain de la Main et du Membre Supérieur, Biarritz, France

Physiopathology

Most fractures of the scaphoid concern the waist of the bone that is narrower and more fragile than the rest of the bone.

The injury is most often due to a trauma in compression/shearing in wrist hyperextension, combined with a radial or ulnar inclination. This explains the variety of the fractures (Segalman and Graham 2004). Several classifications have been described for these fractures, including the Herbert classification (Adams and Steinmann 2010; Herbert 1990) (Fig. 4.1).

This mechanism puts tension on the palmar radio-carpal ligaments that forbid the scaphoid from going frontwards. The bone then suffers the shock from the posterior part of the radius at the level of the waist (Marcuzzi et al. 2014). The radio-scapho-capitate ligament can increase the displacement in flexion of the distal fragment, causing a shortening of the bone (Fig. 4.2).

This mechanism only occurs in fractures of the waist and does not concern the fractures of the proximal part.

The same mechanism puts important constraints on the scapholunate ligament (Geoffroy and Mesplié 2018), as opposed to the differential gliding between the scaphoid and lunate.

That is why in a trauma in hyperextension, we can observe a fracture of the scaphoid, an injury

G. Mesplié (ed.), *Wrist Functional Anatomy and Therapy*,
https://doi.org/10.1007/978-3-031-42879-1_4

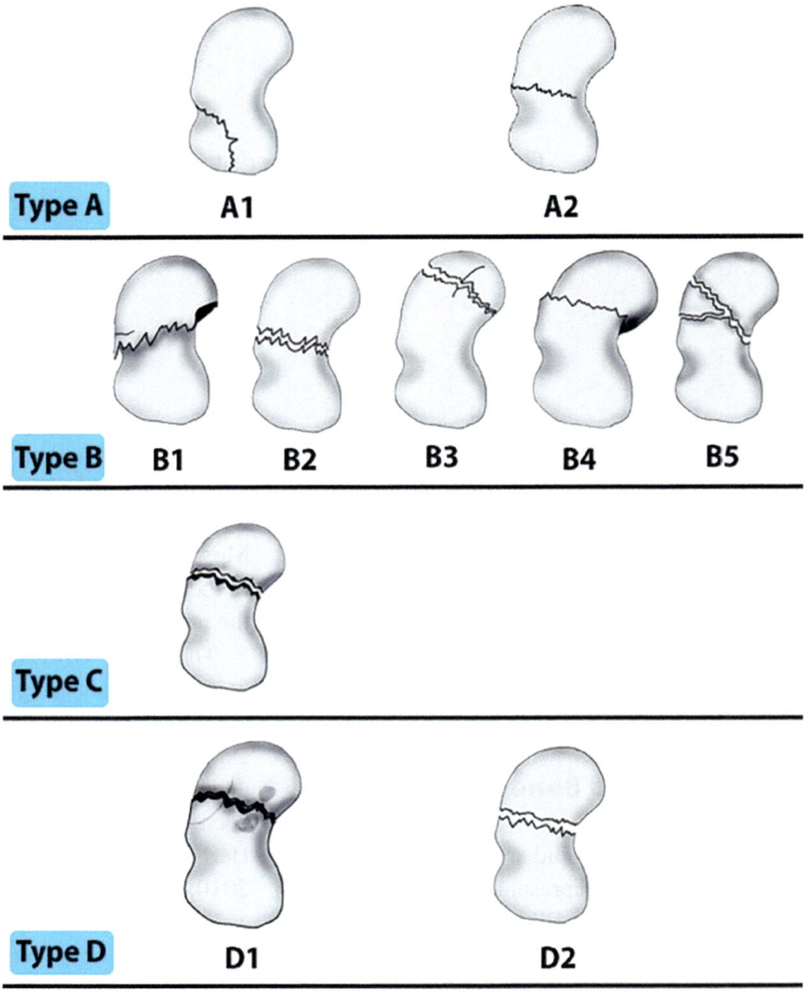

Fig. 4.1 Herbert classification

of the scapholunate ligament or a fracture of the distal radial epiphysis. The combination of these injuries is rare (Fig. 4.3).

Clinical and Paraclinical Signs

With the patient interview only, we can determine if there has been a "risky" trauma.

The most suggestive clinical sign is pain when palpating the anatomical snuffbox (Fig. 4.4), with the wrist in ulnar inclination to increase the palpable surface (Giugale et al. 2015). However, if there is an edema in this area or in the radial side of the wrist and pain when putting a load on the scaphoid, we will have to realize X-rays (Young and Giachino 2009).

Sometimes, the X-rays are clear (Fig. 4.5) and the diagnosis is easy, but in 15–25% of the cases the fracture is not visible on the X-ray on the day of the trauma (Sabbagh et al. 2019).

In those cases, a resting orthosis is realized and kept for 15 days, and then other X-rays are realized to confirm the presence or absence of fracture.

However, we must keep in mind that the decalcification process around the fracture line that allows the detection of a fracture after 15 days is not systematic, especially in proximal fractures. When in doubt, we use MRI and scintigraphy (Schernberg 2005).

Echography also has a certain interest in the diagnosis, but its efficiency is operator dependent.

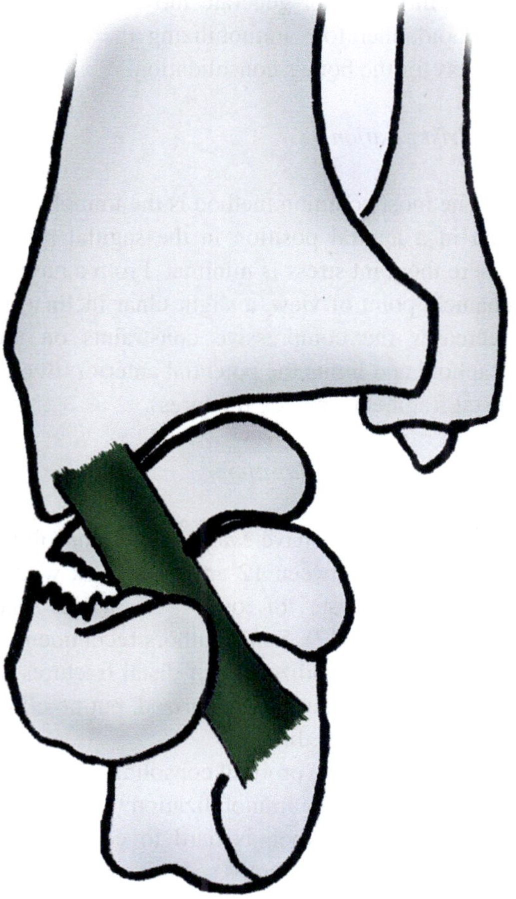

Fig. 4.2 Action of the radioscaphocapitate ligament that can increase the displacement of the distal fragment in fractures of the scaphoid waist

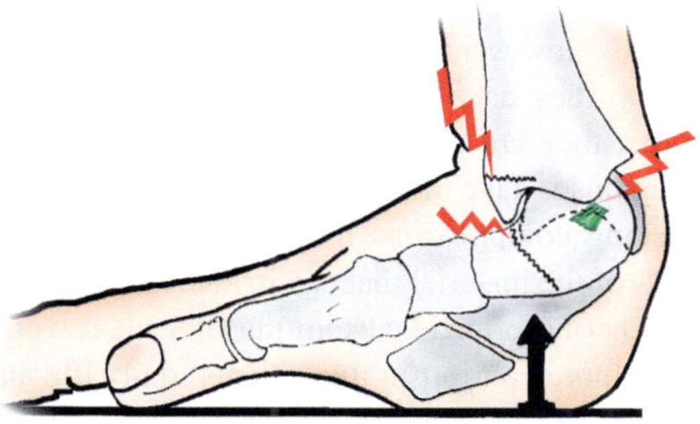

Fig. 4.3 Injury mechanism that can cause a rupture of the scapholunate ligament, a fracture of the scaphoid or the radius

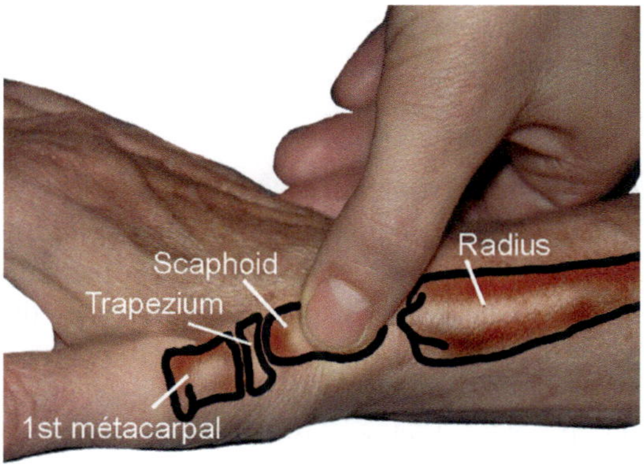

Fig. 4.4 Palpation of the scaphoid in the anatomical snuffbox, between the first extensor gliding and the extensor pollicis longus

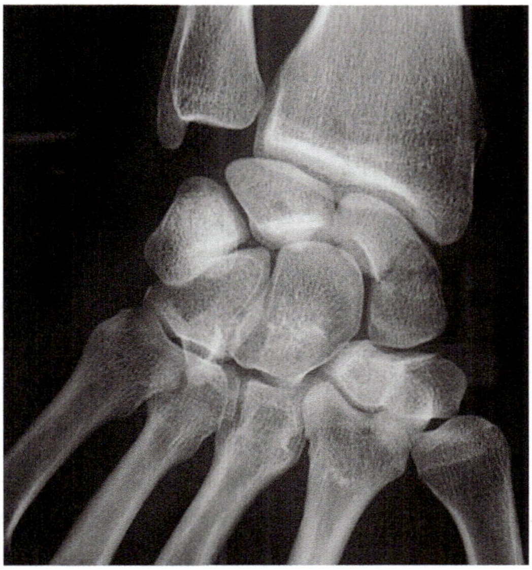

Fig. 4.5 Radiography showing a fracture of the scaphoid waist

Therapeutic Process and Surgical Treatment

The treatment depends on the location of the fracture line (Schernberg 2005; Schernberg et al. 2000), whether the fracture is displaced or not, and the patient's socio-economical and sports context. This treatment can be orthopedic or surgical with conventional screwing, percutaneous technique, simple pin, and more rarely plate or staples.

Orthopedic Treatment

The orthopedic treatment by prolonged immobilization is, according to us, the first-line indication to treat non-displaced fractures of the scaphoid—despite the development of percutaneous osteosynthesis. Several studies agree that there is a high rate of consolidation (more than 90%), however, opinions differ more widely regarding the type of immobilization, the wrist position, and the duration of immobilization.

- *Immobilize the elbow and the thumb?*

The SOFCOT's round table in 1988 gathers a series of 209 recent non-displaced fractures of the scaphoid treated with brachio-palmar immobilization in 41% of the cases and antebrachio-palmar immobilization in 33% of the cases. The 26% left were treated with a combination of the two previous techniques (first brachio-palmar, then antebrachio-palmar). The conclusion of this study does not bring formal statistical elements to confirm the superiority of one treatment or the other.

In 1990, a study showed on 10 subjects that pronosupination does not put constraints on the scaphoid, unlike the flexion/extension and the radial and ulnar inclinations. Only two studies analyze the consolidation rate depending on whether the elbow is in the cast or not, they both conclude that the consolidation is not improved when the elbow is immobilized.

The fact that the thumb must be immobilized in fractures of the scaphoid is deeply rooted in people's minds. In 1943, Watson-Jones recommended blocking the thumb's metacarpophalangeal joint, and we must wait until 1991 for a randomized prospective study to obtain results identical between the group of patients immobilized until the interphalangeal joint and those with the thumb free (Clay et al. 1991). Some more recent biomechanical studies have shown that mobilizing the thumb's metacarpophalangeal joint does not generate movement for the scaphoid, therefore immobilizing the thumb is useless for the bone's consolidation.

- *Wrist position*

The most common method is the immobilization in a neutral position in the sagittal plane, where the joint stress is minimal. From a biomechanical point of view, a slight ulnar inclination decreases the compressive constraints on the scaphoid and limits the potential anterior tilt of a distal fragment (in neck fractures).

- *Immobilization duration*

Several studies have evaluated the consolidation duration between 12 and 15 weeks, with a consolidation rate of over 90% (Dias and Kantharuban 2017). Some authors recommend a two-month immobilization for distal fractures as the distal part is more vascularized, but no clinical study confirms this.

In theory, only a proof of consolidation should allow us to stop the immobilization, but in practice this consolidation is hard to confirm and immobilizing for 3 months seems to be the most scientifically established, and the most prudent approach.

- *Immobilization type*

The cast still seems to be the most used technique. However, the resins have several advantages: they are two to three times lighter than casts, they are more solid and resist water. But they also have disadvantages: poor plasticity making compressions more frequent and hardness of the material that can irritate the skin.

Thermoformed "custom-made" orthoses provide more comfort in the patients' daily life and can be readjusted when the edema disappears.

In conclusion, 2–3 months of immobilization depending on the location of the fracture line, with the wrist in a neutral position and the thumb free in a thermoformed orthosis is the first-line indication in non-displaced fractures of the scaphoid.

Surgery

Displaced and unstable fractures of the scaphoid and delayed bone healing are indications for surgery. In 1968, the screwing with a spongy 4 mm screw has been described in the AO's osteosynthesis manual (*Arbeitsgemeinschaft für Osteosynthesefragen*), but later studies have shown technique difficulties due to the particular anatomy of this bone and the equipment load. Since the beginning of the 80 s and the apparition of Herbert's headless screw (Herbert and Fisher 1984), several screws have been developed to favor compression and make the placement easier.

In this chapter, we will develop the main osteosynthesis techniques with traditional screws, percutaneous screws, and percutaneous pins.

- *Traditional screws*

Screwing can be realized in a retrograde way with an anterior approach (Fig. 4.6), or from proximal to distal with a posterior approach in proximal fractures (Fig. 4.7).

We use an AO stainless steel screw with a 2-mm diameter and a long thread length to allow good compression. Perforated screws avoid multiple drilling but have a wider diameter.

In anterograde screwing from proximal to distal, we prefer screws with a smaller diameter considering the small size of the proximal fragment.

The surgical follow-ups depend on the surgeon and go from no immobilization to a resin cuff for a month. De Chevigné observes a consolidation rate of 100%.

- *Percutaneous screws*

For a few years, minimally invasive surgical techniques have been developed to reduce morbidity and preserve the scaphoid's vascularization, as well as the ligaments surrounding it. Ledoux and coll. Describe in 1995 a series of 23 patients treated with Herbert's screw (percutaneous screwing) (Herbert and Fisher 1984): they were all consolidated and back to work in the seventh week on average (Ledoux 1995).

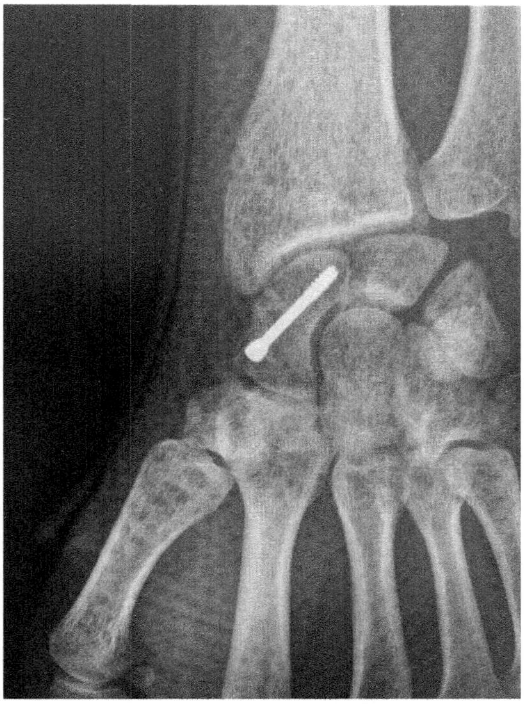

Fig. 4.6 Retrograde screwing with anterior surgical approach

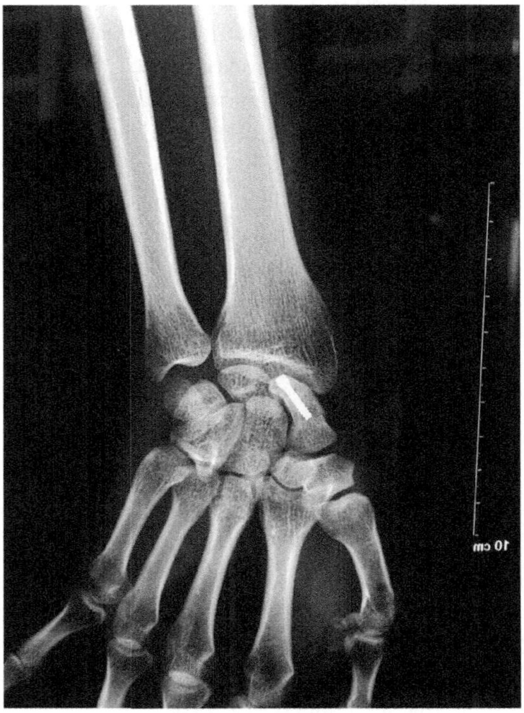

Fig. 4.7 Screwing with posterior surgical approach for proximal fractures

The approach can be palmar or dorsal, and the reduction is controlled with radioscopy or coupled with arthroscopy (Slutsky and Trevare 2014). Wrist arthroscopy allows the control of the fracture's reduction (Fig. 4.8) with a probe and a thumb traction. It also allows the diagnosis of potential combined ligament injuries. The control of the reduction and compression is realized by the medio-carpal and the radio-carpal approach, to check that the screw is not protruding (Mathoulin 2014). This technique uses perforated screws guided by a pin (Fig. 4.9). The diameter of the screw is 2–3 mm depending on the manufacturer.

Osteosynthesis is necessary in unstable or displaced scaphoid fractures. The percutaneous technique is reserved for fractures that are little displaced and is more and more used in non-displaced fractures based on economic, social, professional, and sports factors, as it reduces the duration of immobilization (0–30 days).

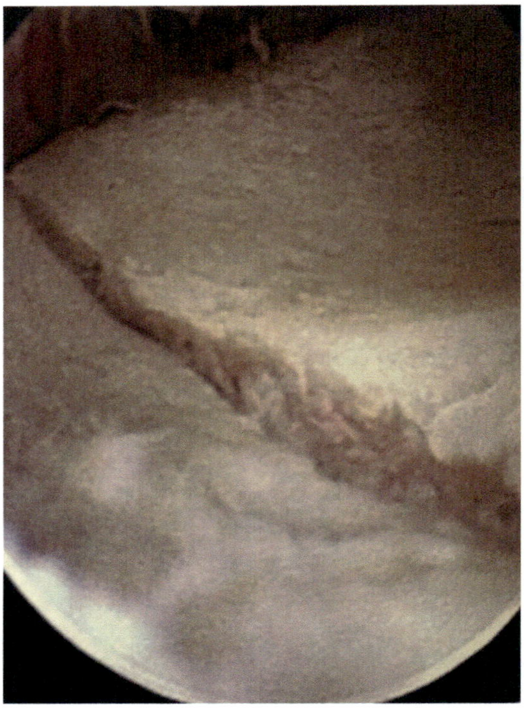

Fig. 4.8 Using arthroscopy to control and reduce the fracture

- *Percutaneous pins*

The pins seem to be the best osteosynthesis technique for the scaphoid, putting compression on the fracture site. However, some authors are now wondering if compression is necessary for the scaphoid. The natural tendency in median fractures is toward flexion so we will have to install a wiring during the synthesis. The pins allow a stable osteosynthesis without shortening the scaphoid and avoid rotation disorders if we place at least three pins with a diameter between 14 and 16.

- Other osteosynthesis systems

The anatomical staple developed by Savornin (Savornin et al. 2000) or the "low profile" plates are rarely used in frequent injuries, but they can be interesting when treating pseudarthrosis with bone graft.

In conclusion, the surgical treatment is justified in non-displaced fractures when:

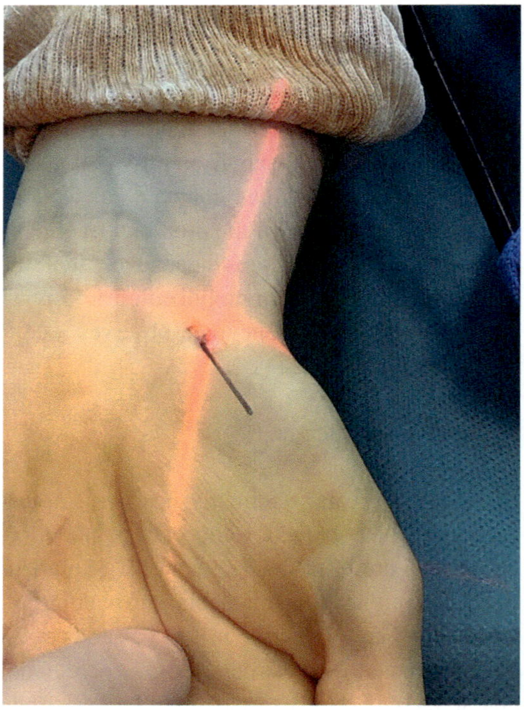

Fig. 4.9 Guiding the screw with a pin under scope control

- The fracture concerns the proximal part.
- There is an associated injury requiring surgery.

– The fracture is open or unstable.
– The patient is a sportsman or motivated worker who wants to quickly go back to his activities.

Rehabilitation and Orthotic Treatment

Rehabilitation can follow surgery or a longer immobilization in case of orthopedic treatment.

The different protocol stages can be modified depending on the bone healing, regularly controlled with X-rays.

In any case, the priorities are regaining physiological amplitudes and strength to restore optimal function, without disturbing the bone's healing.

There are many similar points between this protocol and the one for the fractures of the inferior extremity of the radius, but the concerned patients are usually very different.

The patients with a fracture of the inferior extremity of the radius are usually women of more than 60 years old with osteoporosis, whereas the patients with a fracture of the scaphoid are usually young men who have suffered a high kinetic energy trauma (Dias and Kantharuban 2017; Ibrahim et al. 2011).

Therefore, the rehabilitation goals for these two pathologies are often different, as they are related to the patient's anterior capacities and functional imperatives. The exercises are usually more intense in fractures of the scaphoid, especially the conscious and unconscious neuromuscular proprioception exercises.

Rehabilitation Protocol (Fig. 4.10)

• *Immobilization phase (D0–D15/45 with surgery or D0 to D45/60 without surgery)*

The duration of immobilization after surgery depends on the surgical technique and varies from 15 (percutaneous screws) to 45 days (pins).

During all this phase, rehabilitation is not essential and self-rehabilitation advice are given to the patient, like simple active auto-mobilizations of the metacarpophalangeal joints that tend to stiffen. The patient should do them at home, in a series of short exercises (10–15 repetitions of each exercise) but with a high frequency (3 times in the morning and 3 times in the afternoon). These exercises must be stopped momentarily in case of pain.

The treatment is based on the protocol PRICE that fights against trophic disorders resulting from trauma and surgery:

– P for protection of the fracture line during the whole phase, realized immobilizing the wrist and informing the patient about the tissue fragility in this phase.
– R for rest of the damaged area that must not be solicited during the immobilization phase, aside from self-rehabilitation exercises explained by the therapist.
– I for ice, put cold packs several times a day on the fracture zone. If there is a cast it is impossible, but if there is no wound we immobilize the patient with a thermoformed orthosis, which allows a cold bath against edema.
– C for compression that can be realized in the fingers if they are swollen.
– E for elevation of the wrist to avoid edema.

These exercises are combined with sensorimotor stimulations to maintain body mapping (Roll et al. 2012) and cutaneous receptors.

• *Pre-consolidation phase (D15/45 to D90 with surgery or D45/60 to D120 without surgery)*
• In this phase, we start putting load on the scaphoid and the patient progressively goes back to his daily activities. We fight against pain and trophic disorders if they are still present, try to regain functional amplitudes and start the muscular awakening and reinforcement.
  – *Fight against trophic disorders and pain*

It is essential to start with the other elements of rehabilitation.

We use the same techniques as in fractures of the inferior extremity of the radius:

FRACTURES OF THE SCAPHOID			
	Post-surgery / trauma (A)	**Relative fragility (B)**	**Solidity (C)**
REHABILITATION	<u>Goals:</u> 1 – To reduce trophic disorders 2 – To reduce pain 3 – To prevent the risk of stiffness in the free joints 4 – To maintain the proprioceptive abilities <u>Techniques:</u> 1 – Draining massages and compressive bandage, vacuum therapy for draining, low-frequency electrical currents 2 – Cryotherapy, TENS, TVS (100Hz) 3 – Mobilization of the free joints in passive and active (fingers +++) 4 – TVS (70-80Hz) and varied sensitive stimulation without constraints <u>Risks:</u> Bad healing in case of non-observance	<u>Goals:</u> 1 – Same as in phase A with intensified techniques if necessary 2 – To recover joint mobility 3 – To gradually recover the protective muscles' proprioceptive abilities <u>Techniques:</u> 1 – Pressotherapy for draining, vacuum therapy on the scar, defibrosing massage if the scar is not inflammatory and closed (A1), manipulation of light objects (A4) 2 – Soft mobilizations (instrumental and manual) 3 – Gradual conscious proprioceptive work, conscious neuromuscular rehabilitation for the FCR and then global, NO BALL CLENCHING <u>Risks:</u> Same as phase A + type 1 CRPS	<u>Goals:</u> 1 – Same as in phases A and B with intensified techniques if necessary 2 – Total functional recovery <u>Techniques:</u> 1 – Intensification of the mobilizations with specific joint mobilizations, postures, and electrostimulation (B2) 2 – Unconscious neuromuscular rehabilitation and recovery of normal muscular ratios (B3) 3 – Functional activities adapted to the patient's professional and sports needs <u>Risks:</u> Same as in phases A and B
ORTHOSES	Strict immobilization	Gradual removal	Functional orthosis for resumption of activity
	If surgery D3 to D15/45 **If orthopedic treatment D3 to D/60**	**If surgery D15/54 to D90** **If orthopedic treatment D45/60 to D120**	**If surgery after D90** **If orthopedic treatment after D120**

Fig. 4.10 Rehabilitation protocol (1) and progression pyramid (2)

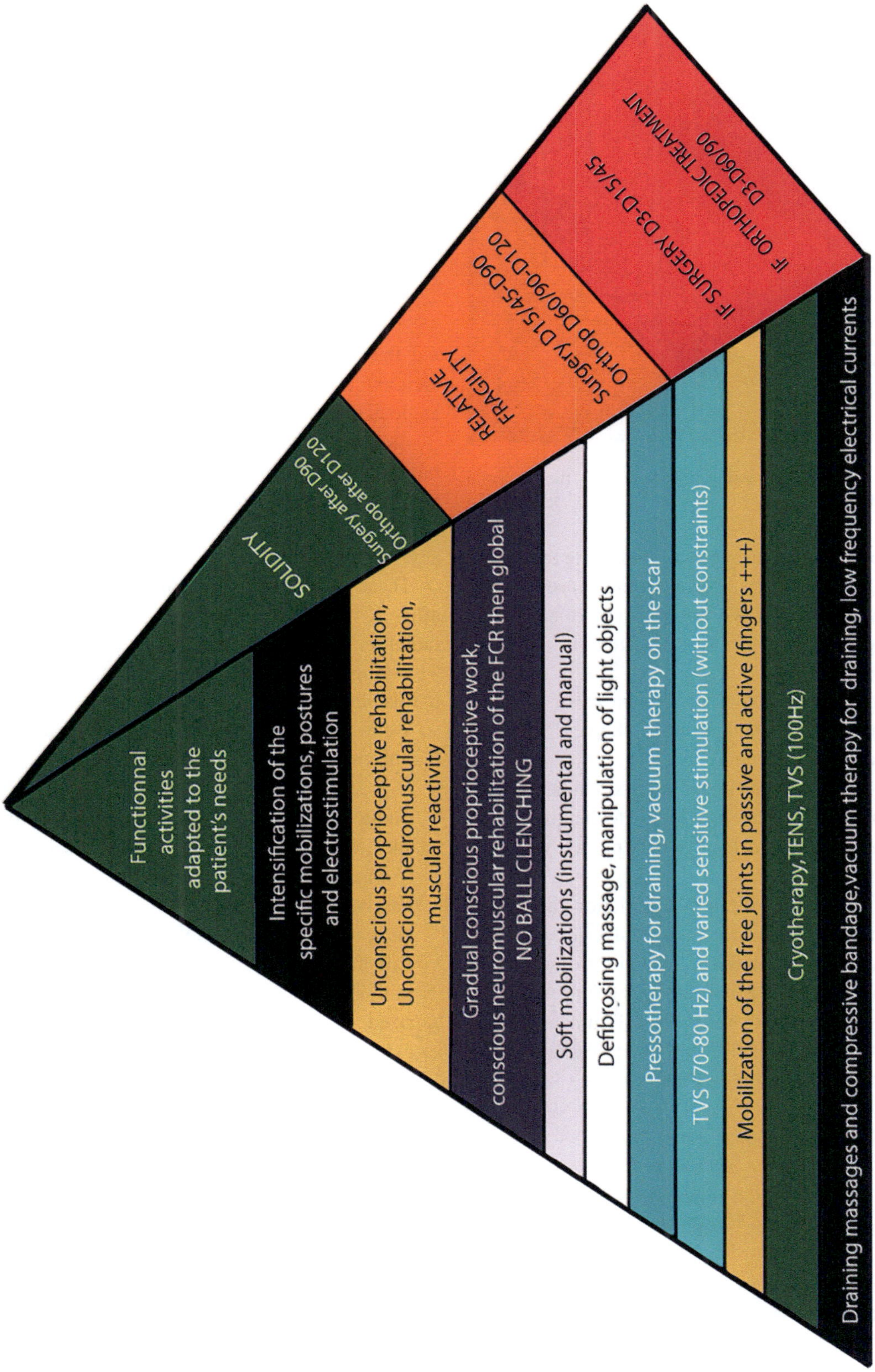

Fig. 4.10 (continued)

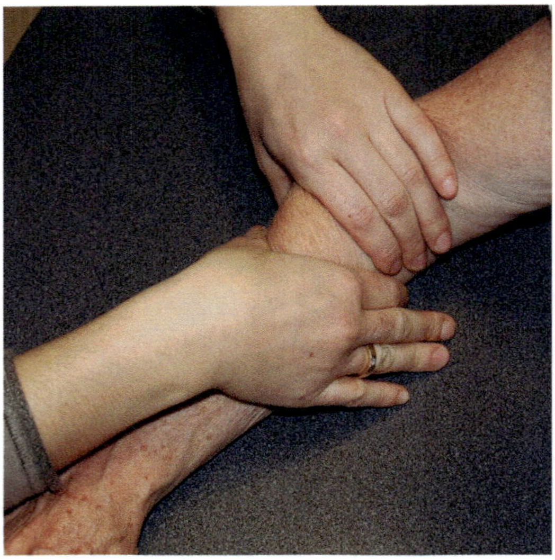

Fig. 4.11 Decontracting massage of the forearm muscles

Draining massages without slackening the scar in case of surgery. Decontracting massages for the forearm if we observe hypertonia in the extrinsic musculature, which is frequent (Fig. 4.11).

Analgesic electrotherapy can be used, with the modalities described in the chapter *"Physical agents"* (volume 1).

Pressotherapy from distal to proximal helps drain the wrist. In this phase, this technique can be badly tolerated by the patient; we will then delay its use.

Transcutaneous vibratory stimulations and infrasound are used for their analgesic and vasomotor effect, with the modalities described in the chapter *"Physical agents"* (volume 1). Vibrations with more than 1 mm amplitude are realized far from the fracture site in order not to disturb the healing process.

– *Regaining functional amplitudes*

It requires a good knowledge of the constraints transmitted to the scaphoid depending on the joint sector.

In flexion-extension, the ligaments are relaxed and the joint pressure is minimal until 20° and becomes significant at 40°. After that, the pressures increase to reach their maximal value of around 80°. After 80°, they become pathogenic (Herbert 1990) (Fig. 4.12).

The normal amplitude in radial inclination is 15°. It induces compressive constraints on the scaphoid that tilts in flexion, which can encourage the formation of a vicious callus, closing the intrascaphoidal sagittal angle (Weber 1980).

The normal amplitude in ulnar inclination is 45°. It creates traction constraints on the scaphoid that tilts in extension. The formation of a vicious callus when the intrascaphoidal sagittal angle is open is rarer but can happen.

As in fractures of the inferior extremity of the radius, these elements allow defining "risky" areas in which the exercises to regain amplitude will have to be realized very cautiously, without any force.

These areas are after 40° in flexion/extension, after 20° in ulnar inclination, and from 5° in radial inclination.

Trying to regain total amplitudes at all costs is, in this phase, useless and dangerous.

We use the same techniques as in fractures of the inferior extremity of the radius:

– Fluidotherapy to relax the muscles and tissues. We use it at the beginning of the session to warm-up the wrist.
– Passive manual mobilizations are basic exercises to regain joint amplitude. They are soft, pain free and can be realized increasing the joint spaces a little. We work in all the authorized sectors, being particularly careful in extension and radial inclination where the constraints on the scaphoid are more important.
– Global active mobilizations are realized after the passive ones, in various finger positions to improve tendinous glidings at the level of the wrist (Fig. 4.13).
– Active-assisted mobilizations can be assisted by an arthromotor. We ask the patient to participate actively in the movements applied by

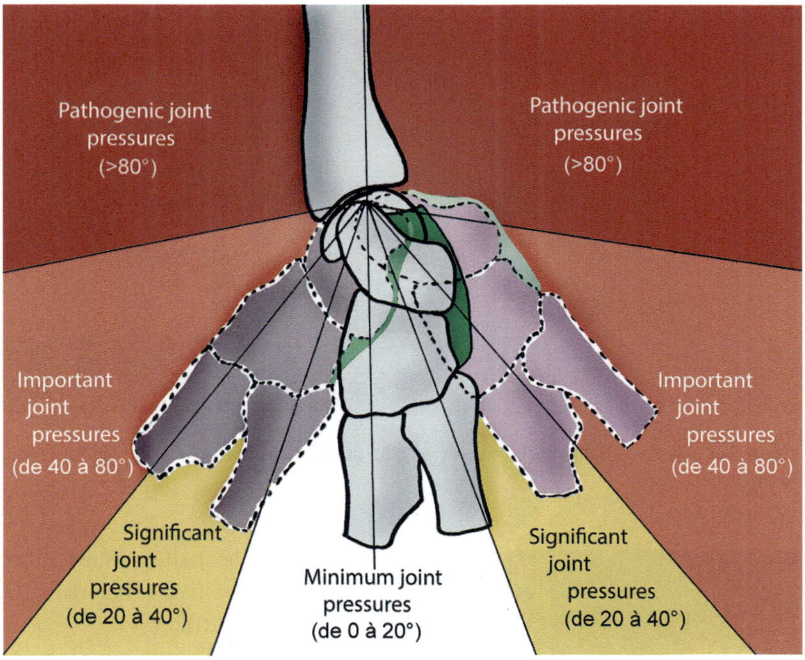

Fig. 4.12 Joint pressures depending on the amplitudes in flexion/extension

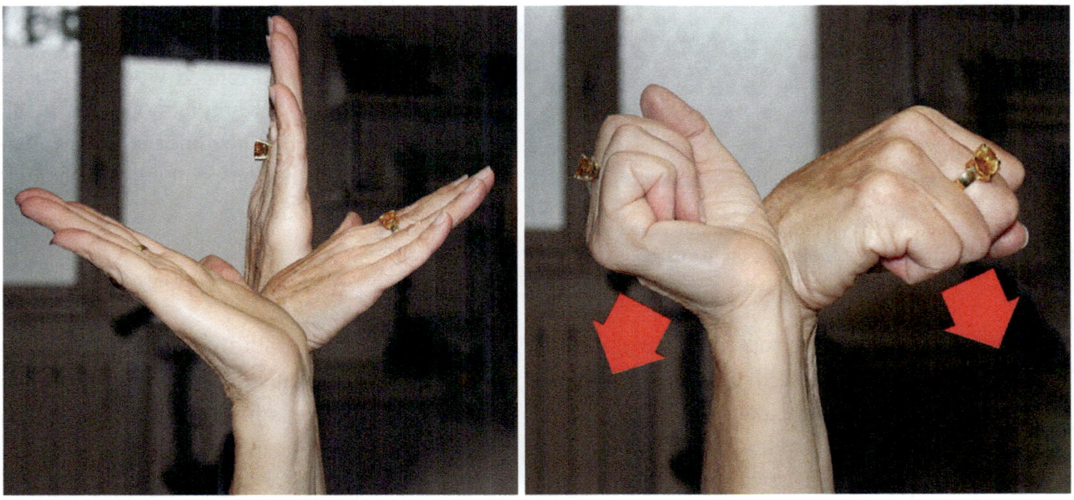

Fig. 4.13 Active mobilizations realized with the fingers extended and a closed fist to improve the tendon glidings in the flexor and extensor systems

the device. This exercise is realized in amplitudes previously regained passively by the therapist. It has an interest at the joint level, but also in draining the edema as it stimulates the "vis a latere". It can be combined with icing (Fig. 4.14).

– Electrostimulation, combined with an active movement (winding the fingers) can help regaining the last degrees of mobility in finger flexion if necessary. The patient mustn't clutch his fingers as it would put important constraints on the scaphoid (Fig. 4.15).

– *Proprioceptive abilities of the wrist*

It is important to propose a coherent evolution for the exercises depending on the healing phase, in order not to disturb the consolidation process.

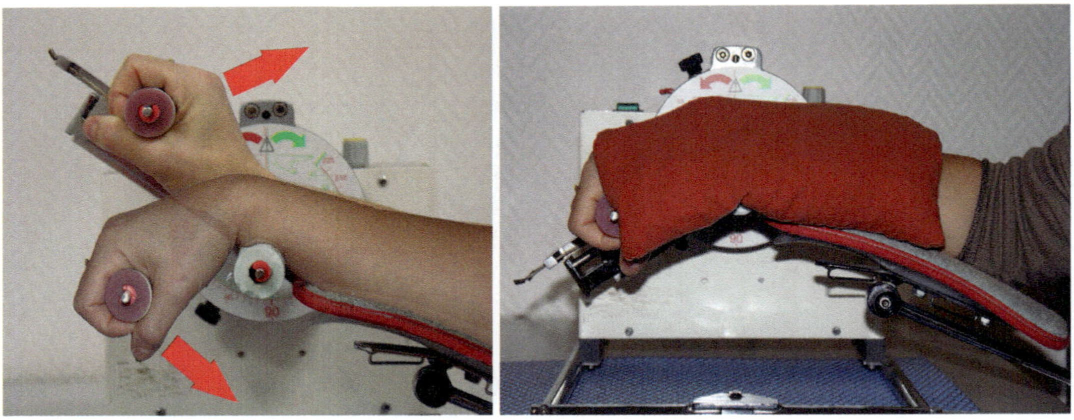

Fig. 4.14 Active-assisted mobilization with an arthromotor without (1) or with (2) ice depending on the trophic state of the wrist

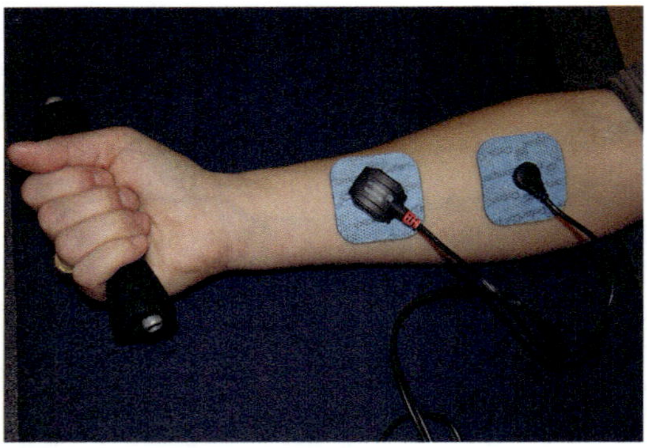

Fig. 4.15 Electroactive winding (without clamping) to avoid putting important constraints on the osseous callus

The recovery stage of the proprioceptive abilities must also be considered so that the patient does not develop compensative pathologies such as tendinopathies or reflex contractures.

- *Perception of joint position (Hagert's stage 3)*

It is defined as the ability to precisely reproduce a given joint angulation (Hagert 2010).

The rehabilitation of this perception is done in three steps. In the first step, the therapist places the patient's wrist in a defined joint position and controls the joint amplitude with a goniometer (Hagert 2010).

In the second step, the wrist is placed in another position, indifferently. In the third step, the patient must place his forearm in the first position (Hagert 2010; Karagiannopoulos et al. 2016).

The exercise is realized with the patient's eyes closed to avoid any visual afference. An error margin of 4° is considered normal in adults (at the level of the wrists).

This test is highly correlated with the wrist's sensorimotor abilities (Karagiannopoulos et al. 2016) and must therefore be done before any evolution of the rehabilitation protocol—especially before Hager's stage 5.

- *Kinesthesia (Hagert's stage 4)*

It is defined as the ability to detect a passive movement. The therapist realizes the movement while the patient keeps his eyes closed and tells him when he perceives the movement.

This exercise is easy to realize at the physiotherapy office or at home but does not allow a precise analysis regarding the patient's perception threshold.

Using an arthromotor device allows analyzing more precisely the movement speed and the studied angular sector.

A laser can also be a very helpful tool to improve conscious proprioceptive abilities. The patient must follow trajectories becoming increasingly complex, going faster and faster (Fig. 4.16).

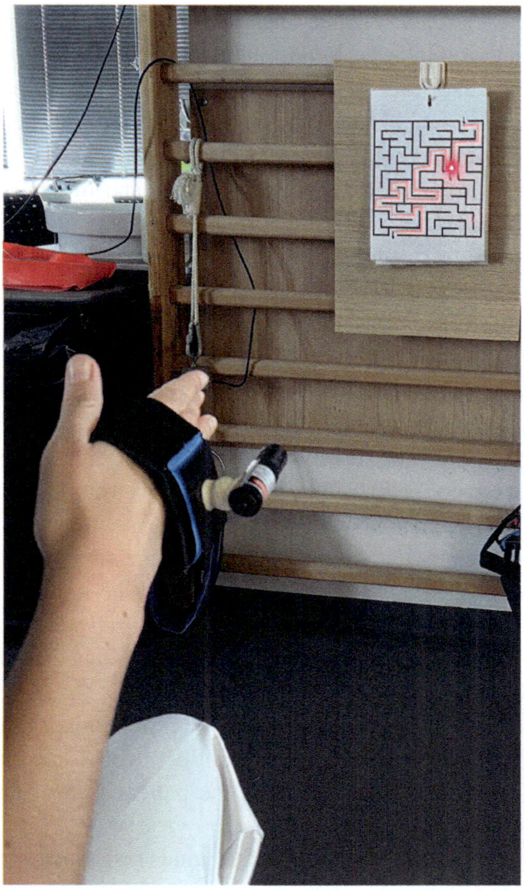

Fig. 4.16 Using a laser to improve conscious proprioceptive abilities

- *Conscious neuromuscular rehabilitation (Hagert's stage 5)*

At this stage, we use muscular awakening techniques and static contractions in four directions, with the same modalities as those described for the fractures of the inferior extremity of the radius.

Muscular awakening is realized with exercises with energy overload, which can be used at first to progressively stimulate atrophic muscles.

"Trigger" muscles are part of the intrinsic musculature to avoid increasing the longitudinal constraints of the carpus on the forearm:

- Abductor pollicis brevis—pronator quadratus (Fig. 4.17).
- Flexor digiti minimi—flexor carpi ulnaris (Fig. 4.18).

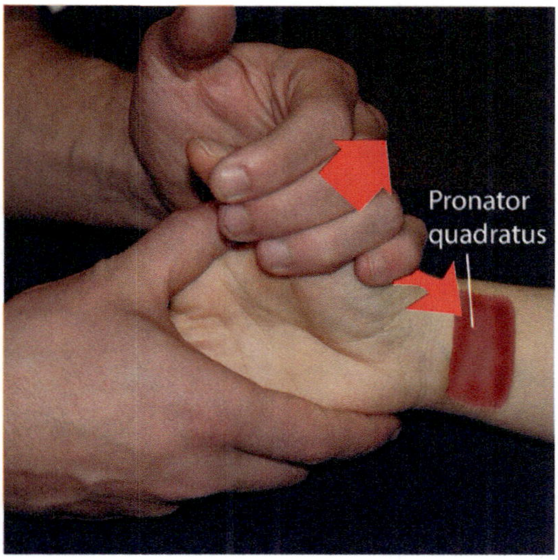

Fig. 4.17 Exercise with energy overload, where the trigger muscle is the abductor pollicis brevis and the target muscle the pronator quadratus

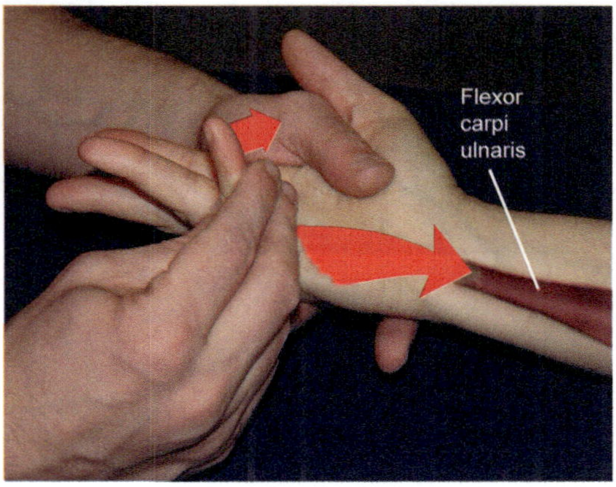

Fig. 4.18 Exercise with energy overload, where the trigger muscle is the flexor digiti minimi brevis and the target muscle is the flexor carpi ulnaris

- Thenar and hypothenar muscles—flexor carpi radialis (Fig. 4.19).
- Abductor digiti minimi and thumb extensors—ulnar and radial carpal stabilizers (Fig. 4.20).

The strengthening protocol itself starts when the previous exercises are easily realized by the patient. All the exercises are performed with the fingers in extension, to limit the axial constraints increased by the contraction of the finger flexors when clamping (Fig. 4.21).

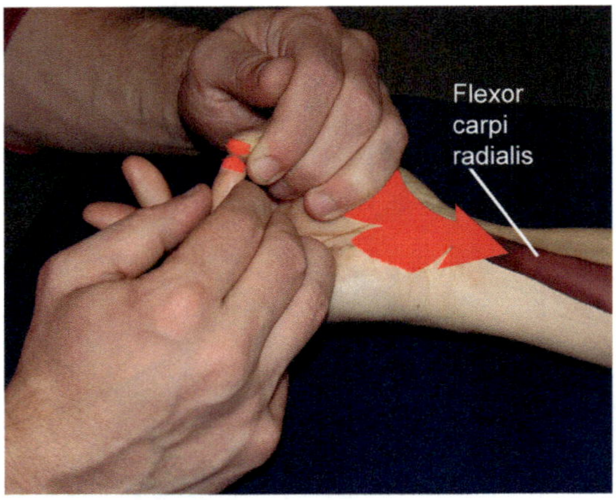

Fig. 4.19 Exercise with energy overload, from the opposition arch to the flexor carpi radialis

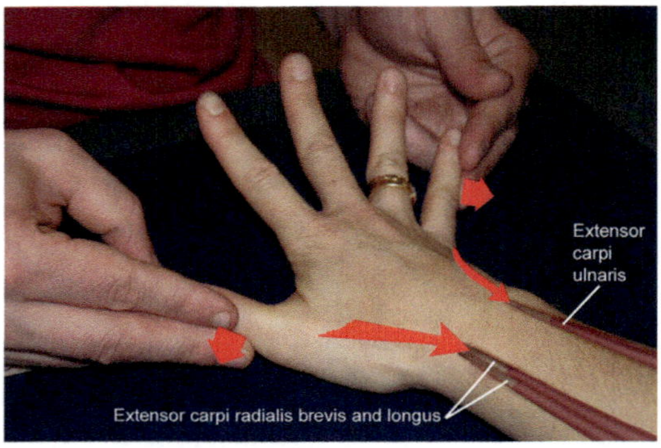

Fig. 4.20 Exercise with energy overload, from the extensors of the thumb and the abductors of the fifth finger to the radial and ulnar stabilizers of the carpus

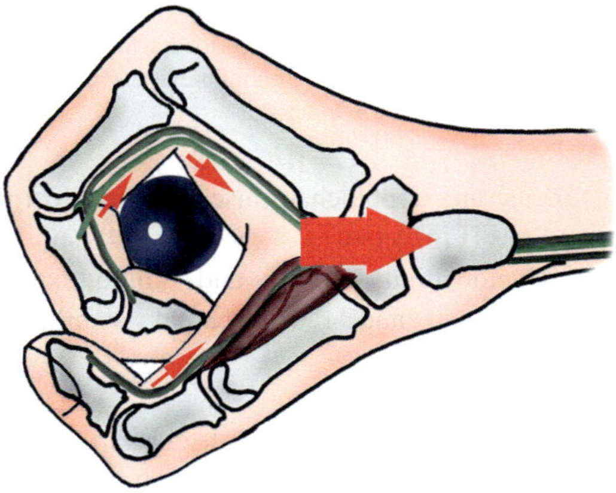

Fig. 4.21 The contraction of the finger flexors when clamping puts compressive constraints on the carpus that can affect the osseous healing of the scaphoid

The first solicited energy system is the aerobic one as it is the least constraining at the muscular and articular level. "Pure" aerobic exercises cannot be realized in this phase as the patient would be asked to realize long contractions (10–15 min!), which in this phase would lead to tendinous and muscular disorders, as well as important pain. Therefore, we use static intermittent exercises adapted to the wrist's functional biomechanics, the relative fragility of the callus and the wrist muscles' physiology.

At the beginning of the phase, we ask for low-intensity static contractions with a series of 30 repetitions, held for 6 s, and with 6 s of rest between the repetitions. The ideal contraction intensity is 20–30% of the maximal strength, but as it cannot be assessed in this phase, it is controlled by the therapist or by a device.

We cannot use the contralateral side to determine the usual strength of the injured side as there are often important differences between the two sides of a patient.

The parameters (number of repetitions, contraction duration, and modalities) evolve during the treatment, adapting to the patient's capacity and osseous consolidation.

A contraction with maximal resistance or clamping is never asked.

Dynamic contractions with wide amplitudes are not in relation to the physiological role of the wrist (orient and stabilize the hand during prehensions). Therefore, they are not included in the reinforcement protocol (except if there is a particular indication).

We realize a static reinforcement of the four sides of the wrist, with the wrist in a neutral position and the fingers in extension:

- *Wrist flexors*: The flexor carpi radialis passes in front of the radial epiphysis and the scaphoid. It avoids the anterior tilt of the distal fragment in neck fractures (Fig. 4.22).

  The flexor carpi ulnaris passes in front of the ulnar head and ends on the pisiform. It produces expansions toward the anterior retinacular ligament, the hamate, and the fourth and fifth metacarpals. It is prolonged along the internal column by the adductor digiti minimi (Fig. 4.23).

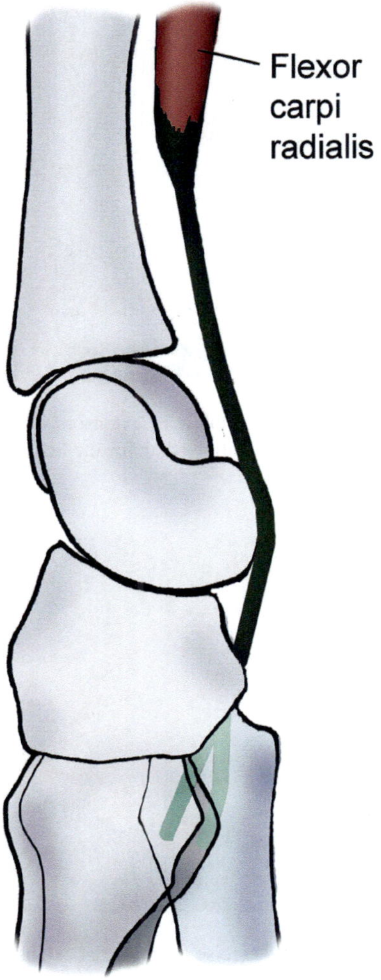

Fig. 4.22 Anatomical disposition of the flexor carpi radialis tendon, forbidding the distal part of the scaphoid to go forward

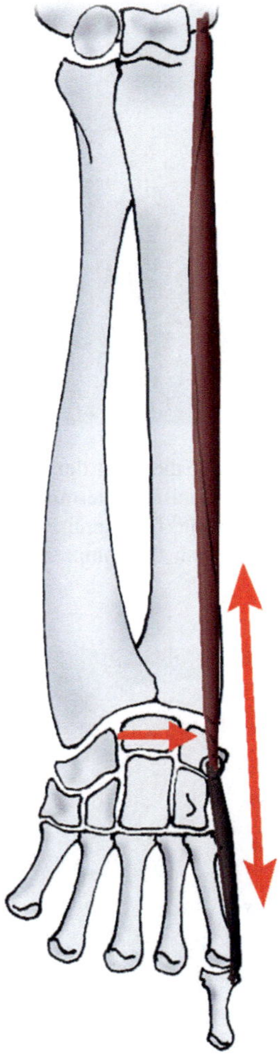

Fig. 4.23 Anatomical disposition of the flexor carpi ulnaris

During these exercises, the flexor carpi radialis and ulnaris work in synergy, and the action of the finger flexors is limited as we place the fingers in extension.

We work with the espalier, with a contraction against an elastic band (moderate resistance). At the beginning of this rehabilitation phase, the patient brings the elastic band in the working position with his contralateral hand, to realize a pure static exercise.

The exercise is then realized only with the damaged side to alternate stato-concentric, static, and stato-eccentric contractions against a controlled resistance.

Visual feedback allows the patient to control the contraction and rest phases (Fig. 4.24).

Manually, the resistance is placed at the level of the palmar side of the metacarpal diaphyses, stabilizing the forearm with the contralateral hand. This grip allows us controlling the osseous callus and limits the compression and shearing constraints imposed on it.

A digital grip with the fingers in extension is also possible (Fig. 4.25).

An ulnar or radial inclination can be asked to work with the flexor carpi ulnaris or radialis.

– *Wrist extensors*: The extensor carpi radialis longus and brevis pass on the posterior side of the radial styloid process and in the anatomical

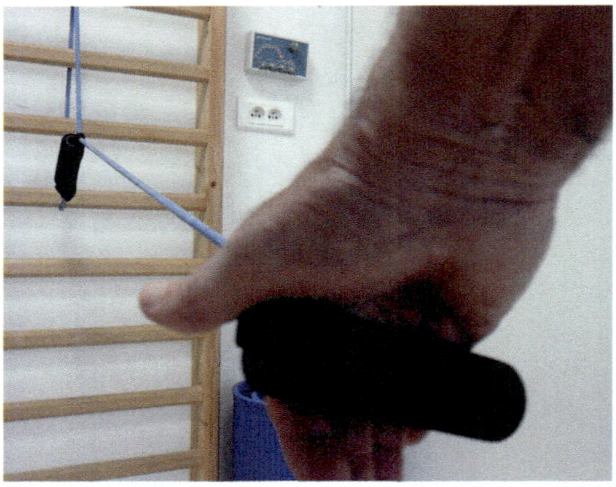

Fig. 4.24 Exercise for the wrist flexors with an espalier and visual feedback precisely determining the contraction time and the resting time. The exercise is realized with the fingers extended to limit the compressive constraints on the scaphoid

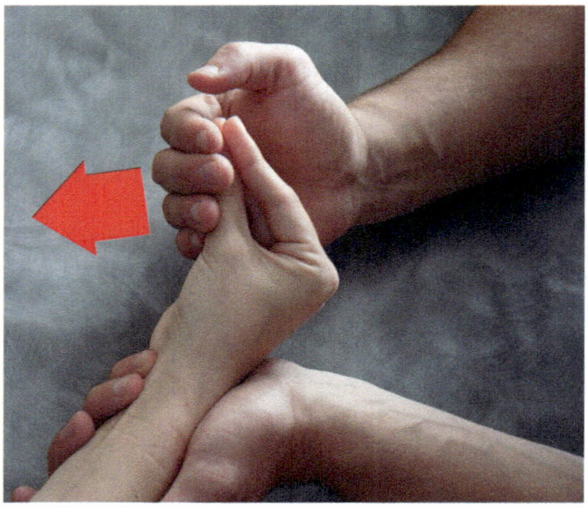

Fig. 4.25 Manual exercise for the wrist flexors with a digital grip. The interphalangeals are extended and the metacarpals are flexed. As the metacarpophalangeal flexion is ensured by the intrinsic system, there is no increase in the compressive constraints on the scaphoid

snuffbox, before ending respectively on the posterior side of the second and third metacarpals. They participate in stabilizing the radial column, along with the flexor carpi radialis.

The extensor carpi ulnaris passes with the extensors between the styloid process and the ulnar head before ending on the fifth metacarpal's postero-internal tubercle. It participates in stabilizing the ulnar column, along with the flexor carpi ulnaris.

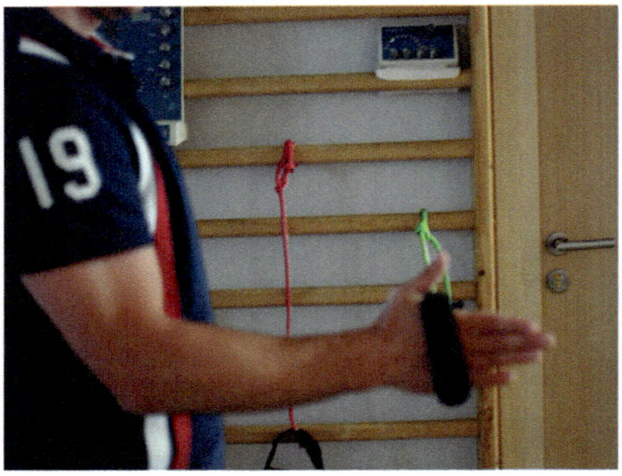

Fig. 4.26 Exercise for the wrist extensors with an espalier, with the same modalities than for the flexors

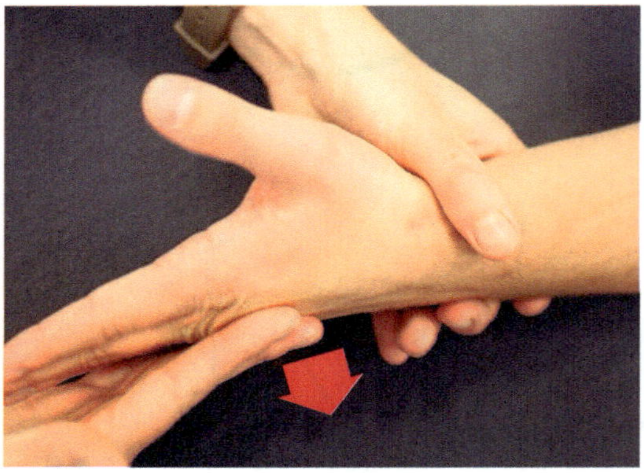

Fig. 4.27 Manual exercise for the wrist extensors

The abductor pollicis longus and extensor pollicis brevis stabilize the radial column, but their analytical contraction is moderate in this phase as there are important risks of tendinopathy.

We use the espalier with an elastic band, according to the same modalities than for the wrist flexors, and always with visual feedback (Fig. 4.26).

Manually, the resistance is placed at the level of the dorsal side of the metacarpal diaphyses, stabilizing the ulnar side of the wrist with the contralateral hand (Fig. 4.27).

As for the reinforcement of the wrist flexors, we can associate a radial or ulnar inclination to work with the extensor carpi radialis or ulnaris.

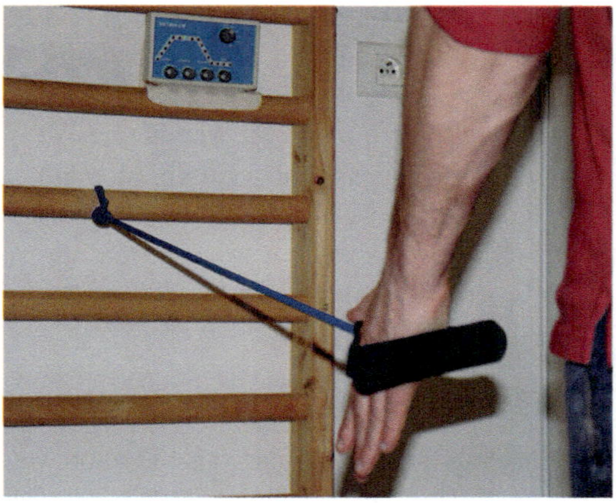

Fig. 4.28 Synergic exercise for the flexor carpi ulnaris and the extensor carpi ulnaris with an espalier

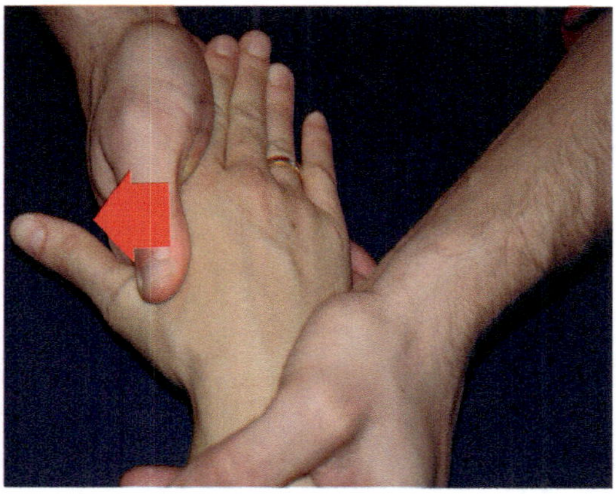

Fig. 4.30 Manual exercise for the radial stabilizers of the carpus with a stabilizing counter-grip on the ulnar compartment. The wrist mustn't be in an important radial inclination to limit the constraints on the scaphoid

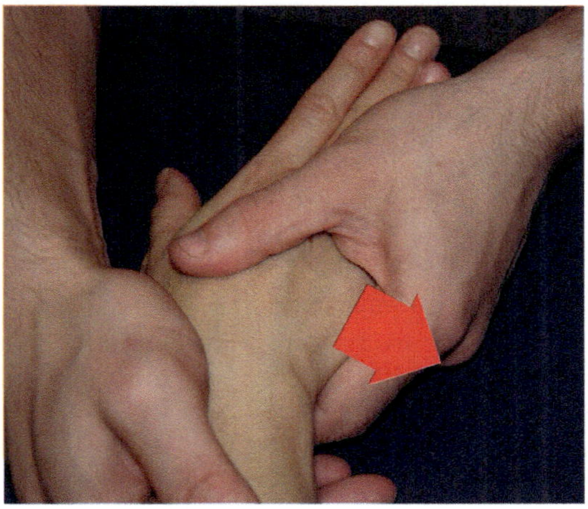

Fig. 4.29 Manual exercise for the ulnar stabilizers of the carpus with a stabilizing counter-grip on the radial compartment

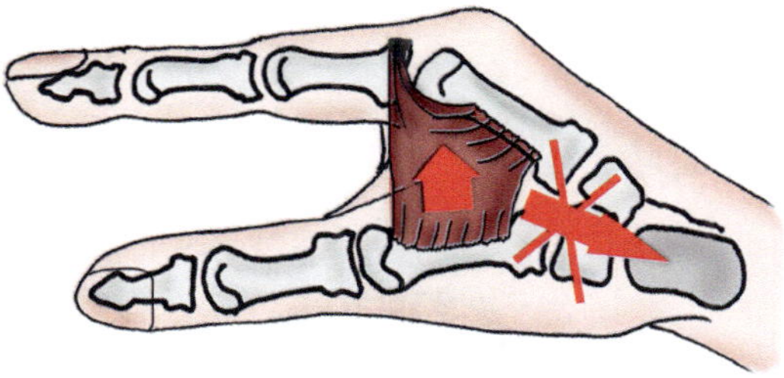

Fig. 4.31 The contraction of intrinsic muscles that don't have a longitudinal orientation does not put important compressive constraints on the scaphoid

- *Ulnar stabilizers*: The extensor and flexor carpi ulnaris can work in synergy in an exercise with the espalier (Fig. 4.28).

  Manually, we can ask for a direct contraction against resistance at the level of the ulnar side of the carpus (triquetrum, hamate, and fifth metacarpal), stabilizing the scaphoid with the contralateral hand (Fig. 4.29).

  Another exercise consists of working with the abductor digiti minimi brevis as it is in continuity with the flexor carpi ulnaris.
- *Radial stabilizers*: The opposite exercise is proposed to solicit preferentially the wrist radial stabilizers. Resistances are placed on the radial side of the second metacarpal to reduce the contraction of the thumb muscles.

  This exercise is realized very carefully, and the patient is forbidden to mobilize his wrist in radial inclination during the contraction (Fig. 4.30).
- *Intrinsic muscles*: The contraction of the intrinsic muscles does not produce important axial constraints, unlike the contraction of the extrinsic muscles (Fig. 4.31).

  We will strengthen preferentially the interossei, the flexor pollicis brevis, and the adductor pollicis.

  We ask the patient to realize a "vise" pinch against resistance, with visual feedback to manage the duration of contraction and rest (Fig. 4.32).

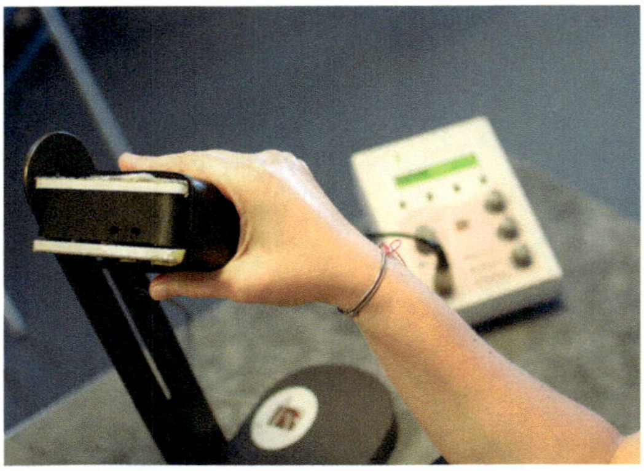

Fig. 4.32 Instrumental contraction exercise for the intrinsic muscles with an intrinsic pinch and visual feedback

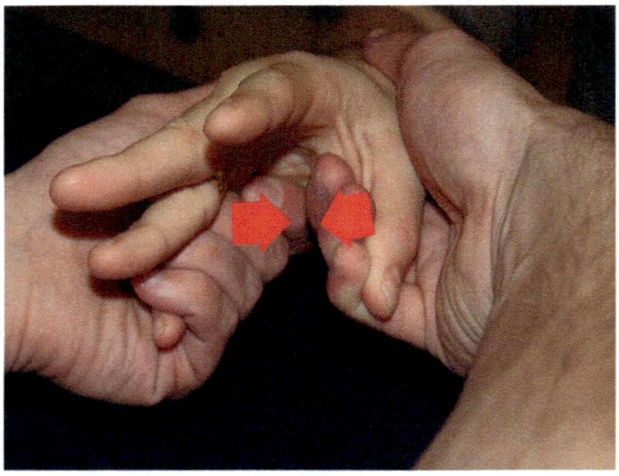

Fig. 4.33 Manual reinforcement of the muscles that are part of the arch of opposition between the thumb and the fifth finger

The same exercise can be realized manually.

The opposition arch between the thumb and the fifth finger can also be solicited manually (Fig. 4.33).

- *Electrostimulation*: Combined with an active contraction of the stimulated muscles, it improves motor recruitment and maintains body mapping, thus participating in active wrist stabilization.

  It can concern intrinsic or extrinsic muscles and follows the principles of progression and protection of the bone callus depending on the consolidation.

- *Unconscious neuromuscular rehabilitation or reflex muscular activation (Hagert's stage 6)*

N.B.: Even if these techniques are the same as in fractures of the inferior extremity of the radius, there are some variations. We will particularly insist on regaining strength in the radial muscles (flexor carpi radialis and radial extensors) that are important stabilizers of the scaphoid, especially in neck fractures.

Conscious neuromuscular rehabilitation voluntarily targets the solicited muscles, whereas unconscious neuromuscular rehabilitation calls upon reflexes to actively stabilize a joint, thus partly compensating its passive instability.

In this phase, the exercises are of moderate intensity in order not to disturb the healing process.

- *Table-tennis racket*

  We ask the patient to maintain the ball on the racket, which implies a good sensorial analysis and a contraction adapted to the received information.

  Progressively, we ask the patient to throw the ball and receive it "softly" on the racket.
- *Exercises with a plastic ball*

  We use a light plastic ball and ask the patient to pass it from one hand to the other, to throw and catch it.

- *Prehensions*

We work on prehensions to improve coordination and dexterity and therefore improve functional capacities in daily activities.

These exercises are realized without clamping or putting excessive constraints on the scaphoid.

For example, clamping a ball is forbidden (Fig. 4.34).

In this phase, these exercises are performed only if there are no pain or trophic disorders. They improve the patient's proprioceptive abilities without taking any risks regarding bone healing.

- *Consolidation (after D90 with surgery, after D120 without surgery)*

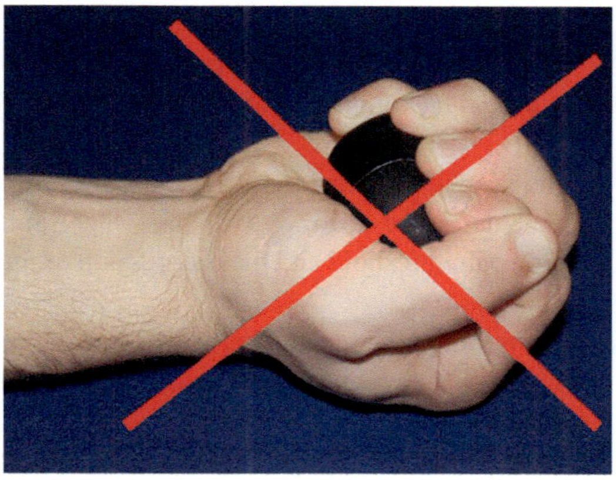

Fig. 4.34 Clamping a ball, forbidden during the healing phase as it puts compressive constraints on the scaphoid

When the scaphoid is solid, we can start more intensive techniques (never aggressive).

In this phase, we aim to regain strength and wrist amplitudes. Rebalancing force ratios between the different muscular groups limits the risks of secondary tendinopathy.

Prehension and proprioception exercises help the patient regain the functionality he will need in his work and sports activities.

– *Regaining wrist amplitudes*

We keep realizing techniques from the previous phase and intensify them if necessary (pain free) to completely regain the wrist amplitudes.

We use specific peri-scaphoidal mobilization techniques:

- *Stretching*

  If the mobility limitation depends on the position of the fingers, we add stretching techniques for the forearm muscles: the wrist flexors in case of stiffness in extension and the wrist extensors in case of stiffness in flexion.
- *Specific mobilizations*

  They require a good knowledge of the morpho-palpatory anatomy and the intracarpal biomechanics. Tractions-glidings are performed between the radius and the first carpal row, between the first and second carpal row, and between the scaphoid and the adjacent bones, insisting on the lunate with which it forms a pair essential in the good functioning of the wrist (Wolfe 2001; Garcia-Elias 2013).

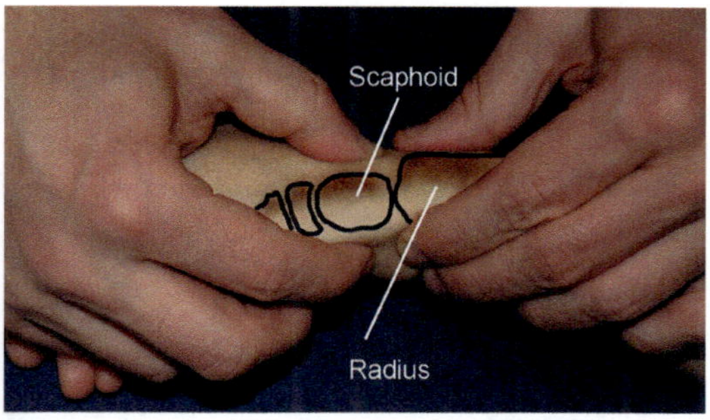

Fig. 4.35 Analytical mobilization of the scaphoid with respect to the radius, wrist in a neutral position

We realize mobilizations between the radius and the carpus and between the two carpal rows (described in the chapter *"Recent fractures of the inferior extremity of the radius"*), to which we add analytical mobilizations between the scaphoid and the adjacent bones.

- *Mobilization scaphoid/radius*

  The patient keeps his wrist in a neutral position to avoid limiting mobility with the reduction of the space between the trapezo-trapezoidal joint and the radius during radial inclination, or the tension in radial ligaments during ulnar inclination.

  The scaphoid is maintained between the therapist's thumb and index, with the thumb on the scaphoid's tubercle and the index on the posterior side of the proximal part.

  The other hand maintains the radius, and we apply antero-posterior glidings on the scaphoid (Fig. 4.35).
- *Mobilization scaphoid/lunate*

  The wrist is still in a neutral position; the patient places his forearm in pronation.

  The scaphoid is maintained by the radial hand between the thumb (dorsal side of the proximal part) and the index (tubercle). The lunate is maintained by the ulnar hand between the thumb (dorsal side) and the pulp of the other fingers (palmar side). Each hand applies an opposite gliding to obtain maximal movement (Fig. 4.36).
- *Mobilization scaphoid/trapezium*

  In the same position as for the mobilization scaphoid/lunate, the scaphoid is maintained the same way and the trapezium is between the thumb (dorsal side) and the index (palmar side). We apply a differential gliding on each bone in a direction oblique backward and outward or frontward and inward, with the scaphoid oriented frontward and outward.

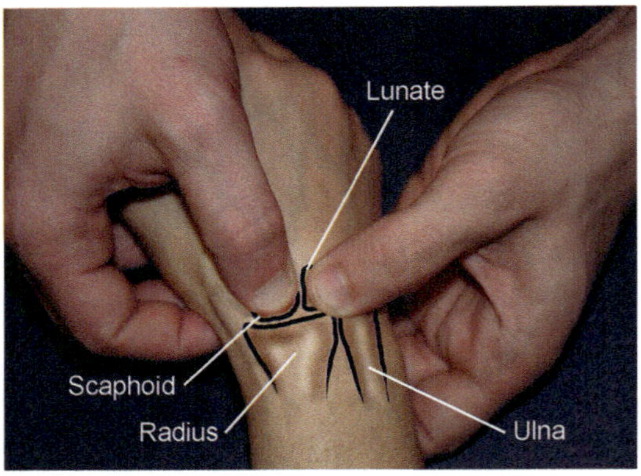

Fig. 4.36 Scapholunar mobilization with opposed glidings of the two mobilizing hands

- *Total proprioceptive recovery*
- *Intensifying conscious neuromuscular rehabilitation techniques (Hagert's stage 5)*

The scaphoid is healed so the muscular reinforcement can be realized with no other limit than the pain threshold and the progression of the techniques.

We use the same techniques as in the previous phase with more important loads, to regain strength comparable to the sane side.

Chain work is realized according to the patient's functional needs (Fig. 4.37).

The assessment of the muscular ratios is essential, and we often observe weakness in the radial and extrinsic elements in relation to the ulnar and intrinsic ones. This difference is prob-

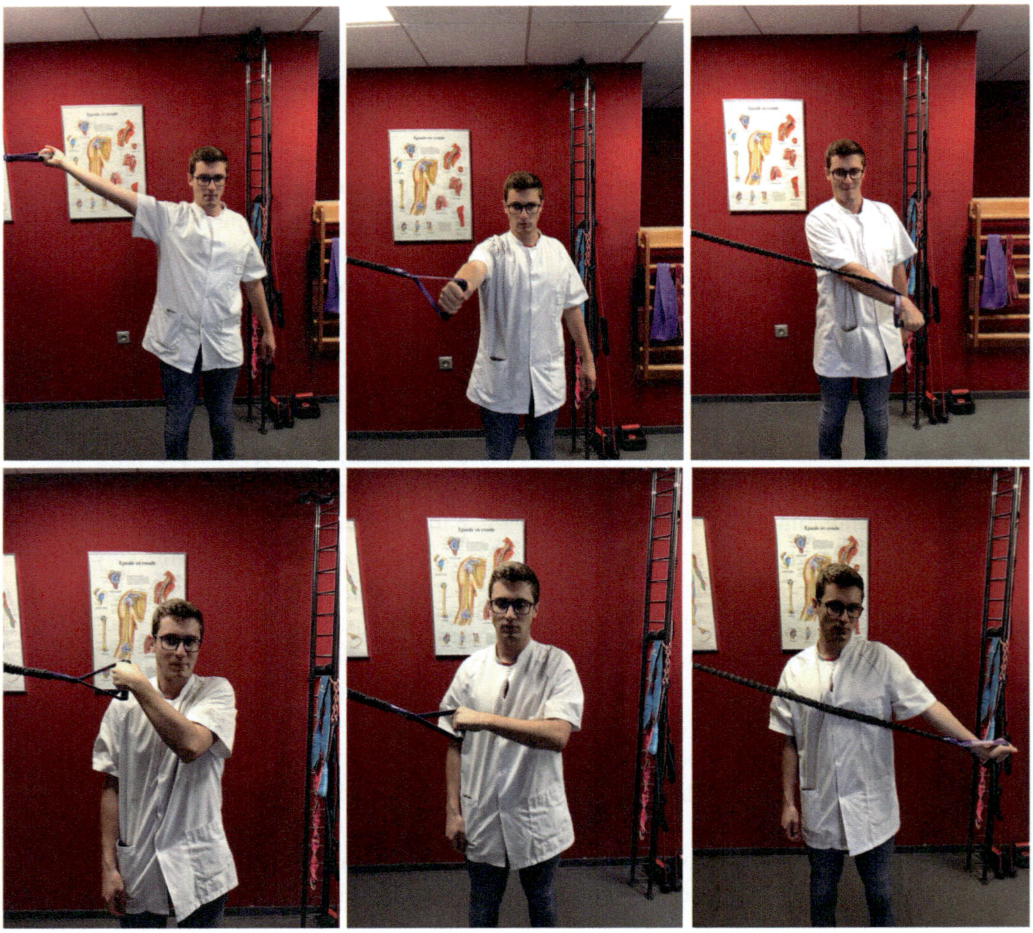

Fig. 4.37 Example of an exercise in chain for the whole superior limb. The aim is to find exercises close to the patient's functional needs

ably related to the limits imposed in the other phases to protect the scaphoid.

The exercises and protocols are like the ones for the fractures of the distal extremity of the radius:

- Using a load cell and visual feedback allows for accurately targeting the solicited energy system, modifying the load and duration of contraction and rest. The reinforcement is realized in flexion-supination and extension-pronation to improve muscular capacities and regain muscular balance, comparable to the sane side (Fig. 4.38). If a comparison with the sane side cannot be done, our experience has determined that strength in flexion-supination is 1.8 times more important than strength in extension-pronation in men, and 2.6 times in women.
- Using a dynamometer combined with a device allows for regulating the duration of contraction and rest, with visual feedback to target the solicited energy system, reinforce and rebalance the pronators and supinators (Fig. 4.39).
- Global exercises for the superior limb can be done too, realizing a controlled contraction with visual feedback of the ulnar (Fig. 4.40) or radial stabilizers, and the wrist flexors (Fig. 4.41) and extensors.
- Using weights solicits flexors/extensors in half-open chain (Fig. 4.42). It allows alternating concentric, static, and eccentric contractions whose parameters evolve depending on the patient's functional needs.
- Using a hammer solicits pronators/supinators in half-open chain (Fig. 4.43). Like with weights, we can alternate different contraction modes and the parameters evolve depending on the patient's functional needs and progress.
- Using a minibike in active mode improves the wrist flexors and extensors' endurance. The resistance and exercise duration evolve, adapting to the patient's needs and capacities (Fig. 4.44).
- Support exercises to work in closed chain (Fig. 4.45).

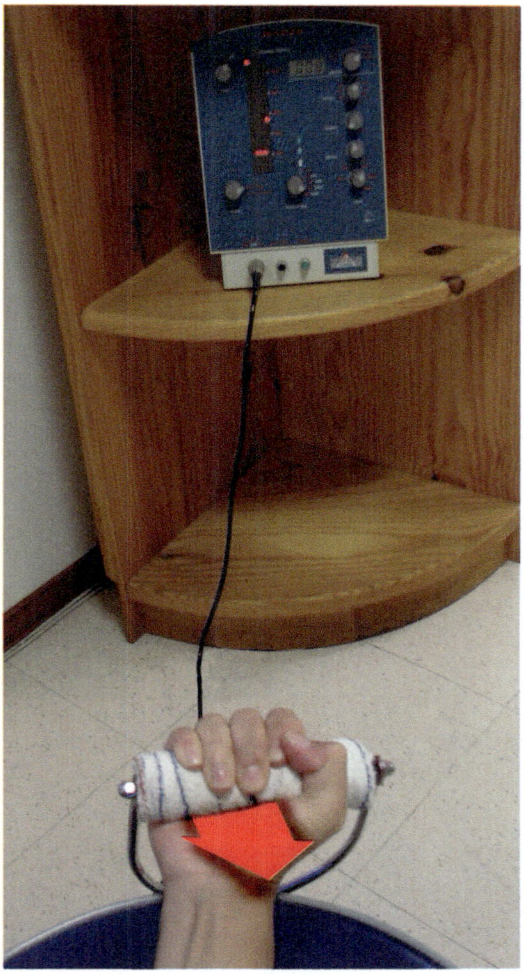

Fig. 4.38 Reinforcement exercise for the wrist flexors with the forearm supinated, with load cell and visual feedback

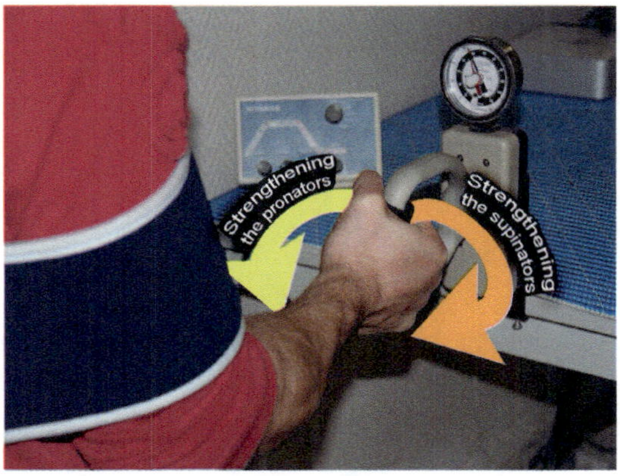

Fig. 4.39 Exercise for the pronators and supinators with dynamometer and a device regulating the contraction and rest duration, and visual feedback

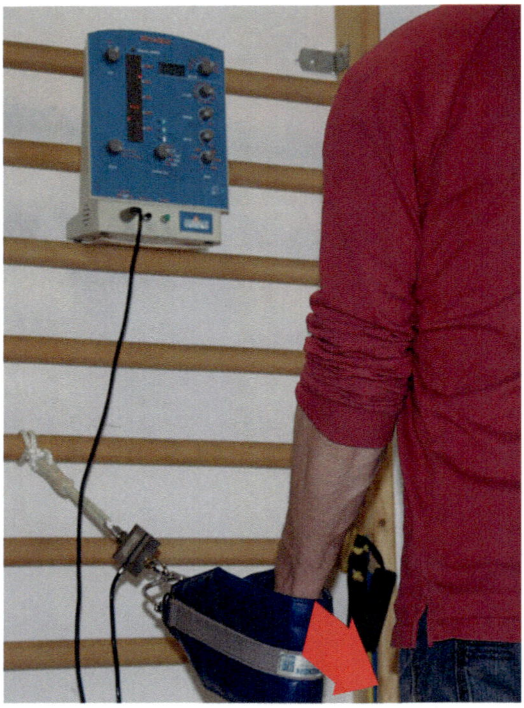

Fig. 4.40 Exercise for the ulnar stabilizers of the wrist with load cell and visual feedback

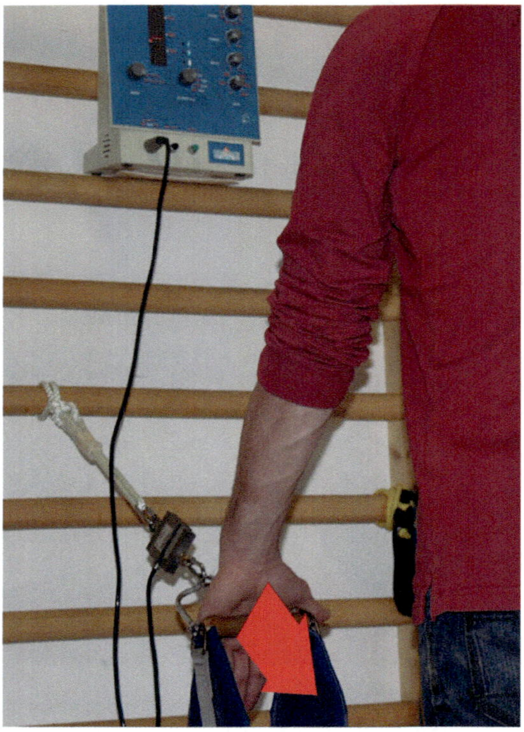

Fig. 4.41 Exercise for the wrist flexors with load cell and visual feedback

– Techniques using digito-antebrachial chains can be realized manually or instrumentally (Fig. 4.46).
– Electrostimulation can be associated with every exercise previously described; adapting the program to the energy system we want to work with (see chapter *"Physical agents,"* volume 1).

- *Intensifying unconscious neuromuscular rehabilitation or reflex muscle activation (Hager's stage 6)*

It is essential in the functional recovery of the wrist and can be realized manually or with instrumental techniques.

We use exercises with oscillating poles, medicine balls, and rhythmical stabilization, described in chapter *"Proprioception"* (volume 1).

– Multidirectional proprioception and feedforward pressing on a plastic ball first poorly inflated and then progressively more inflated (Fig. 4.47).
– Rhythmical stabilization with an oscillating pole (Fig. 4.48).
– Exercises passing a weighted ball from one hand to the other, throwing and receiving it. We progressively increase the weight (Fig. 4.49).

– *Prehensions*

We realize exercises to improve the types of prehensions the patient will need in his daily activities, work, and sports.

Orthotic Treatment

The orthotic treatment evolves along with the rehabilitation protocol.

– *Immobilization*

It can be a cast or made of resin, but we prefer using perforated thermoformable plastic (2,4 mm thick) to realize a non-removable orthosis.

We obtain a precise immobilization, eight times lighter than with resin, that can go in water (if there is no wound), radiolucent, and with perforations that allow the skin to "breathe."

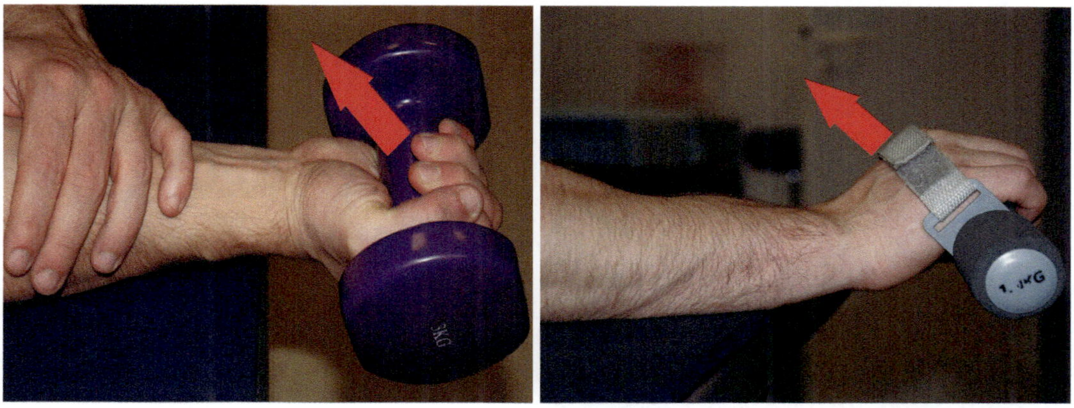

Fig. 4.42 Exercise for the flexors (1) and extensors (2) with weights. It allows alternating concentric, static, and eccentric contractions whose parameters evolve depending on the patient's progresses

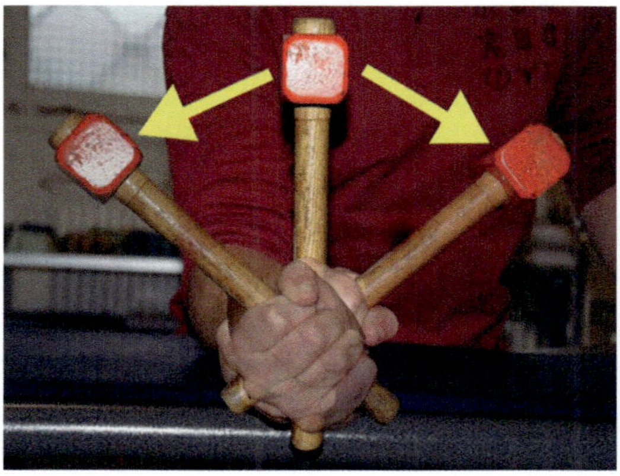

Fig. 4.43 Auxotonic exercise for the pronators and supinators

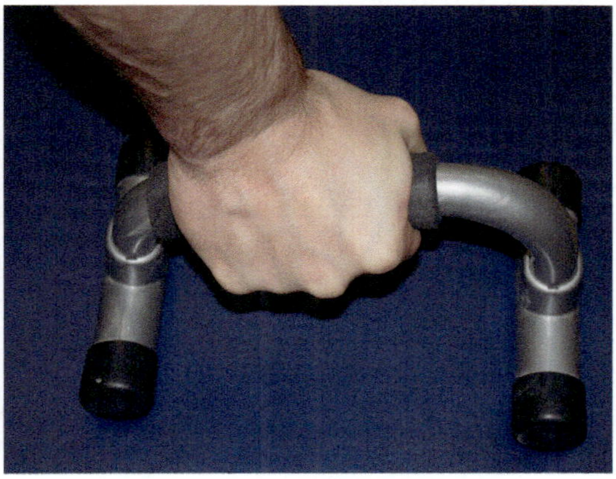

Fig. 4.45 Support exercise allowing working in a closed chain. Destabilizing maneuvers can be added to obtain an interesting proprioceptive exercise

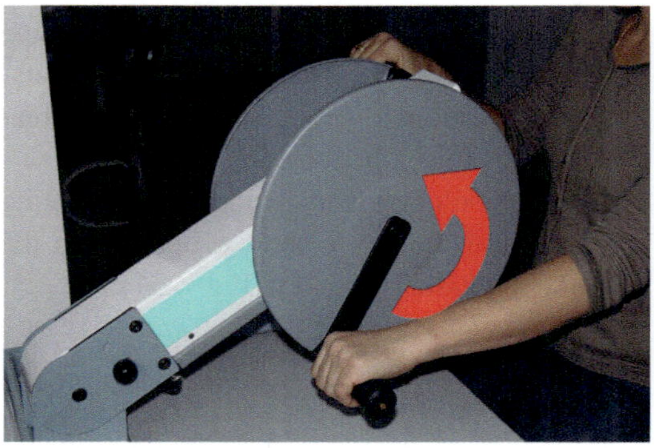

Fig. 4.44 Endurance exercise setting the resistance, speed and duration

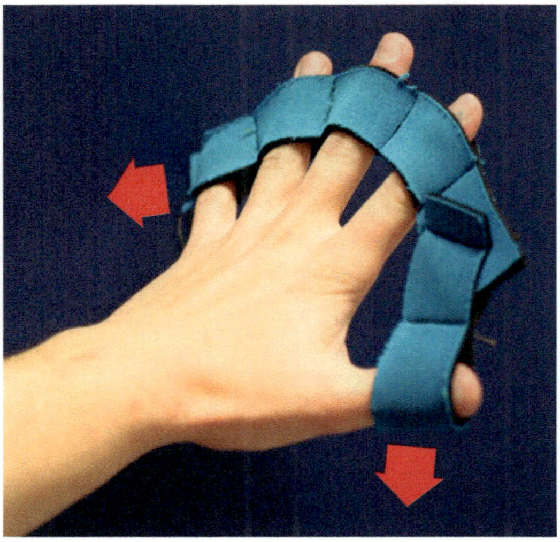

Fig. 4.46 Exercise for the digito-antebrachial chains

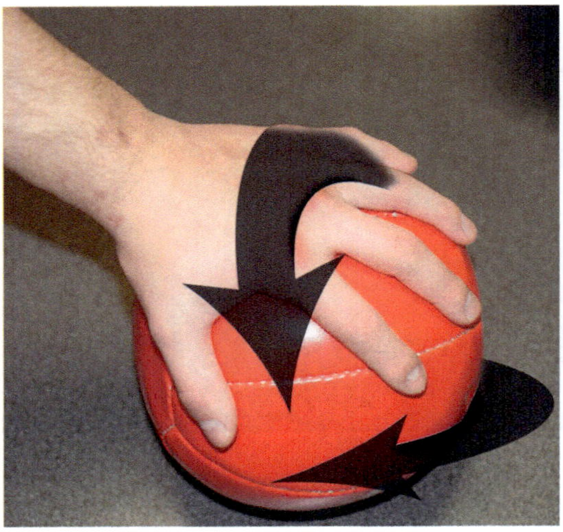

Fig. 4.47 Proprioceptive exercise pressing on a ball more or less inflated

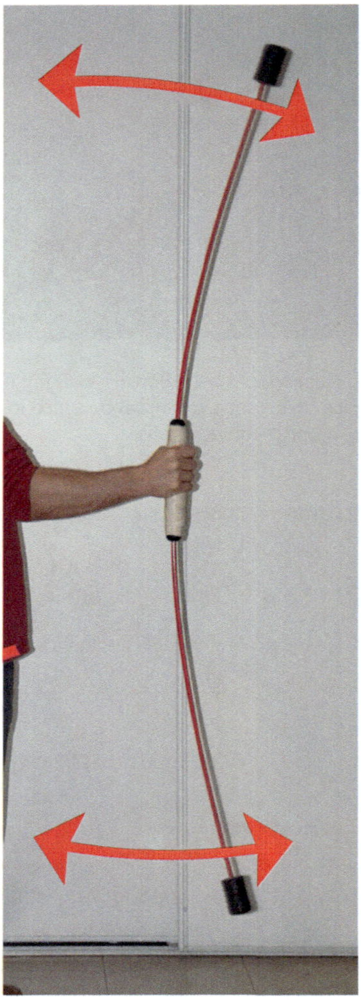

Fig. 4.48 Rhythmical stabilization exercise with an oscillating pole

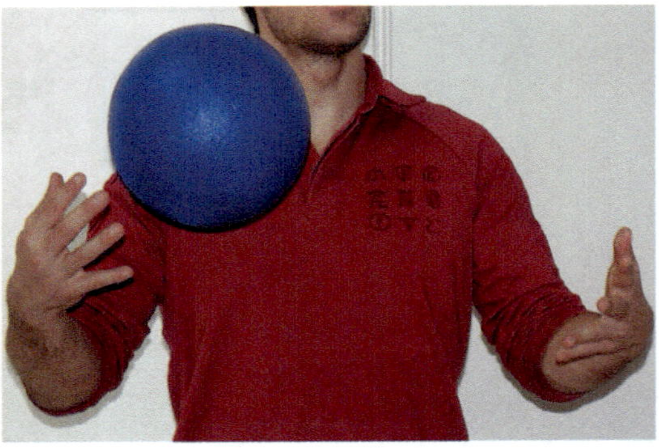

Fig. 4.49 Proprioceptive exercise with weighted balls, increasing the weight depending on the patient's progresses

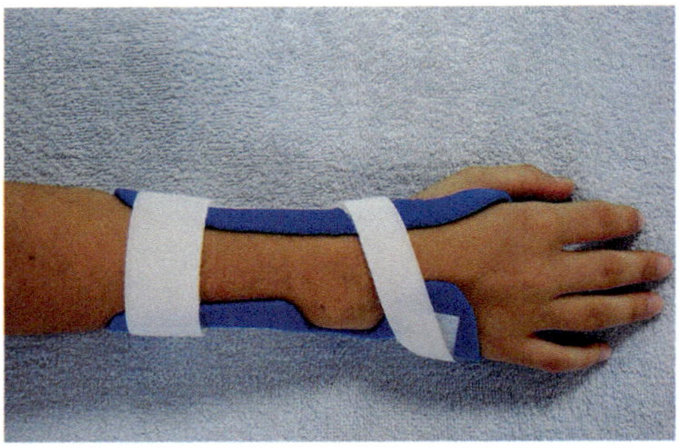

Fig. 4.50 Immobilization orthosis for the scaphoid. Some studies are questioning the interest of the thumb's immobilization

As described in the paragraph about immobilization, recent studies tend to demonstrate that letting the thumb free does not affect the healing process. Therefore, we realize orthoses leaving the thumb free, with the wrist straight in the sagittal plane, combined with a slight ulnar inclination in case of neck fracture (Fig. 4.50).

New technologies using scans and 3D printing can also offer quality orthoses, optimizing the patient's functional recovery (Fig. 4.51).

– *Pre-consolidation*

It is not done all the time, but a resting orthosis can be useful in case of nocturnal pain or in daily activities.

However, we make sure the patient gets progressively rid of the orthosis without impeding his functional evolution.

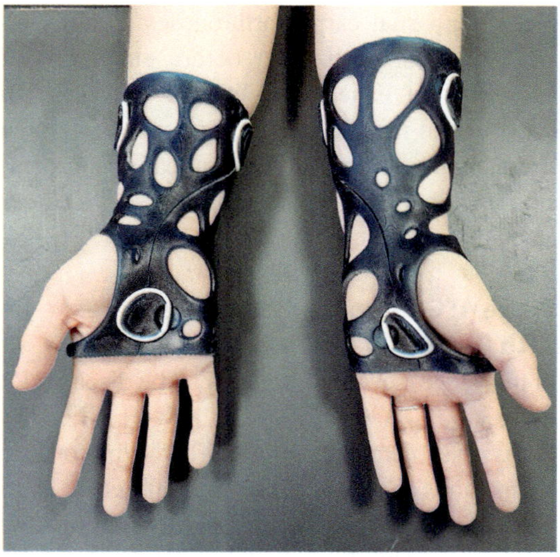

Fig. 4.51 Orthosis made with a 3D-printer and the Xkelet © technology

The orthosis lets the thumb free and maintains the wrist in a neutral position. The plastic is perforated, and its thickness depends on the patient's morphology.

– *Consolidation*

A neoprene orthosis can be made to go back to professional or sports activities. It protects the wrist from shocks, and has an interesting contention effect, useful at a proprioceptive level and in the patient's apprehension. It is most of the time a wrapped-on cuff and thermoformed plastic reinforcements can be added depending on the indications (Fig. 4.52).

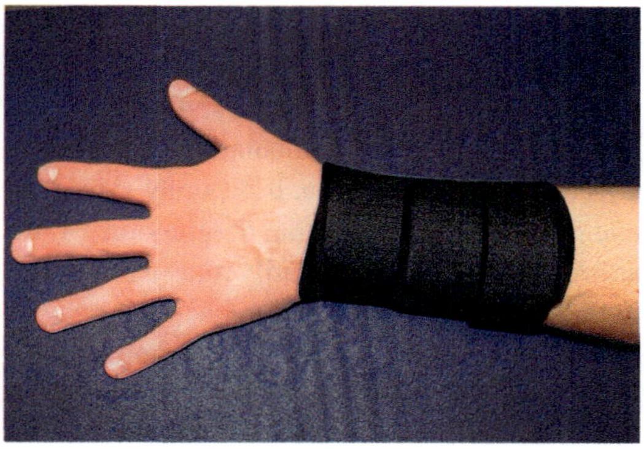

Fig. 4.52 Neoprene wrap-around cuff to restart sports and force activities. Plastic reinforcement can be added to increase the rigidity of the orthosis if needed

Complications

Other than the usual complications related to surgery and immobilization, pseudarthrosis is the main complication in scaphoid fractures (Waitayawinyu et al. 2010).

They are more frequent in case of insufficient initial treatment, displaced fractures, or fractures localized in the proximal part, which vascularization is precarious.

The treatment for pseudarthrosis is surgical, most often realizing a bone graft from the hip bone or the radial epiphysis (Pinder et al. 2015). The goal is to avoid the evolution toward a degenerative wrist. The rehabilitation after a graft uses the same principles as in simple fractures, modifying the durations depending on the case and the surgeon's indications.

In case of inadequate treatment (or no treatment at all), the wrist can evolve toward a degenerative wrist, or Scaphoid Nonunion Advanced Collapse (SNAC). The treatment is surgical, palliative, and identical to the one proposed in the case of Scapho-Lunate Advanced Collapse (SLAC) that happens after a mistreated or untreated scapholunate instability.

There are:

- SNAC wrists, described by Watson (Scaphoid Nonunion Advanced Collapse) and related to a scaphoid fracture poorly consolidated with arthrosis.
- SLAC wrists (Scapho-Lunate Advanced Collapse) are related to a scapholunate disjunction in its last stage of arthrosis.

Once the arthrosis is here, the etiological treatment (scaphoid graft in SNAC wrists and scapholunate ligamentoplasty in SLAC wrists) is no longer relevant: putting more stress on the arthrosic interline can increase the damage.

In SNAC and SLAC wrists, arthrosis appears because of the joint's lack of congruence.

The evolution over time is fairly stereotypical; we can describe four stages, each with its own therapeutical options.

Stage I: Isolated Radio-Styloid Arthrosis

In this stage, an arthroscopic styloidectomy is possible. It is a minimal ambulatory surgery, with a loco-regional anesthesia. It is purely symptomatic and will not stop the progression of the arthrosis, but it can temporarily relieve the patient with a simple surgery.

Then there are a few days of immobilization, and the rehabilitation can start.

Stage II: Complete Radio-Scaphoid Arthrosis

The solution of choice in this stage is a proximal row carpectomy (Richou et al. 2010). It is an ambulatory surgery, performed under loco-regional anesthesia, with a dorsal approach. The surgeon resects the three bones of the first carpal row, removing the painful micromovements in the radio-scaphoid interline. This surgery stops the arthrosic evolution: the capitate will now articulate with the radius' lunate facet.

After a 10-day period of immobilization, the rehabilitation can start. It usually lasts a few months, as strength takes time to recover. Early mobilization is essential for optimal results (Edouard et al. 2010). The patients recover functional mobilities. On the X-rays, the capitate's head changes to look like the lunate joint surface.

The resection of the scaphoid alone cannot be done as it can result in a Dorsal Intercalated Segment Instability (DISI).

Stage III: Stage II with Midcarpal (Capito-Lunate) Damage

A proximal row carpectomy cannot be done, so the surgeon will have to resect the scaphoid and perform a midcarpal arthrodesis. The movement will happen in the healthy radio-lunate interline.

The most described techniques are Watson's arthrodesis of the four internal bones (Traverso et al. 2017), and more recently the shortening arthrodesis of the three wrist bones (ARTOP) (Delattre et al. 2015) that improves the ulnar inclination by resecting the triquetrum. However, this last technique has a lower consolidation ratio.

Those partial carpus arthrodeses require 3–4 weeks of immobilization before starting with rehabilitation. The rehabilitation process also lasts several months, with a long work stoppage for manual workers. It can even lead to a professional reclassification or retraining, and a career change.

Stage 4: Generalized Arthrosis with Damaged Radio-Lunate Interline

In this stage, several options must be discussed:

- A wrist denervation is purely symptomatic and aims at cutting the painful afferences (Van de Pol et al. 2006). The surgery and follow-ups are simple but the result of pain is random.
- A total carpus arthrodesis with screwed plate or screwed iliac graft. The immobilization is long (between a month and a half and three months), with only pronosupination allowed. There is often residual pain, preventing the patient from going back to a manual job.
- A pyrocarbon implant (Amandys) (Bellemere 2018) is a recent solution (Bellemere et al. 2012). Rehabilitation follows a three-week immobilization. The outcome is often long to obtain, but the patient can keep some mobility. If this does not work, a total carpus arthrodesis is possible, but often difficult because of the loss of bone substance.

Fractures of Other Carpal Bones

Even though the scaphoid fractures are the most frequent carpal bones fractures, other bones are frequently broken (Garcia-Elias 2001; Auffray 1970; Snodgrass 1937) (Fig. 4.53), with specific risks and particularities that should be known by hand therapists.

Fractures of the Triquetrum

The most frequent fractures of the triquetrum are those of the posterior cortical (Fig. 4.54). There are two distinct mechanisms of injury:

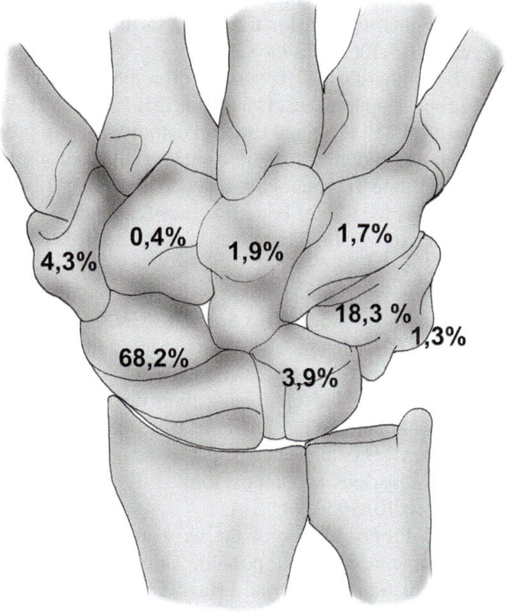

Fig. 4.53 Fractures frequency depending on the carpal bone (according to Garcia-Elias)

- One after a fall on the wrist in hyperextension, producing compressive constraints from the ulna on the triquetrum.
- The other is after a fall on the wrist in hyperflexion, tearing the dorsal radio-triquetral ligament.

In the case of a compressive traumatism, an immobilization in neutral wrist position allows bone healing. In case of injury of the dorsal radio-triquetral ligament, a palmo-dorsal press should be added on the pisiform to avoid the deformation of the first carpal row in supination, and let the ligament heal.

From a rehabilitation point of view, if the dorsal radio-triquetral ligament tears the dorsal cortical, the neuromuscular rehabilitation of the extensor carpi ulnaris will be preponderant as it produces an intracarpal pronation that protects the injured ligament.

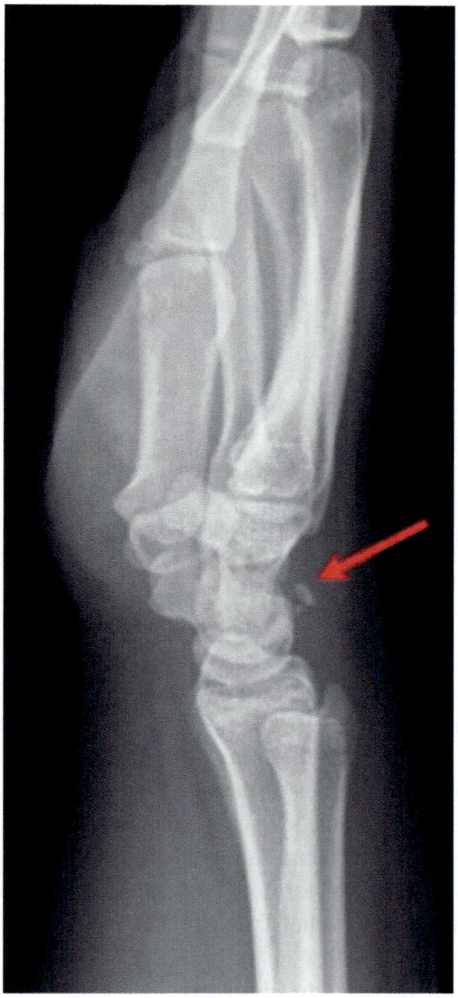

Fig. 4.54 Fracture of the posterior cortical of the triquetrum

Other Fractures

Fractures of the Trapezium

They are often related to mechanisms in compression localized on the insertion of the anterior retinacular ligament, or the body of the bone.

Fractures of the Hamate

They are mainly fractures of the hamate's hook. Their incidence is higher in. sports activities such

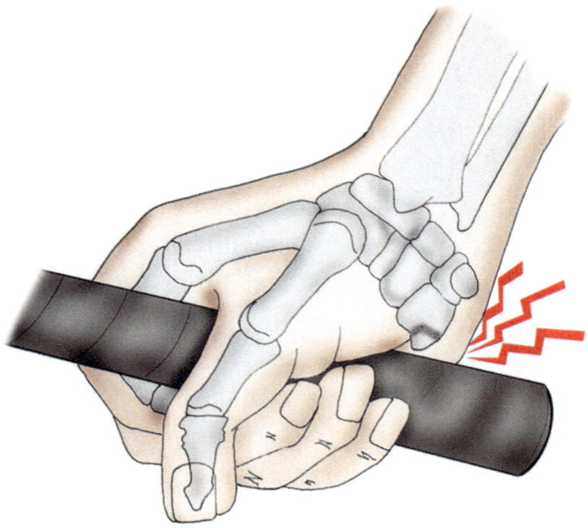

Fig. 4.55 Orientation of the racket handles or the golf clubs favoring a fracture of the hamate's hook

as bike, golf, or tennis: the handlebars or the racket handle come into contact with the hook and can cause its fracture due to repetitive constraints (Papp 2010; Sennwald 2004) (Fig. 4.55).

In this type of injury, we should check for combined injuries of the ulnar nerve as it passes near the hamate's hook and goes around it to innervate the ulnar lumbrical muscles, the interossei, the adductor pollicis, and the deep bundle of the flexor pollicis brevis.

Fractures of the Pisiform

They represent less than 2% of carpal fractures (Garcia-Elias 2001) but can cause arthrosis between the pisiform and the triquetrum if they are not treated correctly. This arthrosis will be treated by excision of the pisiform.

Bibliography

Adams JE, Steinmann SP. Acute scaphoid fractures. Hand Clin. 2010;26(1):97–103.

Auffray Y. Les fractures du pyramidal. Acta Orthop Belg. 1970;36:313–45.

Bellemere P. Pyrocarbon implants for the hand and wrist. Hand Surg Rehabil. 2018;37(3):129–54.

Bellemere P, et al. Amandys((R)) implant: no- vel pyrocarbon arthroplasty for the wrist. Chir Main. 2012;31(4):176–87.

Clay N, et al. Need the thumb be immobilised in scaphoid fractures ? J Bone Joint Surg. 1991;73-B(5):828–32.

Delattre O, et al. Three-corner arthrodesis with scaphoid and triquetrum excision for wrist arthritis. J Hand Surg Am. 2015;40(11):2176–82.

Dias J, Kantharuban S. Treatment of scaphoid fractures: European approaches. Hand Clin. 2017;33(3):501–9.

Edouard P, et al. Proximal row carpectomy: is early post-operative mobilisation the right rehabilitation protocol? Orthop Traumatol Surg Res. 2010;96(5):513–20.

Garcia-Elias M. Carpal bone fractures (excluding scaphoid fractures). In: The wrist, W.H. Weinberg, Editor. 2001. p. 174–181.

Garcia-Elias M. Understanding wrist mechanics: a long and winding road. J Wrist Surg. 2013;2(1):5–12.

Gelberman RH, Menon J. The vascularity of the scaphoid bone. J Hand Surg. 1980;5A(5):508–13.

Geoffroy C, Mesplié G. Rééducation des ins- tabilités scapho-lunaires. Kinésithérapie, la Revue. 2018;18:29.

Giugale JM, et al. The palpable scaphoid surface area in various wrist positions. J Hand Surg Am. 2015;40(10):2039–44.

Hagert E. Proprioception of the wrist joint: a review of current concepts and possible implications on the rehabilitation of the wrist. J Hand Ther. 2010;23(1):2–16. quiz 17

Herbert T. The fractured scaphoid. St. Louis (MO): Quality Medical Publishing; 1990.

Herbert T, Fisher W. Management of the fractured scaphoid using a new bone screw. J Bone Joint Surg. 1984;66-B(1):114–23.

Ibrahim T, et al. Surgical versus nonsurgical treatment of acute minimally displaced and undisplaced scaphoid waist fractures: pairwise and network meta-analyses of randomized controlled trials. J Hand Surg Am. 2011;36(11):1759–1768 e1.

Karagiannopoulos C, et al. Responsiveness of the active wrist joint position sense test after distal radius fracture intervention. J Hand Ther. 2016;29(4):474–82.

Ledoux P. Ostéosynthèse percutanée du sca- phoïde par vis de Herbert. Acta Belgica Orthop. 1995;61:43–7.

Lephart S, et al. The role of proprioception in the management and rehabilitation of athletic injuries. Am J Sports Med. 1997;25:130–7.

Marcuzzi A, Ozben H, Russomando A. The use of a pyrocarbon capitate resurfacing implant in chronic wrist disorders. J Hand Surg Eur. 2014;39(6):611–8.

Mathoulin C. Arthroscopie du poignet : Techniques. Sauramps Medical; 2014.

Papp S. Carpal bone fractures. Hand Clin. 2010;26(1):119–27.

Pinder RM, et al. Treatment of scaphoid nonunion: a systematic review of the existing evidence. J Hand Surg Am. 2015;40(9):1797–1805 e3.

Richou J, et al. Proximal row carpectomy: long-term results. Chir Main. 2010;29(1):10–5.

Roll R, et al. Illusory movements prevent cortical disruption caused by immobilization. NeuroImage. 2012;62(1):510–9.

Sabbagh MD, Morsy M, Moran SL. Diagnosis and management of acute scaphoid fractures. Hand Clin. 2019;35(3):259–69.

Savornin C, Esling F, N'Guyen L. Pseudarthrose du scaphoïde carpien : résultat de la stabilisation par "agrafe anatomique". À propos de 60 cas. Journal de traumatologie du sport. 2000;896(3).

Schernberg F. Fractures récentes du scaphoïde (moins de trois semaines). Chir Main. 2005;24(3–4):117–31.

Schernberg F, Harisboure A, Gaston E. Fractures des os du carpe. EMC - Appareil locomo- teur. 2000:14–46.

Segalman KA, Graham TJ. Scaphoid proximal pole fractures and nonunions. J Am Soc Surg Hand. 2004;4(4):233–49.

Sennwald G. Carpal bone fractures other than the scaphoid. In: Berger RA, Weiss AP, editors. Hand surgery. Philadelphia: Lippincott Williams & Wilkins; 2004. p. 418.

Slutsky DJ, Trevare J. Use of arthroscopy for the treatment oj scaphoid fractures. Hand Clin. 2014;30:90–103.

Snodgrass L. Fractures of the carpal bones. Am J Surg. 1937;38:539–48.

Traverso P, et al. Ten-year minimum follow-up of 4-corner fusion for SLAC and SNAC wrist. Hand (N Y). 2017;12(6):568–72.

Van de Pol GJ, et al. Innervation of the wrist joint and surgical perspectives of denervation. J Hand Surg Am. 2006;31(1):28–34.

Waitayawinyu T, et al. Management of scaphoid nonunions. Hand Clin. 2010;26(1):105–17.

Weber E. Biomechanical implications of scaphoid waist fractures. Clin Orthop. 1980;149:83–9.

Wolfe SW. Scapholunate instability. J Am Soc Surg Hand. 2001;1(1):45–60.

Young DK, Giachino A. Clinical examination of scaphoid fractures. Phys Sportsmed. 2009;37(1):97–105.

5 Carpal Instabilities

Grégory Mesplié

Wrist traumas are frequent and can cause carpal instability, resulting in disturbed sports and work activities. It can also lead to a degenerative wrist if the injury is mistreated (Garcia-Elias 2011) (see Chap. 4).

Treating these injuries requires a good knowledge of the elements involved, as well as their precise role in carpal stability.

Carpal instabilities can be divided into several categories depending on their chronicity, etiology, location, and direction.

The dissociative instabilities correspond to a disturbed cohesion between the bones of the first carpal row.

Radiologically speaking, when the lunate tilts in flexion, there is a Ventral Intercalated Segment Instability (VISI). This instability corresponds to an injury of the lunotriquetral ligament that no longer ensures the link between the lunate and the triquetrum. The lunate follows the scaphoid and tilts in flexion (Fig. 5.1) (see Chap. 1).

When the lunate tilts in extension, there is a Dorsal Intercalated Segment Instability (DISI) that corresponds to an injury of the scapholunate ligament. The lunate follows the triquetrum and tilts in extension (Fig. 5.2).

Non-dissociative instabilities correspond to a disturbed cohesion between the two carpal rows, without any modification of their intrinsic stability.

There are several non-dissociative instabilities: palmar, dorsal, complex, and adaptive. The palmar ones are the most frequent in sport traumatology. They correspond to a palmar subluxation of the midcarpal joint, with a combined radiological VISI as the first carpal row tilts in flexion.

Dorsal non-dissociative instabilities correspond to a dorsal subluxation of the midcarpal joint with a radiological DISI caused by the tilt in extension of the first carpal row.

Combined or complex non-dissociative instabilities correspond to a palmar collapse of the carpus, that can be seen with a visual inspection. It can look like a palmar non-dissociative instability, but the dorsal instability tests are also positive, with a dorsal subluxation visible with video fluoroscopy.

Adaptive instabilities are the only non-dissociative instabilities corresponding to a carpal instability caused by abnormal extrinsic factors (radial vicious callus, for example).

G. Mesplié (✉)
ISAMMS, Biarritz, France

G. Mesplié (ed.), *Wrist Functional Anatomy and Therapy*,
https://doi.org/10.1007/978-3-031-42879-1_5

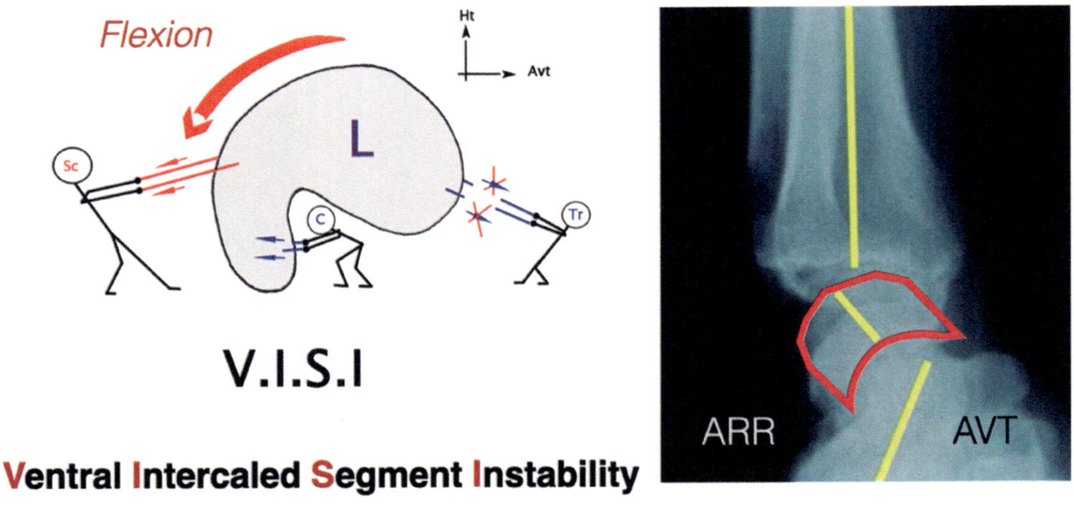

Fig. 5.1 VISI deformation (the lunate tilts in flexion)

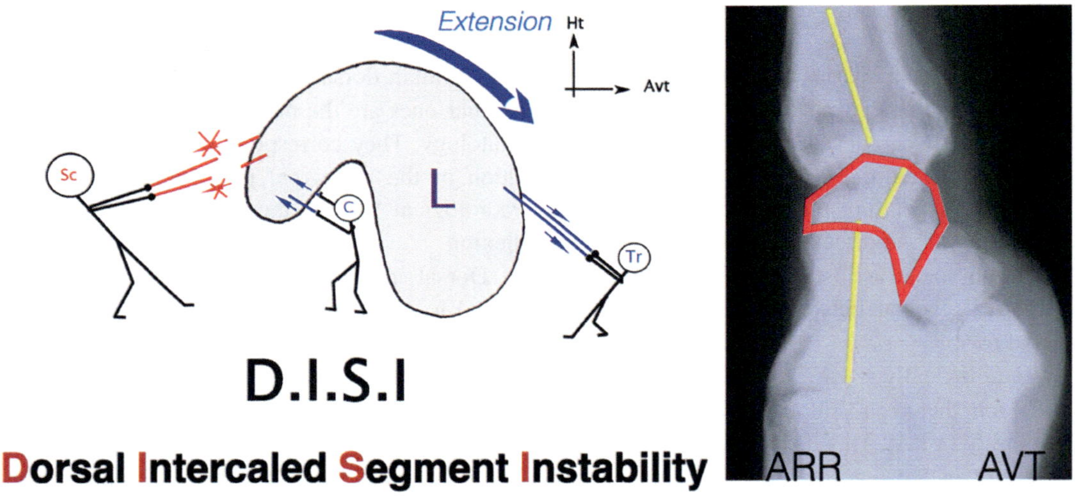

Fig. 5.2 DISI deformation (the lunate tilts in extension)

Dissociative Instabilities

Scapholunate Instabilities

Injuries of the scapholunate ligament are the most frequent intracarpal ligamentous injuries.

They lead to instability in the carpus, evolving toward a Scapho Lunate Advanced Collapse (SLAC) wrist.

Physiopathology

The injury mechanism is related to trauma in hyperextension/radial inclination, most often because of a fall on the thenar eminence.

In these conditions, the scaphoid is under two opposite constraints, toward the extension because of the wrist extension and toward the flexion because of the combined radial inclination (Fig. 5.3).

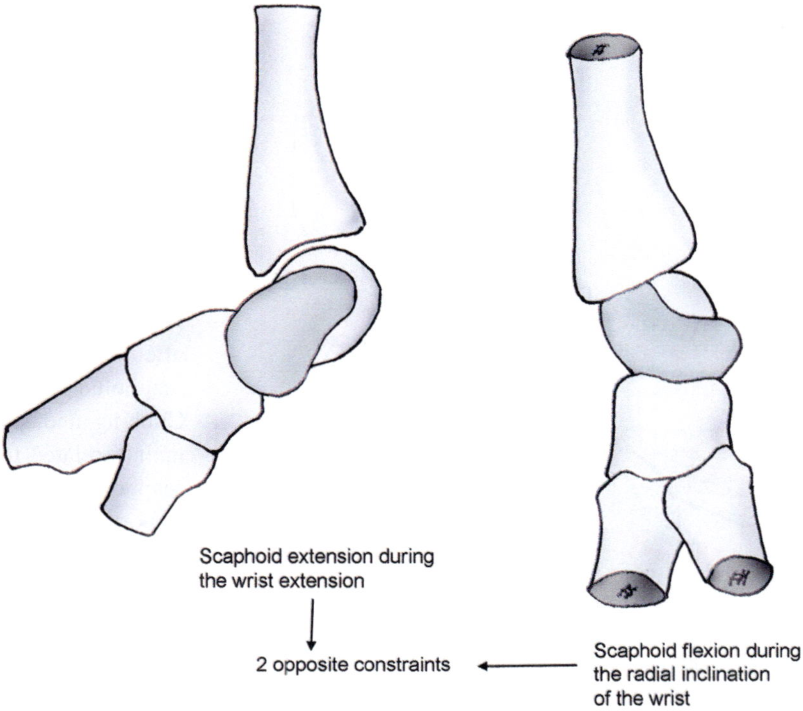

Fig. 5.3 A combination of wrist extension and radial inclination leads to opposed constraints on the scaphoid

The posterior part of the radius presses on the scaphoid that then transmits important constraints on the scapholunate ligament. This ligament opposes the palmar displacement of the scaphoid's proximal part (Fig. 5.4).

The first carpal row is like a "mobile meniscus" that absorbs axial constraints as long as it forms a coherent set (Fig. 5.5).

When the scapholunate ligament breaks, the first carpal row is disunited and the whole carpal stability is compromised:

- The scaphoid goes to flexion because of longitudinal constraints.
- The lunate goes to extension because of the triquetrum (Dorsal Intercalated Segment Instability).
- The scapholunate space increases, creating a scapholunate diastasis (Fig. 5.6).

However, these evolutions of the carpal architecture only appear if the essential extrinsic systems do not play their part anymore (Raja et al. 2022; Short et al. 2005).

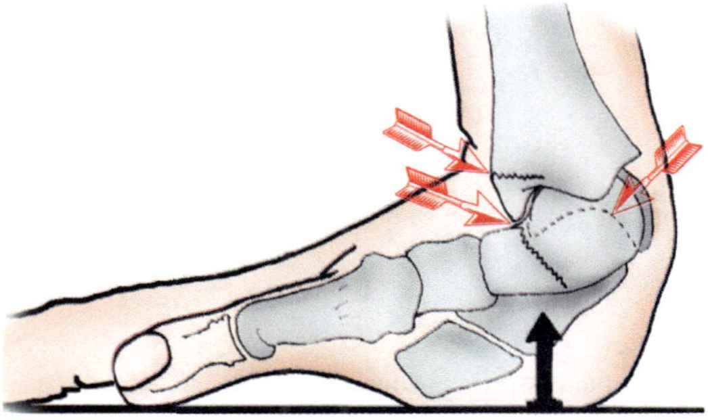

Fig. 5.4 The extension and radial inclination of the injury mechanism put constraints on the radius, the scaphoid, and the scapholunate ligament. In this mechanism, the scapholunate ligament forbids the proximal part of the scaphoid from going to palmar

Therefore, a DISI will be associated with an injury or secondary slacking of the dorsal intercarpal and long radio-lunate ligaments (Fig. 5.7).

The biomechanical changes in the wrist after this type of injury lead to degenerative phenomena, even if it is difficult to predict when they are going to appear.

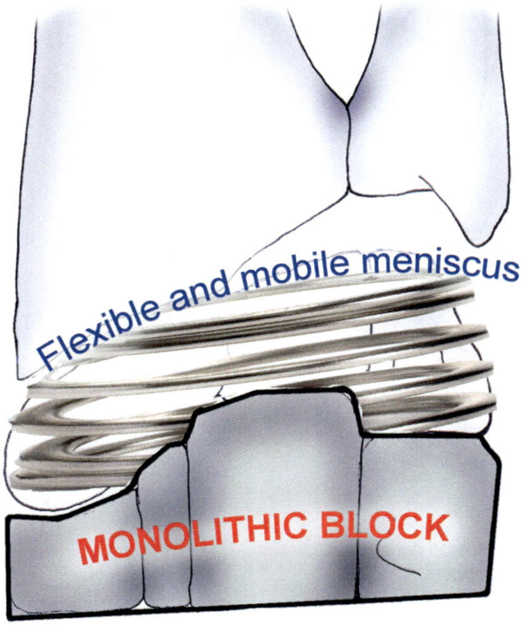

Fig. 5.5 The first carpal row plays the role of a "flexible and mobile meniscus" that absorbs the longitudinal constraints from the carpus

Clinical and Paraclinical Signs

An early diagnosis is a crucial factor for the patient's recovery as surgery is more difficult with an old injury.

- *Clinical signs*

  The clinical exam allows finding several elements that, unfortunately, are not specific to injuries of the scapholunate ligament:
  - Pain on the radial side of the wrist, most often with intense pain when palpating the scapholunate interline (Fig. 5.8).
  - Clicking and snapping when mobilizing, mainly related to the disconnection of the scaphoid and lunate.
  - Important strength loss.
  - Mobility loss (later).

  There also exist some clinical tests that can help the assessment:

- *Scapholunate instability test*

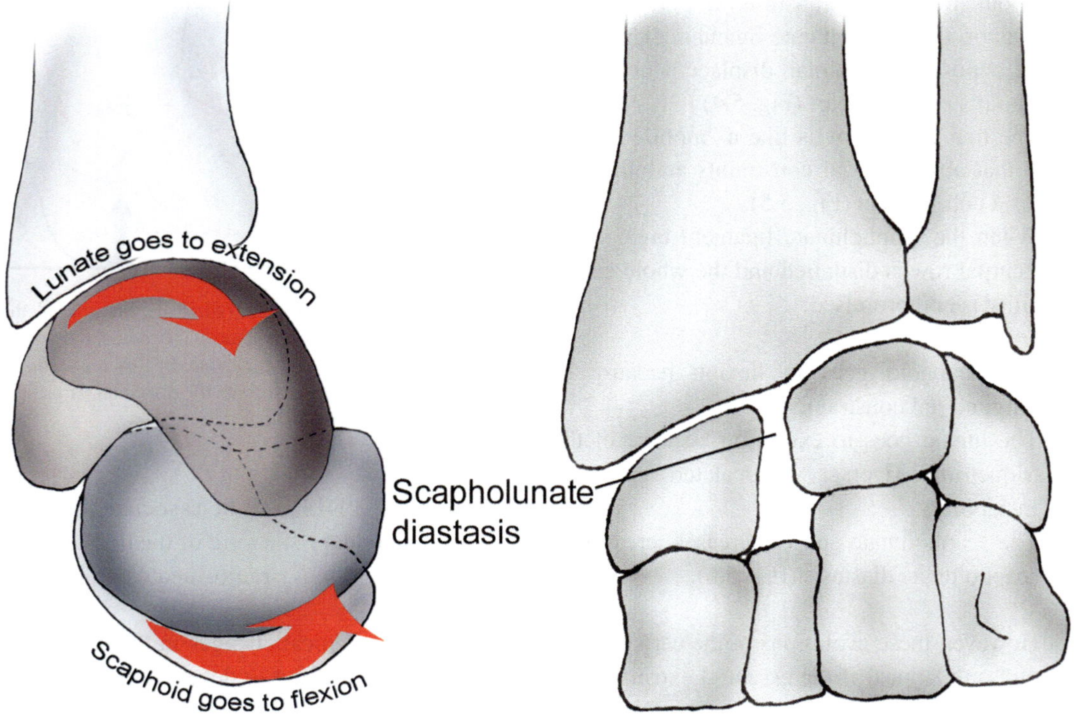

Fig. 5.6 The rupture of the scapholunate ligament results in the scaphoid tilting in flexion, the lunate/triquetrum tilting in extension, and in a scapholunate diastasis

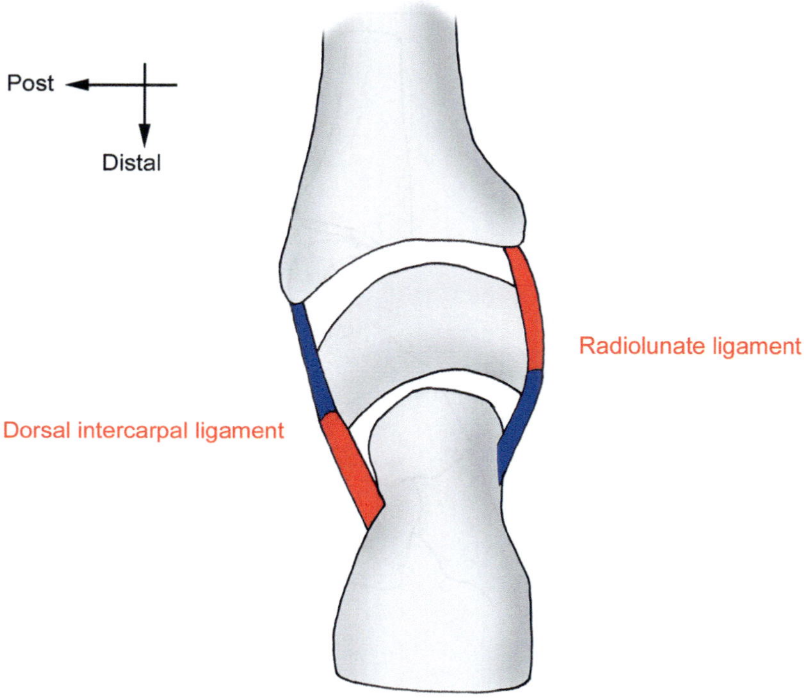

Fig. 5.7 Extrinsic ligaments allowing the DISI to happen if they do not perform their function

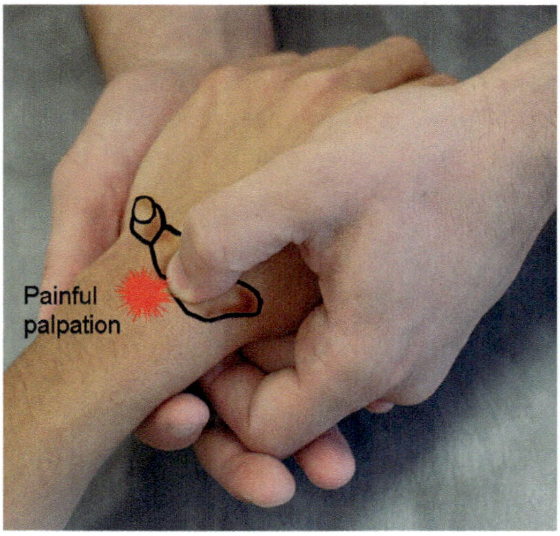

Fig. 5.8 Palpation of the scapholunate interline

It consists in applying opposite glidings on the scaphoid and the lunate. Pain or abnormal movements guide the therapist toward an injury of the scapholunate ligament (Fig. 5.9).

– *Evaluation of the scaphoid dynamic (bell sign)*

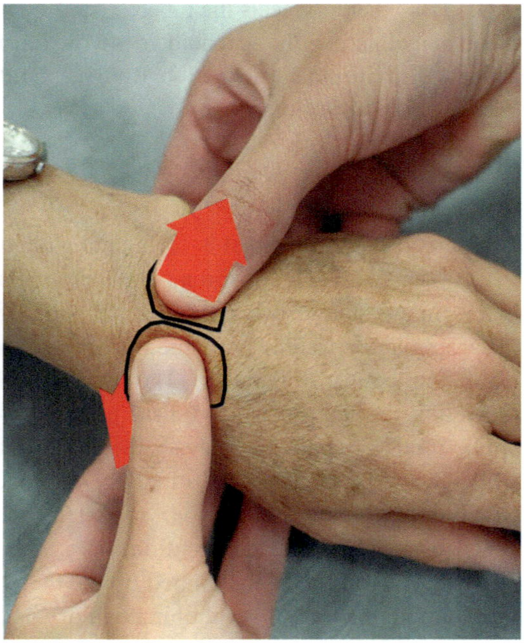

Fig. 5.9 Scapholunate instability test

It consists of assessing the scaphoid's mobility with the wrist in radial and ulnar inclination. The therapist places his thumb at the level of the

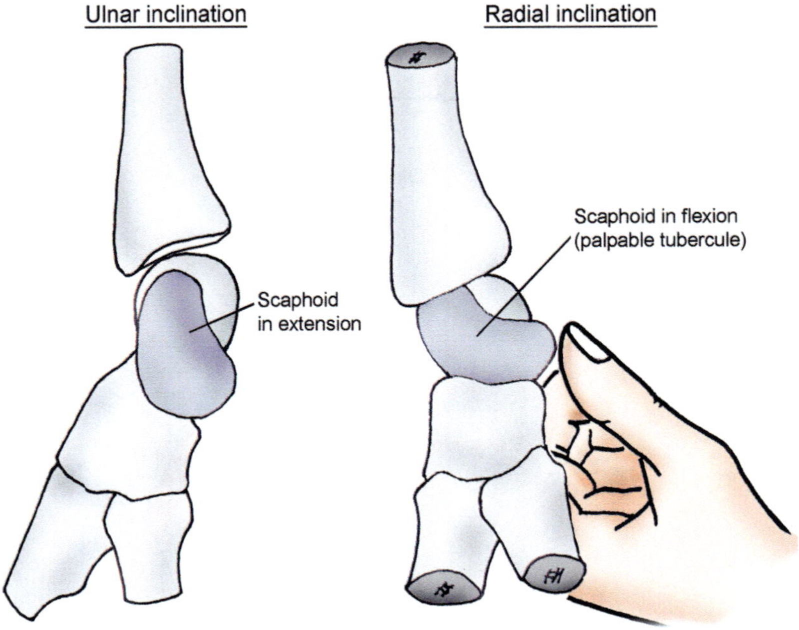

Fig. 5.10 Evaluation of the scaphoid dynamic

scaphoid's tubercle and applies radial and ulnar inclinations in the wrist. If the scaphoid dynamic is good, the therapist feels the tubercle sticks out in radial inclination (the scaphoid goes to flexion) and goes in in ulnar inclination (the scaphoid goes to extension) (Fig. 5.10).

– *Watson's test (scaphoid shear test)*

In this test, the therapist is facing the patient in an "arm wrestling" position. The therapist's index fingers are placed on the dorsal side of the scaphoid's proximal part, and his/her thumb is on the palmar tuberosity. The other hand maintains the metacarpals. A firm pressure is applied on the palmar side of the scaphoid while the wrist is placed in ulnar inclination, which makes the scaphoid go to extension. When passing in radial inclination, the scaphoid cannot flex as it is maintained by the therapist's thumb. In case of scapholunate injury and in patients with great laxity, the scaphoid tends to go backward under the posterior part of the radius, and therefore contacts with the therapist's index which revives pain. Pain can be present on its own or be associated with snapping. When pressure is released, the scaphoid gets back to its normal position, sometimes with an audible "thunck." In some cases, the lack of mobility in comparison to the sane side can express an oedematous and synovial reaction. To avoid false positives that are still too frequent, we must first put pressure on the posterior side of the scaphoid and see if there is spontaneous pain.

• *Paraclinical signs*

After a complete clinical exam, these signs will confirm or reject the injury of the scapholunate ligament, and its stage.

– *X-ray*

• *Static*

Frontal X-rays assess:
  - The scapholunate diastasis (or gap), greater than 3 mm in case of injury.
  - The ring-sign that means the scaphoid tilts in flexion.
  - The carpal height that can be reduced as the scaphoid tilt in flexion and the lunate tilt in extension decrease their working distance.

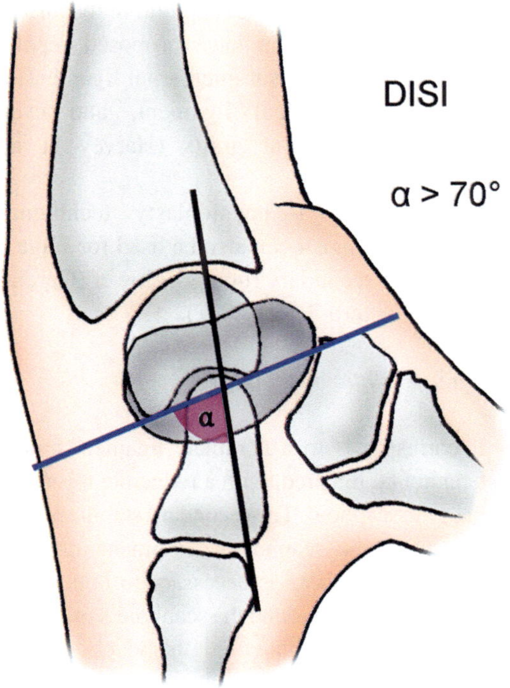

Fig. 5.11 Scapholunate angle superior to 70° that shows an injury of the scapholunate ligament

Lateral X-rays assess:

- The scapholunate angle is normally lower than 70° (Fig. 5.11).
- The displacement of the lunate in extension or DISI (Dorsal Intercalated Segment Instability).

• *Fist closed*

The patient clutches his/her fingers with the maximal intensity, which makes the capitate go toward the scapholunate space. If the scapholunate ligament is ineffective, it creates a diastasis between the scaphoid and the lunate (Fig. 5.12).

• *Dynamic*

Dynamic X-rays in flexoextension and inclinations of the wrist highlight injuries of the scapholunate ligament with rupture of the Gilula's lines, which don't appear on static X-rays. We talk about dynamic scapholunate instability.

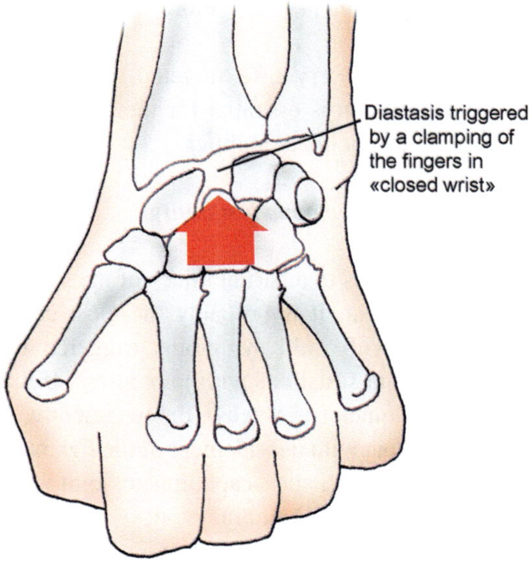

Fig. 5.12 An X-ray of the clamping hand can show a scapholunate diastasis

- *Arthrogram*

  It is a preferred technique that highlights chondral and ligamentous damage to the carpus. However, there are false negatives (ligamentous perforation filled with scar tissue) and false positives (gap without instability, degenerative injury), and localization is often difficult. Therefore, arthroscopy stays important.
- *Arthroscopy*

  It is essential and allows to precisely evaluate the state of the ligamentous and cartilaginous injuries of the carpus.
- *Other exams*

  The arthro-MRI obtains a diagnosis comparable to the arthrogram, but its price and availability are important disadvantages.

The MRI results in this area are subject to controversy.

Therapeutical Process and Surgical Treatment

The therapeutic process and surgical treatment will depend on the injury stages described by Marc Garcia-Elias (Garcia-Elias et al. 2006). The arthroscopy helps us treat these injuries efficiently from the early stages, and the importance of conservative treatment is more and more questioned.

However, in every case, targeted proprioceptive rehabilitation is essential for the patients to recover their functional abilities.

- *Stage 1 (pre-dynamic instability)*

It corresponds to a partial injury of the scapholunate ligament. It is probably the most common stage, with mild symptoms triggered by maneuvers and situations with joint stress. If the diagnosis is quick (<6 weeks), the treatment will be arthroscopic with debridement of the ligament and a pin through the scapholunate joint, followed by a 6-week immobilization.

An older instability, often combined with an injury of the Dorsal Capsulo-Scapholunate Septum (DCSS) (Overstraeten et al. 2013), can be treated by repairing the DCSS. This can be enough to recover good carpal stability, probably because the dorsal intercarpal ligament is pressed against the lunate and the scaphoid, stabilizing them (Raja et al. 2022). Immobilization after a repair of the DCSS alone can be shortened to 3 weeks, but it seems very interesting to do an adapted proprioceptive rehabilitation before the surgery (Garcia-Elias and Cantero-Tellez 2021).

- *Stage 2 (pre-dynamic or dynamic instability)*

It corresponds to a complete but fixable ligament injury. In these cases, the direct repair of the ligament followed by putting a pin through the scapholunate joint is the recommended treatment in the absence of bone avulsion.

If there is a bone avulsion, open surgery will be inevitable, with a ligament reinsertion followed by putting a pin through the scapholunate joint. This surgery can be combined with a dorsal capsulodesis in some cases.

- *Stage 3 (dynamic instability)*

It corresponds to a complete ligament injury, that cannot be repaired, but with the scaphoid well-aligned. The secondary stabilizers (dorsal intercarpal ligament, DCSS, long radio-lunar ligament, scapho-trapezio-trapezoidal ligaments) are enough to maintain the scaphoid in its normal position. Some authors have proposed repairs from pieces of the dorsal intercarpal ligament or the dorsal radiocarpal ligament, and even ligament-bone-ligament grafts (Harvey et al. 2007).

However, the ligamentoplasty techniques described for stage 4 can also be used for stage 3 as the risk of secondary rupture is lower (Garcia-Elias and Cantero-Tellez 2021).

- *Stage 4 (static instability)*

It corresponds to a complete ligament injury, that cannot be repaired, with a reducible misalignment of the scaphoid. The secondary stabilizes cannot maintain the scaphoid's alignment anymore and a ligamentoplasty is necessary to oppose the scapholunate diastasis and the scaphoid's misalignment. Two techniques are used: the Scapho-Lunate and dorsal Inter-Carpal ligamentoplasty (SLIC) (Athlani et al. 2017; Athlani et al. 2018) (Fig. 5.13) and the "three ligaments" tenodesis (Garcia-Elias et al. 2006; Athlani et al. 2018) (Fig. 5.14).

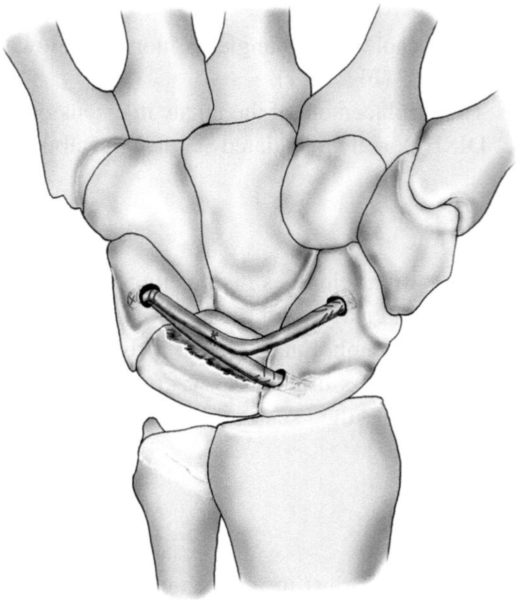

Fig. 5.13 The "SLIC" ligamentoplasty uses the palmaris longus and has two segments: a scapho-luno-triquetral correcting the scapholunate diastasis, and a triquetro-luno-scaphoid correcting the DISI and the scaphoid's tilt in flexion/pronation

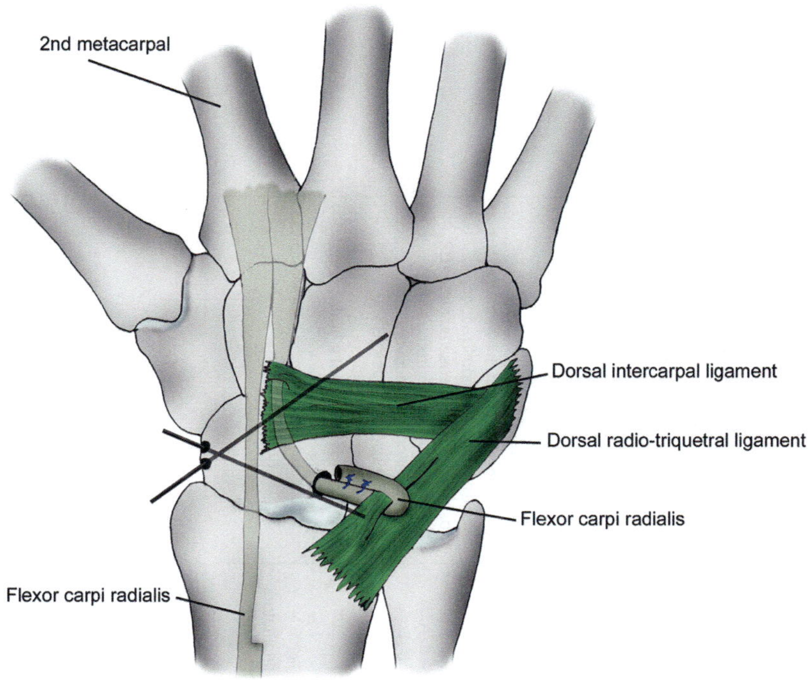

Fig. 5.14 The "three ligaments" tenodesis uses part of the flexor carpi radialis that passes through a trans-osseous tunnel in the scaphoid, crossing the scapholunate joint to tie the dorsal radio-triquetral ligament before being sutured on itself

- *Stage 5 (complete ligament rupture)*

It corresponds to a complete rupture, that cannot be repaired, with the scaphoid misaligned (normal cartilage). The areas around the scaphoid are fibrosed but the cartilage is not injured yet (especially the proximal part of the scaphoid).

These injuries are treated with an arthrodesis, most often at the scapho-trapezo-trapezoid level. There can also be a scapholunate or scapho-capitate arthrodesis (Garcia-Elias and Cantero-Tellez 2021).

- *Stage 6 (degenerative wrist or SLAC wrist)*

It corresponds to a SLAC wrist when it occurs after a scapholunate injury that has been poorly or not treated. Its treatments and specific rehabilitation are described in Chap. 4.

Rehabilitation and Orthotic Treatment

The rehabilitation of scapholunate injuries must allow regaining a good wrist stability and avoiding evolution toward a SLAC wrist.

Immobilization can last between 45 and 60 days depending on the surgery, except for the arthroscopic repair of the DCSS alone where the recommended immobilization duration is 3 weeks.

- *Rehabilitation protocol* (Fig. 5.15)

– *Immobilization phase (D0-D45/60)*

As in other wrist injuries, rehabilitation is not essential in this phase. Self-rehabilitation advice is given to the patient.

The treatment is based on the protocol PRICE that fights against trophic disorders resulting from trauma and surgery:

- P for protection of the fracture line during the whole phase, realized immobilizing the wrist and informing the patient about the tissue fragility in this phase.
- R for rest of the damaged area that must not be solicited during the immobilization phase, aside from self-rehabilitation exercises explained by the therapist.
- I for ice, put cold packs several times a day on the fracture zone. If there is a cast it is impossible, but if there is no wound we immobilize the patient with a thermoformed orthosis, which allows a cold bath against oedema.

DISSOCIATIVE INSTABILITIES (WITH SURGERY)			
	Post-surgery (A)	**Relative fragility (B)**	**Solidity (C)**
REHABILITATION	**Goals:** 1 – To reduce trophic disorders 2 – To reduce pain 3 – To prevent the risk of stiffness in the free joints 4 – To maintain the proprioceptive abilities **Techniques:** 1 – Draining massages and compressive bandage, vacuum therapy for draining, low-frequency electrical currents 2 – Cryotherapy, TENS, TVS (100Hz) 3 – Mobilization of the free joints in passive and active (fingers +++) 4 – TVS (70-80Hz) and varied sensitive stimulation without constraints **Risks:** Bad healing in case of non-observance	**Goals:** 1 – Same as in phase A with intensified techniques if necessary 2 – To recover joint mobility (except flexion if capsulodesis) 3 – To gradually recover the protective muscles' proprioceptive abilities **Techniques:** 1 – Pressotherapy for draining, vacuum therapy on the scar, defibrosing massage if the scar is not inflammatory and closed (A1), manipulation of light objects (A4) 2 – Soft mobilizations (instrumental and manual) 3 – Gradual conscious proprioceptive work, then conscious neuromuscular rehabilitation for the carpal supinators (if SL ligament) and the ECU (if lunotriquetral ligament), **NO EXERCISE FOR THE "HARMFUL" MUSCLES, no exercise in the harmful pronosupination position (depending on the ligament), NOBALL CLENCHING** **Risks:** Same as phase A	**Goals:** 1 – Same as in phases A and B with intensified techniques if necessary 2 – Total functional recovery **Techniques:** 1 – Intensification of the mobilizations with specific joint mobilizations, postures, and electrostimulation (B2) 2 – Unconscious neuromuscular rehabilitation and recovery of normal muscular ratios (B3) 3 – Functional activities adapted to the patient's professional and sports needs **Risks:** Same as in phases A and B
ORTHOSES	Orthosis realized in the protective pronosupination position: - Strict immobilization (limiting the rehabilitation options) - Removable orthosis	Gradual removal	Functional orthosis for resumption of activity
	D3 to D45/60	**D45/60 to D90**	**After D90**

Fig. 5.15 Rehabilitation protocol (1) and progression pyramid (2)

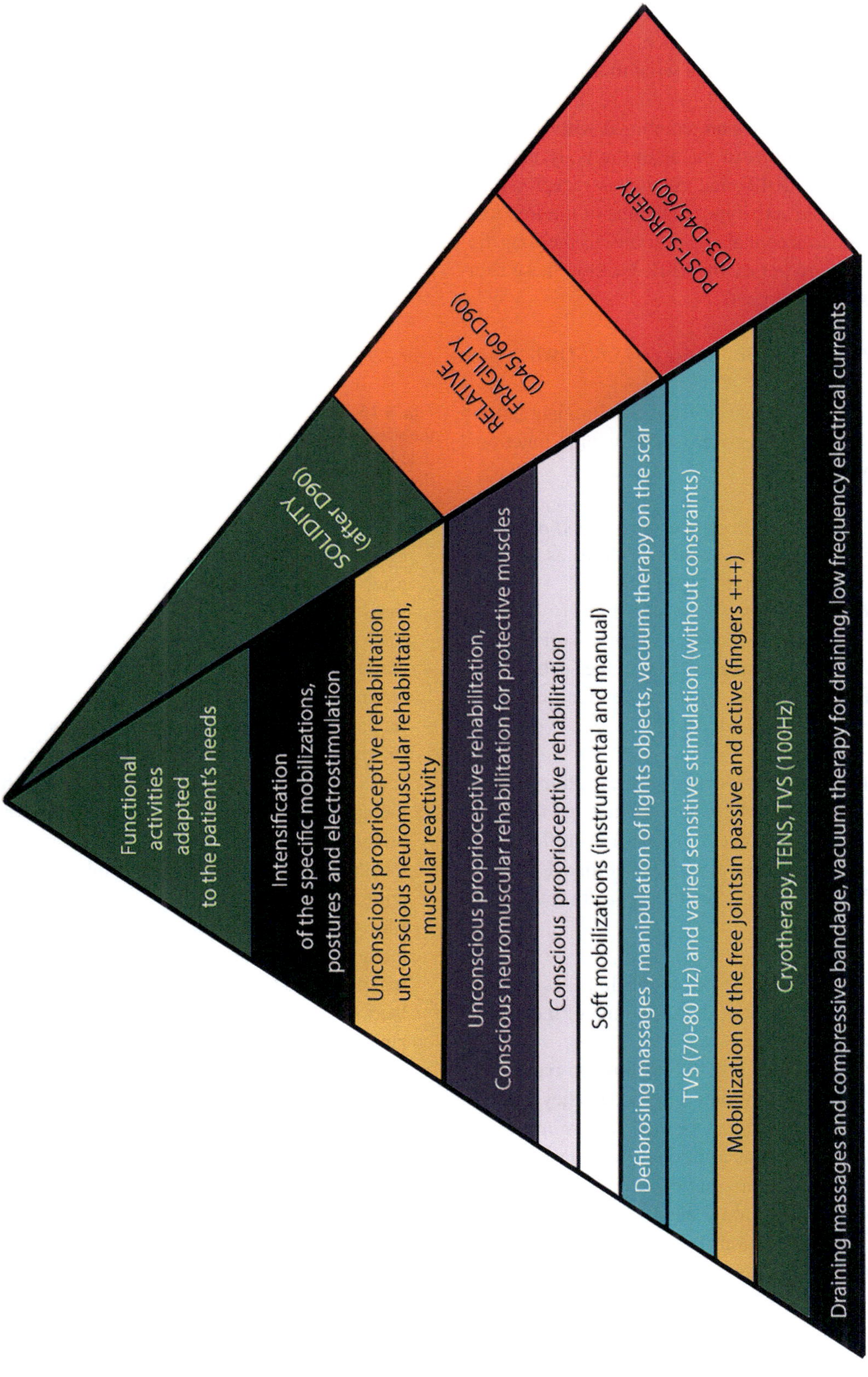

Fig. 5.15 (continued)

- C for compression that can be realized in the fingers if they are swollen.
- E for elevation of the wrist to avoid oedema.

These exercises are combined with sensorimotor stimulations to maintain the body mapping (Roll et al. 2012) and cutaneous receptors, and with simple active mobilizations of the free joint (the metacarpophalangeal joints in the long fingers tend to get easily stiff). We stop these exercises if pain appears.

- *Relative fragility phase (D45/60-D90)*

The goal in that phase is to eliminate pain in the wrist and recover stability and functional mobility.

- *Fight against trophic disorders and pain*
  We apply the same modalities as for other traumatic injuries of the wrist.
- *Recovering functional amplitudes*
  Wrist mobilizations must be soft to avoid putting excessive tension on the scapholunate ligament. These tensions are significant after 30° of flexion/extension.

If surgery is associated with capsuloplasty, the wrist mobility in flexion is limited and the therapist must not "force" on the wrist in flexion, as there is a risk of recreating instability (Fig. 5.16).

We use the same techniques as in fractures of the scaphoid:

- Fluidotherapy to relax the muscles and tissues. We use it at the beginning of the session to warm-up the wrist.
- Passive manual mobilizations are basic exercises to regain joint amplitude. They are soft, pain free, and can be realized by increasing the joint spaces a little. To begin, we work in the joint sectors that cause less stress (30° in flexion/extension), and then toward greater ranges of motion if it does not cause pain or trophic disorders.

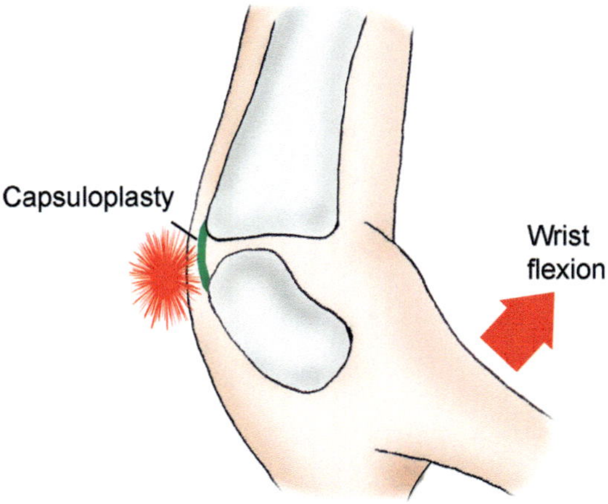

Fig. 5.16 Realizing a capsuloplasty allows stabilizing the scaphoid in the sagittal plane but can limit the amplitude in flexion. Therefore, the therapist mustn't "force" in flexion

- Global active mobilizations are performed after the passive ones, in various finger positions to improve tendinous glidings at the level of the wrist.
- Active-assisted mobilizations can be assisted by an arthromotor. We ask the patient to participate actively in the movements applied by the device. This exercise is realized in amplitudes previously regained passively by the therapist. It has an interest at the joint level, but also in draining the edema as it stimulates the "vis a latere." It can be combined with icing.
- Electrostimulation, combined with an active movement (winding the fingers) can help regain the last degrees of mobility in finger flexion if necessary. The patient must not clutch his fingers as it would put important constraints on the scaphoid.

In this stage, specific radiocarpal mobilizations are forbidden as they can be bad for the ligament's healing process.

- *Proprioceptive abilities of the wrist: perception of joint position (Hagert's stage 3)*

It is important to propose a coherent evolution for the exercises depending on the healing phase, in order not to disturb the consolidation process. The recovery stage of the proprioceptive abilities must also be considered so that the patient does not develop compensative pathologies such as tendinopathies or reflex contractures.

Hagert's stage 3 is defined as the ability to precisely reproduce a given joint angulation (Hagert 2010). The rehabilitation of this perception is done in three steps. In the first step, the therapist places the patient's wrist in a defined joint position and controls the joint amplitude with a goniometer (Hagert 2010).

In the second step, the wrist is placed in another position, indifferently. In the third step, the patient must place his forearm in the first position (Hagert 2010; Karagiannopoulos et al. 2016).

The exercise is realized with the patient's eyes closed to avoid any visual afference. An error margin of 4° is considered normal in adults (at the level of the wrists).

This test is highly correlated with the wrist's sensorimotor abilities (Karagiannopoulos et al. 2016) and must therefore be done before any evolution of the rehabilitation protocol—especially before Hager's stage 5.

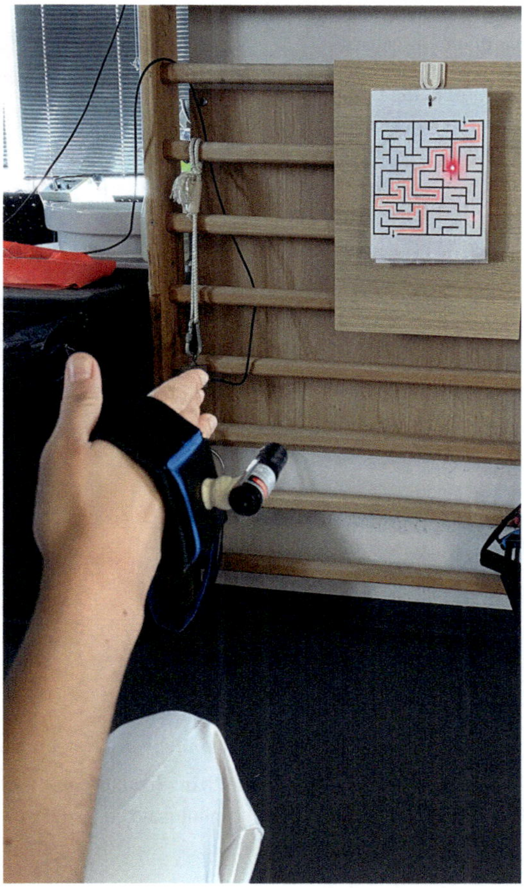

Fig. 5.17 Using a laser to improve conscious proprioceptive abilities

- *Proprioceptive abilities of the wrist: Kinesthesia (Hagert's stage 4)*

It is defined as the ability to detect a passive movement. The therapist realizes the movement while the patient keeps his eyes closed and tells him when he perceives the movement.

This exercise is easy to realize at the physiotherapy office or at home but does not allow a precise analysis regarding the patient's perception threshold.

Using an arthromotor device allows for analyzing more precisely the movement speed and the studied angular sector.

A laser can also be a very helpful tool to improve conscious proprioceptive abilities. The patient must follow trajectories becoming increasingly complex, going faster and faster (Fig. 5.17).

- *Proprioceptive abilities of the wrist: conscious neuromuscular rehabilitation (Hagert's stage 5)*

At this stage, we use muscular awakening techniques and static contractions of the muscles that protect the scapholunate ligament. We avoid working on the extensor carpi ulnaris as it does an intracarpal pronation that is bad for the ligament's healing process (Fig. 5.18).

Depending on the type of instability, the physiotherapist must strengthen protective muscles

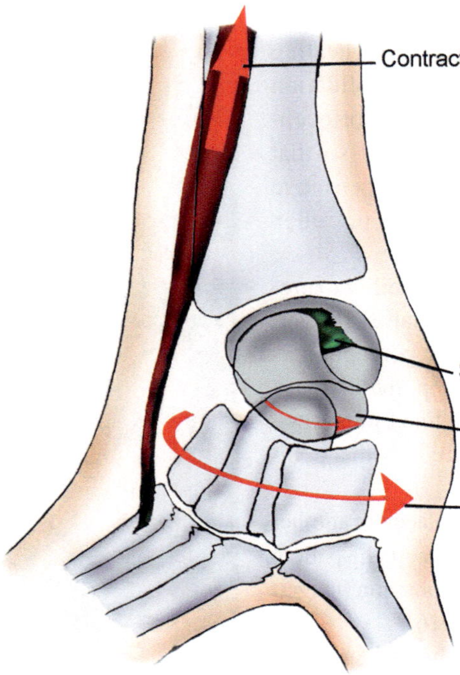

Fig. 5.18 The extensor carpi ulnaris causes an intracarpal pronation, harmful to the healing of the scapholunate ligament

Table 5.1 Types of frequent instabilities, main stabilizing ligaments, and protective and harmful muscles

Type of instability	Main stabilizing ligaments	Muscles to use	Muscles to not use
Scapholunate instability	Dorsal scapholunate ligament	Extensor carpi radialis longus Extensor carpi radialis brevis Abductor pollicis longus Flexor carpi radialis	Extensor carpi ulnaris
Lunotriquetral instability	Palmar lunotriquetral ligament	Extensor carpi ulnaris Flexor carpi radialis	Extensor carpi radialis longus Extensor carpi radialis brevis Abductor pollicis longus
Palmar midcarpal instability	Palmar triquetro-hamato-capital and dorsal radio-triquetral ligaments	Extensor carpi ulnaris Flexor carpi ulnaris Flexor carpi radialis	Extensor carpi radialis longus Extensor carpi radialis brevis Abductor pollicis longus

and avoid harmful muscles during the healing phase (Table 5.1).

Muscular awakening is realized with exercises with energy overload, which can be used at first to progressively stimulate atrophic muscles.

The "trigger" muscles used aim at producing a contraction of the muscles protecting the scapholunate ligament: flexor digiti minimi brevis—flexor carpi ulnaris (Fig. 5.19), and thenar and hypothenar muscles—flexor carpi radialis (Fig. 5.20).

The strengthening protocol itself starts when the previous exercises are easily realized by the patient. All the exercises are performed with the fingers in extension, to limit the axial constraints increased by the contraction of the finger flexors when clamping (Fig. 5.21).

The first solicited energy system is the aerobic one as it is the least constraining at the muscular and articular level. "Pure" aerobic exercises cannot be realized in this phase as the patient would be asked to realize long contractions (10–15 min!), which in this phase would lead to tendinous and muscular disorders, as well as important pain. Therefore, we use static intermittent exercises adapted to the wrist's functional biomechanics, the relative fragility of the callus and the wrist muscles' physiology.

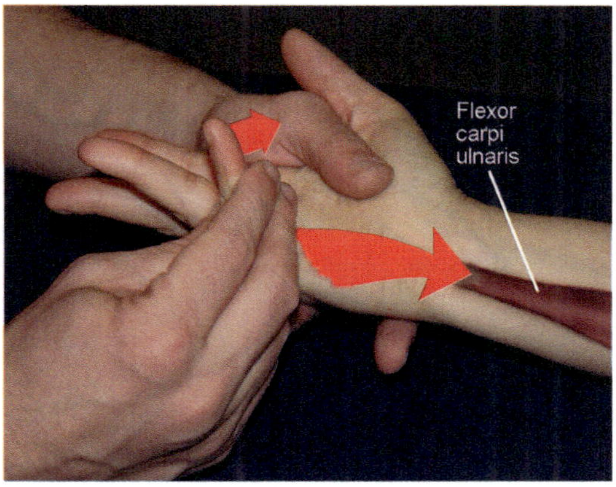

Fig. 5.19 Exercise with energy overload, where the trigger muscle is the flexor digiti minimi brevis and the target muscle is the flexor carpi ulnaris

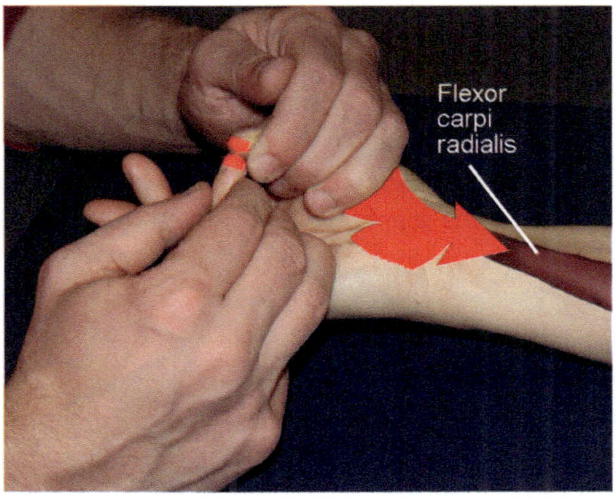

Fig. 5.20 Exercise with energy overload, from the opposition arch to the flexor carpi radialis

At the beginning of the phase, we ask for low-intensity static contractions with a series of 30 repetitions, held 6 s, and with 6 s of rest between the repetitions. The ideal contraction intensity is 20–30% of the maximal strength, but as it cannot be assessed in this phase, it is controlled by the therapist or by a device.

We cannot use the contralateral side to determine the usual strength of the injured side as there are often important differences between the two sides of a patient.

The parameters (number of repetitions, contraction duration, and modalities) evolve during the treatment, adapting to the patient's capacity and osseous consolidation.

A contraction with maximal resistance or clamping is never asked.

Dynamic contractions with wide amplitudes are not in relation to the physiological role of the wrist (orient and stabilize the hand during prehensions). Therefore, they are not included in the reinforcement protocol (except if there is a particular indication).

We realize a static reinforcement of the flexor carpi ulnaris and the extensor carpi radialis brevis and longus, with the wrist in a neutral position and the fingers in extension. During the first sessions, the forearm is placed in a neutral position or in pronation, as the supination creates huge constraints on the scapholunate ligament (Esplugas et al. 2018):

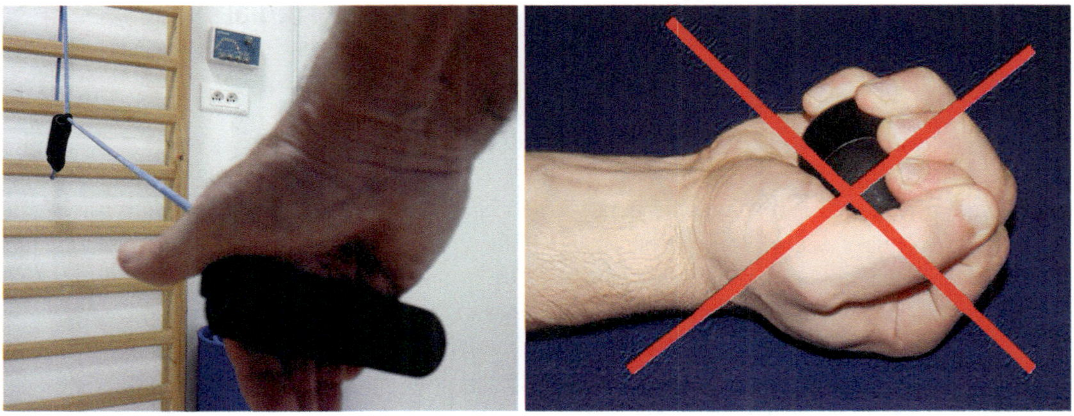

Fig. 5.21 Muscular awakening and reinforcement exercises are realized with the fingers extended during the healing phase of the scapholunate ligament (1). Kneading and clamping a ball is forbidden during the healing phase (2)

- *Flexor carpi radialis and flexor carpi ulnaris*: The flexor carpi radialis causes pronation of the second row on the first row, tensioning the scapholunate ligament. However, its tendon passes in front of the scaphoid's tubercle and opposes the tilt in flexion/pronation of the scaphoid. It also coapts the scapholunate space (Fig. 5.22). The flexor carpi ulnaris passes in front of the ulnar head and ends on the pisiform. It produces expansions toward the anterior retinacular ligament, the hamate, and the fourth and fifth metacarpals. It causes a supination of the second row on the first row, protecting the scapholunate ligament. We work with the espalier, with the fingers in extension and a contraction against an elastic band (moderate resistance). At the beginning of this rehabilitation phase, the patient brings the elastic band in the working position with his contralateral hand, to realize a pure static exercise. The exercise is then realized only with the damaged side to alternate stato-concentric, static, and stato-eccentric contractions against a controlled resistance. Visual feedback allows the patient to control the contraction and rest phases (Fig. 5.21(1)). During these exercises, the flexor carpi radialis and ulnaris work in synergy, and the action of the finger flexors is limited as we place the fingers in extension. Manually, the resistance is placed at the level of the palmar side of the metacarpal diaphyses, stabilizing the forearm with the contralateral hand. This grip allows us controlling the ligament and limits the compression and shearing constraints imposed on it. A digital grip with the fingers in extension is also possible (Fig. 5.23).
- *Extensor carpi radialis brevis and longus*: They pass on the posterior side of the radial styloid process and in the anatomical snuffbox, before ending respectively on the posterior side of the second and third metacarpals. They participate in stabilizing the radial column, along with the flexor carpi radialis. They are also intracarpal supinators and therefore protect the scapholunate ligament (Fig. 5.24).

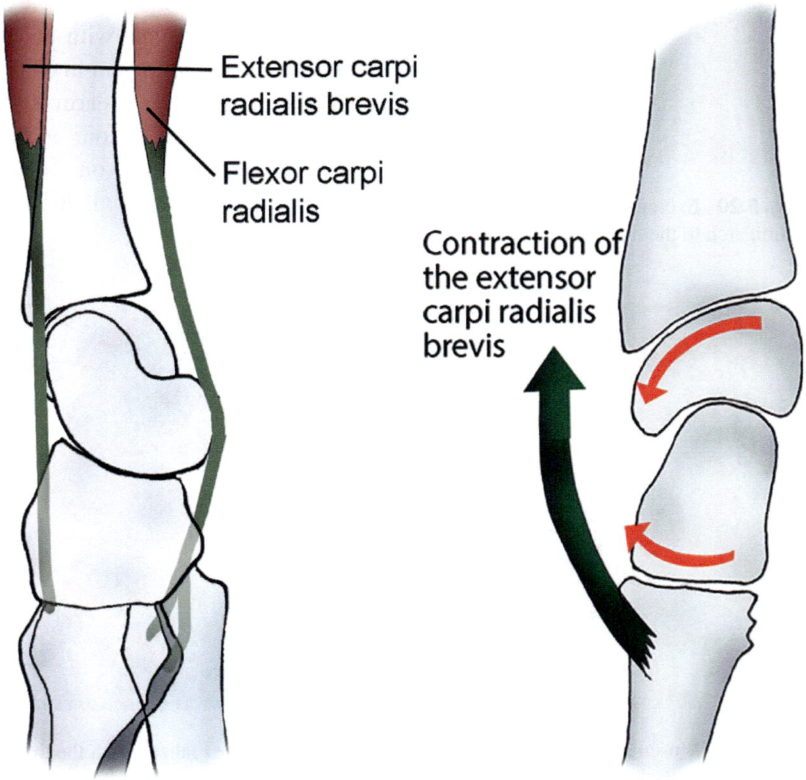

Fig. 5.22 Strengthening of the flexor carpi radialis, preventing the distal part of the scaphoid from going frontward with its tendon (1), and the extensor carpi radialis brevis that prevents the posterior tilt of the lunate (2)

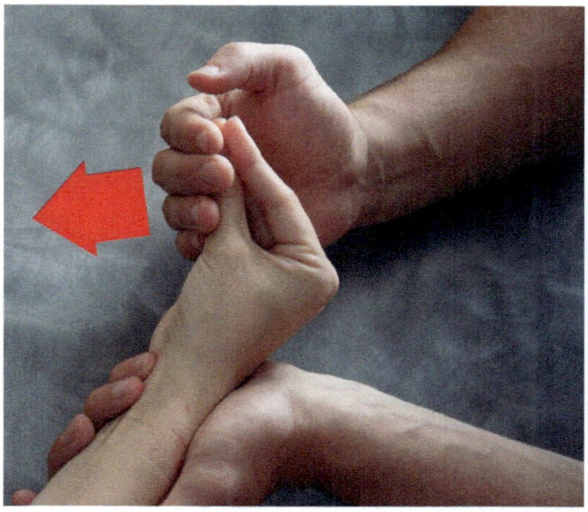

Fig. 5.23 Manual exercise for the wrist flexors with a digital grip. The interphalangeals are extended and the metacarpals flexed. As the metacarpophalangeal flexion is ensured by the intrinsic system, there is no increase in the compressive constraints on the scaphoid

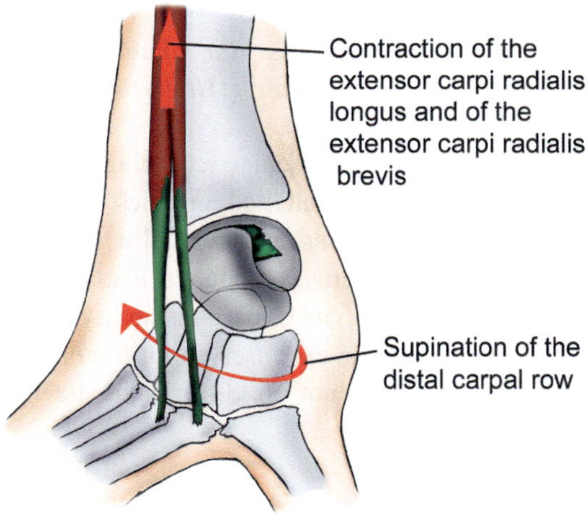

Fig. 5.24 Intracarpal supination during the contraction of the ECRL and ECRB

In the sagittal plane, the extensor carpi radialis brevis opposes the lunate's posterior tilt (DISI) through the capitate (Fig. 5.22 (2)). The abductor pollicis longus and extensor pollicis brevis stabilize the scapholunate area, but their analytical contraction is moderate in this phase as there are important risks of De Quervain tenosynovitis. We use the espalier with an elastic band, according to the same modalities as for the wrist flexors, and always

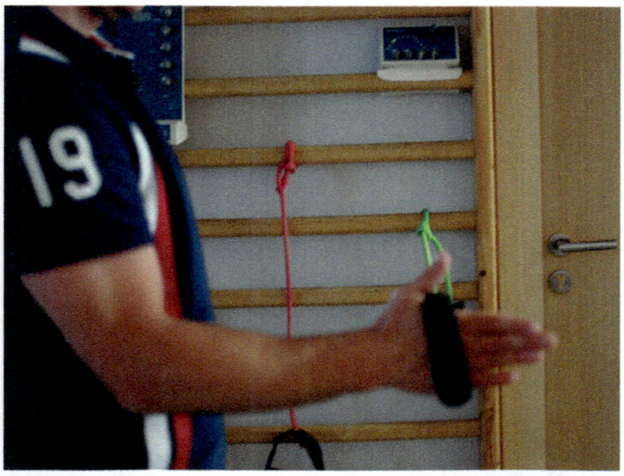

Fig. 5.25 Exercise for the wrist extensors with an espalier, with the same modalities as for the flexors. During this exercise, the extensor carpi ulnaris does not do much work, as its action occurs mainly in the frontal plane (ulnar inclination)

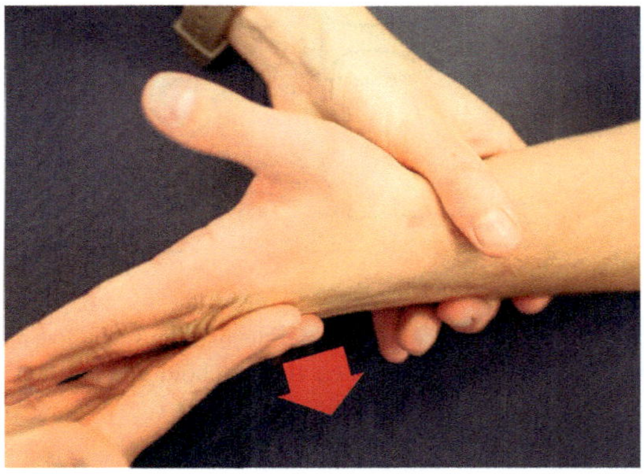

Fig. 5.26 Manual exercise for the wrist extensors

with visual feedback (Fig. 5.25). Manually, the resistance is placed at the level of the dorsal side of the metacarpal diaphyses, stabilizing the ulnar side of the wrist with the contralateral hand (Fig. 5.26). As for the reinforcement of the wrist flexors, we can associate a radial inclination to work with the extensor carpi radialis.

– *Radial stabilizers*: We can work with the extensor carpi radialis brevis and longus in synergy, with the espalier. The resistances are placed on the radial side of the second metacarpal to limit the contraction of the thumb's muscles. This exercise is realized very carefully, and the patient is forbidden to mobilize

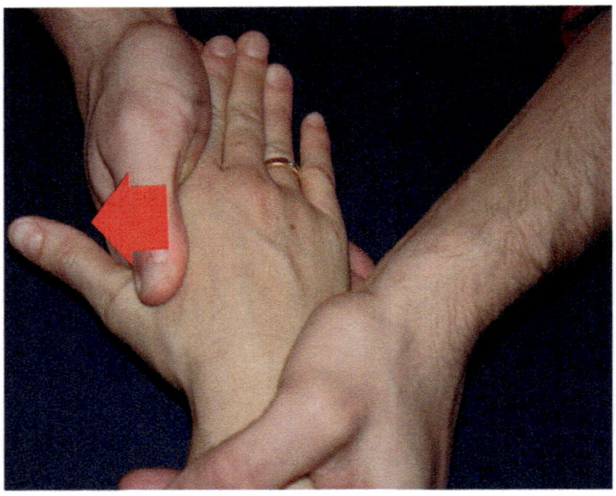

Fig. 5.27 Manual exercise for the radial stabilizers of the carpus with a stabilizing counter-grip on the ulnar compartment. The wrist mustn't be in an important radial inclination to limit the constraints on the scaphoid

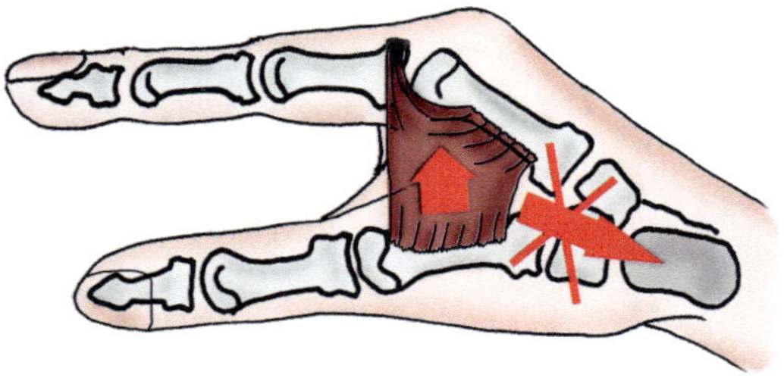

Fig. 5.28 The exercise for the intrinsic muscles doesn't produce axial constraints on the scaphoid as they don't have a longitudinal orientation

his wrist in radial inclination during the contraction (Fig. 5.27).

- *Intrinsic muscles*: The contraction of the intrinsic muscles does not produce important axial constraints, unlike the contraction of the extrinsic muscles (Fig. 5.28). We will strengthen preferentially the interossei, the flexor pollicis brevis, and the adductor pollicis. We ask the patient to realize a "vise" pinch against resistance, with visual feedback to manage the duration of contraction and rest (Fig. 5.29). The same exercise can be performed manually. The opposition arch between the thumb and the fifth finger can also be solicited manually.
- *Electrostimulation*: Combined with an active contraction of the stimulated muscles, it improves motor recruitment and maintains body mapping, thus participating in active wrist stabilization. It can concern intrinsic or extrinsic muscles and follows the principles of progression and protection of the ligament depending on its healing phase.

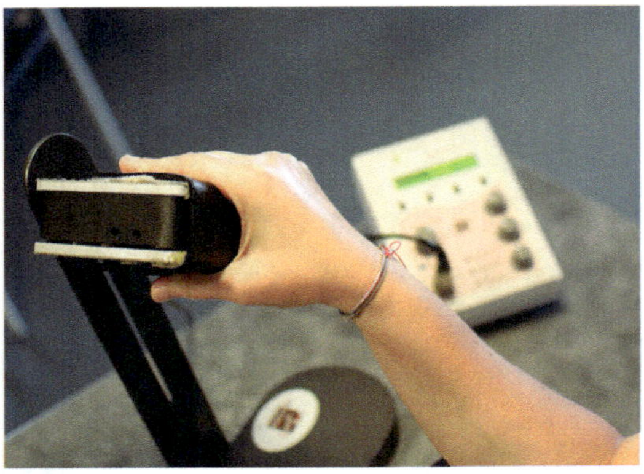

Fig. 5.29 Instrumental contraction exercise for the intrinsic muscles with an intrinsic pinch and visual feedback

- *Unconscious neuromuscular rehabilitation or reflex muscular activation (Hagert's stage 6)*

Conscious neuromuscular rehabilitation voluntarily targets the solicited muscles, whereas unconscious neuromuscular rehabilitation calls upon reflexes to actively stabilize a joint, thus partly compensating its passive instability.

In this phase, the exercises are of a moderate intensity in order not to disturb the healing process:

- *Table-tennis racket*: We ask the patient to maintain the ball on the racket, which implies a good sensorial analysis and a contraction adapted to the received information. Progressively, we ask the patient to throw the ball and receive it "softly" on the racket.
- *Exercises with a plastic ball*: We use a light plastic ball and ask the patient to pass it from one hand to the other, to throw and catch it.

- *Prehensions*

We work on prehensions to improve coordination and dexterity and therefore improve functional capacities in daily activities.

These exercises are realized without clamping or putting excessive constraints on the scaphoid.

For example, clamping a ball is forbidden.

In this phase, these exercises are performed only if there is no pain or trophic disorders. They improve the patient's proprioceptive abilities without taking any risk regarding ligament healing.

– *Solidity phase (after D90)*

Healing is acquired and the goal is to recover a functional wrist allowing the patient to go back to his normal activities.

The exercises performed are comparable to the ones used in fractures of the scaphoid, but there are a few points to remember.

- *About regaining functional amplitudes*

Working on mobility must be done globally and analytically to regain good scaphoid dynamic if it is not acquired yet.

We must not try to regain mobility "at all costs" as it can create scapholunate instability.

- *About muscular reinforcement*

Muscular reinforcement is intensified and controlled with dynamometers and visual feedback, which allows for regaining muscular balance and strength comparable to those of the sane side.

- *About proprioception and prehensions*

These exercises help regaining good neuromuscular coordination and go back to professional and sports activities.

- *Orthotic treatment*

It evolves with ligamentous healing.

– *Immobilization*

It can be a cast or made of resin, but we prefer using perforated thermoformable plastic (2.4 mm thick) to realize a non-removable orthosis. The wrist is placed in a neutral flexoextension and slight ulnar inclination; the fingers are free (Fig. 5.30).

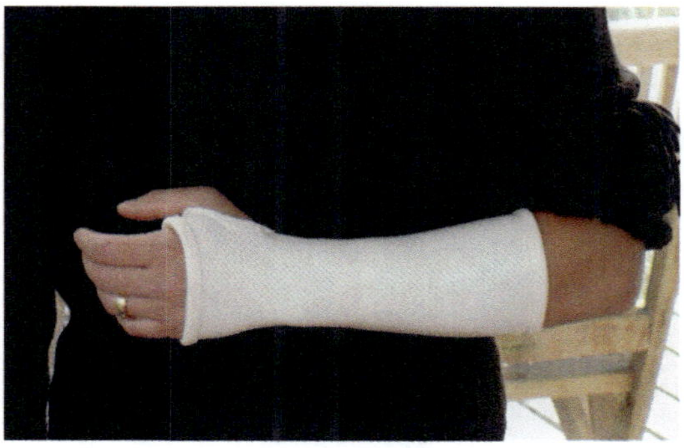

Fig. 5.30 Immobilization orthosis after repair of the scapholunate ligament

The orthosis is made in a pronation position to limit the forearm supination during the first 3 weeks, as this position can tension the scapholunate space (Esplugas et al. 2018).

With this technique, we get a precise immobilization, 8 times lighter than with resin, that can go in water (if there is no wound), radiolucent, and with perforations allowing the skin to "breathe."

New 3D technologies can also create quality orthoses that help optimize the patients' functional recovery (Fig. 5.31).

The Dart Thrower's Motion (DTM) orthosis only allows the movement between radial extension and ulnar flexion. It could seem interesting in this type of pathology as this movement only happens in the midcarpal joint, with no mobility in the first carpal row. However, in complete ligament injuries, the scaphoid acts as a bone of the second row. Complementary studies should be performed to determine if actual surgeries are strong enough to allow the use of this type of orthosis in the post-surgery phase.

– *Relative fragility phase*

Even if it is not realized all the time, a removable resting orthosis can be useful in case of nocturnal pain or in daily activities. The wrist is placed in the same position as in the previous phase (Fig. 5.32).

However, we make sure the patient gets rid of the orthosis without impeding his functional evolution.

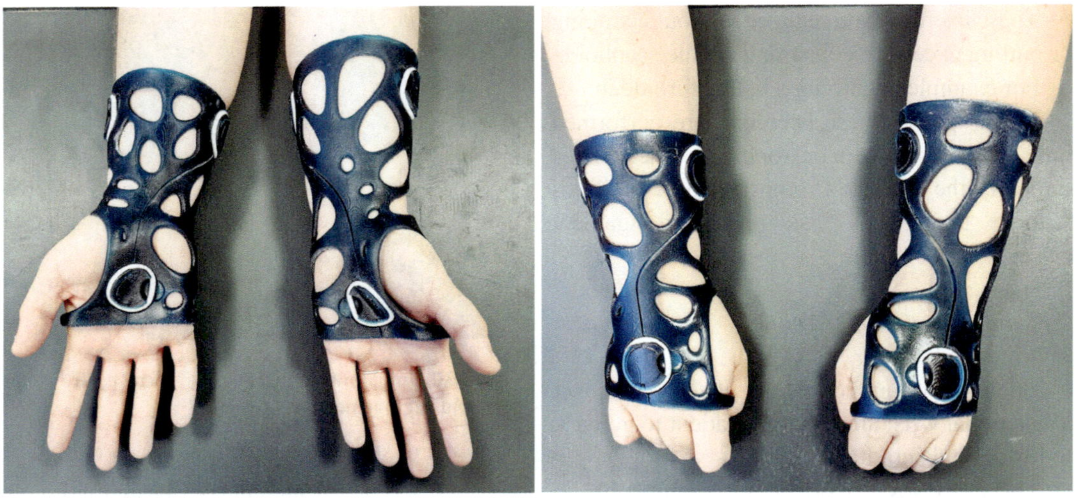

Fig. 5.31 Orthosis made with a 3D-printer and the Xkelet © technology

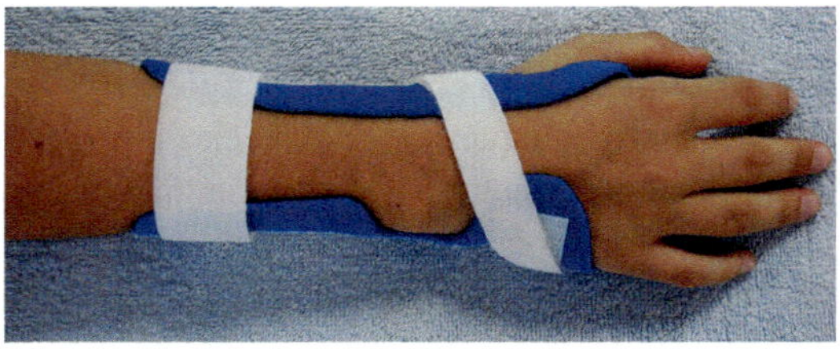

Fig. 5.32 Resting orthosis used after the immobilization phase during the night, and in case of pain. It must be taken off rapidly in order not to hinder the functional evolution

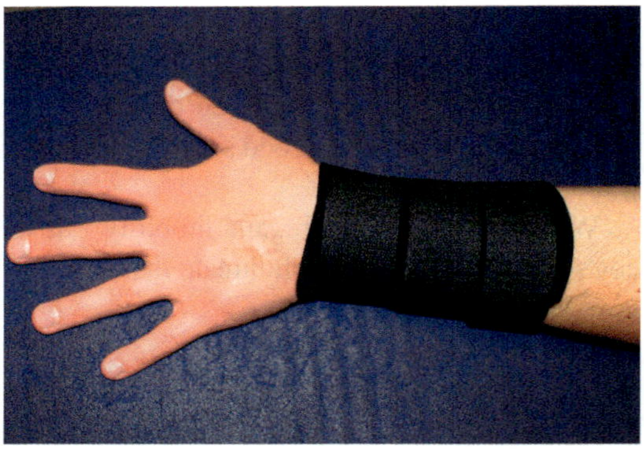

Fig. 5.33 Neoprene wrap-around cuff to restart sports and force activities

The orthosis leaves the thumb free and maintains the wrist in a neutral position. The plastic is perforated, and its thickness depends on the patient's morphology.

– *Consolidation*

A neoprene orthosis (Fig. 5.33) can be realized to go back to professional or sports activities, to protect the wrist against shocks. It also has an interesting contention effect, useful at a proprioceptive level and in the patient's apprehension. It is most often a wrap-around cuff and thermoformed plastic reinforcements can be added depending on the indications.

Complications

Complications related to the injuries of the scapholunate ligament are mainly the evolution toward a SLAC wrist when the cohesion of the first carpal row is compromised. This evolution must be avoided as the treatment for a SLAC wrist is complex and has uncertain results, especially in advanced stages.

This type of complication can also be found in mistreated or non-treated fractures of the scaphoid (see Chap. 4).

Lunotriquetral Instabilities

Whether we talk about physiopathology or clinical management, radial wrist instability has historically been more cared for than other carpal instabilities. However, lunotriquetral instabilities are the frequent origin of ulnar symptomatology. Unfortunately, awareness of this issue has been belated, and correct diagnosis and appropriate treatment are still delayed in many cases.

Physiopathology

We usually think that the exact injury mechanism is multifactorial when the isolated injury of the lunotriquetral ligament is usually the result of a fall with the arm in external rotation and the wrist in extension and radial inclination. This kind of trauma causes a dorsal translation of the triquetrum that is already in extension. The lunate, held by the radio-lunate ligament, does not follow (van de Grift and Ritt 2016).

The rupture of the lunotriquetral ligament is responsible for a dissociative instability with the scaphoid and lunate tilting in flexion and the triquetrum tilting in extension: there is a VISI on the X-ray (Fig. 5.34).

Clinical and Paraclinical Signs

They vary and depend on the stage of the injury. As in scapholunar injuries, an early diagnosis is key for the patient's recovery as surgery is all the more difficult as the injury is old.

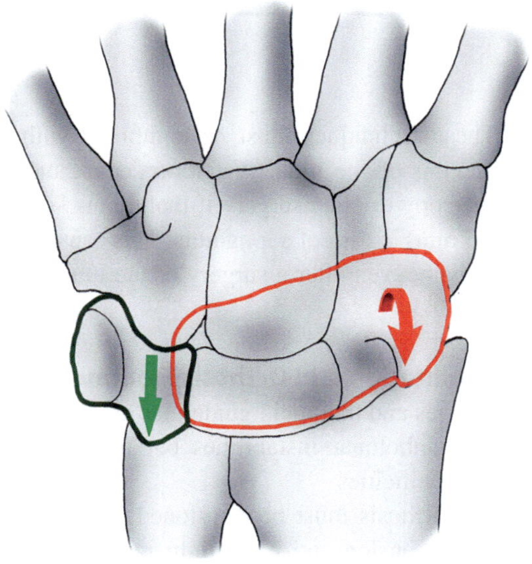

Fig. 5.34 The rupture of the lunotriquetral ligament causes a dissociative instability, with the scaphoid/lunate tilting in flexion and the triquetrum tilting in extension

- *Clinical signs*

Clinically, in acute injuries, there is pain on the ulnar side of the wrist, oedema, strength loss (especially in forearm pronation), or mobility loss (in ulnar inclination). In chronic injuries, the patients often feel ulnar "jumps" and instability (van de Grift and Ritt 2016). This clinical picture also varies depending on the degree of injury: from pain and strength loss for partial injuries, to wrist deformation with total functional loss for complete injuries.

Reagan's test, also known as the lunotriquetral ballottement test, is often used to complete clinical observations, even if its sensitivity and specificity are low (sensitivity 0.64 and specificity 0.44) (Rhee et al. 2014).

The Derby test consists of a simple question: "do you feel like your wrist is unstable, as if it were about to fall off?" The question is followed by a series of three tests (Rhee et al. 2014) (Fig. 5.35). Some authors describe a sensitivity of 0.77 and a positive predictive value of 0.89 to detect lunotriquetral dissociations (confirmed by arthroscopy) (Christodoulou and Bainbridge 1999).

- *Paraclinical sings*

Static X-rays are normal in isolated lunotriquetral instabilities, but the associated slacking or rupture of the extrinsic stabilizers disturbs the Gilula's lines and causes a flexion of the lunate (VISI).

As in scapholunar injuries, dynamic X-rays (in ulnar and radial inclinations) are interesting in this type of injury.

The arthrogram or MRI can be used to confirm the diagnosis.

An arthroscopy should be considered as it can help make the diagnosis and treat the injury, as well as combined injuries in the ulno-triquetral joint and the TFCC.

Therapeutic Process and Surgery

This process must be adapted to the patient's functional needs and social environment.

In chronic injuries, a conservative treatment should be proposed first, with an adapted immo-

Ask the patient: do you feel like your wrist is unstable, as if it were about to fall off?

↓

Proceed to each part of the Derby Relocation Test, successively

A positive Derby Relocation Test includes a subjective acceleration sensation of the wrist at the above interrogation and a positive answer to the 3 parts of the exam

↓

Part 1		
Position	Maneuver	Response
Elbow in a 90° flexion on the table Wrist in pronation, extension, and radial inclination	Place the thumb on the palmar side of the pisiform and apply a pressure in a dorsal direction while bringing the wrist in a neutral position	A positive test will resolve the subjective wrist instability and improve the strength or the duration of the supported prehension

↓

Part 2		
Position	Maneuver	Response
Mobilize the wrist until the sensation of instability comes back The wrist is in pronation, neutral flexion, and radial inclination	A dorso-palmar pressure is applied on the dorsal side of the triquetrum, while the wrist is in ulnar inclination	Positive test if pain appears when the wrist is in ulnar inclination

↓

Part 3		
Position	Maneuver	Response
Mobilize the wrist until the sensation of instability comes back The wrist is in pronation, neutral flexion, and radial inclination	The thumb is placed on the palmar side of the pisiform A pressure is applied in a dorsal direction while the wrist is in ulnar inclination	Positive test if pain decreases during the ulnar inclination (maneuver tested in part 2)

Fig. 5.35 Derby's maneuver in three steps

bilization for 6 weeks followed by a progressive proprioceptive rehabilitation (first targeting the protective muscles, then global).

In acute injuries an arthroscopic treatment is recommended, combining a debridement of the ligament and a pin through the lunotriquetral joint. This treatment is often associated with an assessment and treatment of other carpal ligaments or the TFCC (Badia and Khanchandani 2009).

If those techniques do not work, more invasive techniques can be considered, such as a ligamentoplasty using a piece of the extensor carpi ulnaris, or a lunotriquetral arthrodesis (Garcia-Elias and Cantero-Tellez 2021; Ennaciri and Beaudouin 2016).

These techniques must be combined with a shortening of the ulna (wafer procedure under arthroscopy or open surgery if the ulna is longer than 3 mm) in case of a long ulna. This can create ulnar pain, even after a surgery of the lunotriquetral joint.

Rehabilitation and Orthotic Treatment

The stages and treatment guidelines are the same as in scapholunar instabilities but must follow some specificities.

The orthosis must be positioned in a neutral flexion/extension and in a slight radial inclination. It should be realized in forearm supination to limit the compressive constraints of the ulna on the lunotriquetral space that happens in pronation (Garcia-Elias 2011).

During the relative fragility phase, the therapist must strengthen in priority the extensor carpi ulnaris and the flexor carpi ulnaris as they are intracarpal pronators and therefore protect the lunotriquetral joint. The therapist should also avoid working with the extensor carpi radialis brevis and longus and the flexor carpi ulnaris as they are intracarpal supinators and increase the tensions on the lunotriquetral space (Table 5.1).

Non-dissociative Instabilities

Description

These instabilities correspond to a dysfunction between the distal and proximal carpal rows. The cohesion between the bones of one row is preserved. Depending on the midcarpal instability, we will talk about palmar, dorsal, combined, or adaptive non-dissociative instabilities.

Palmar Instability

The most frequent instability is the palmar one, where the first row goes in flexion and the second row in extension (Fig. 5.36).

Clinically, the patients show pain when palpating the ulnar side of the carpus, more precisely at the level of the triquetro-hamate joint, and a painful "jump" in wrist ulnar inclination. This jump can be avoided if the therapist presses the palmar side of the pisiform during the inclination movement, realigning the first row in extension.

Physiologically speaking, this instability is related to an injury of the triquetro-hamato-capital ligament that no longer transmits the constraints from the hamate to the triquetrum, and therefore leaves the first row under the scaphoid's dominance. The scaphoid tends to bring the first row unflexion because of the axial constraints imposed on it by the second row.

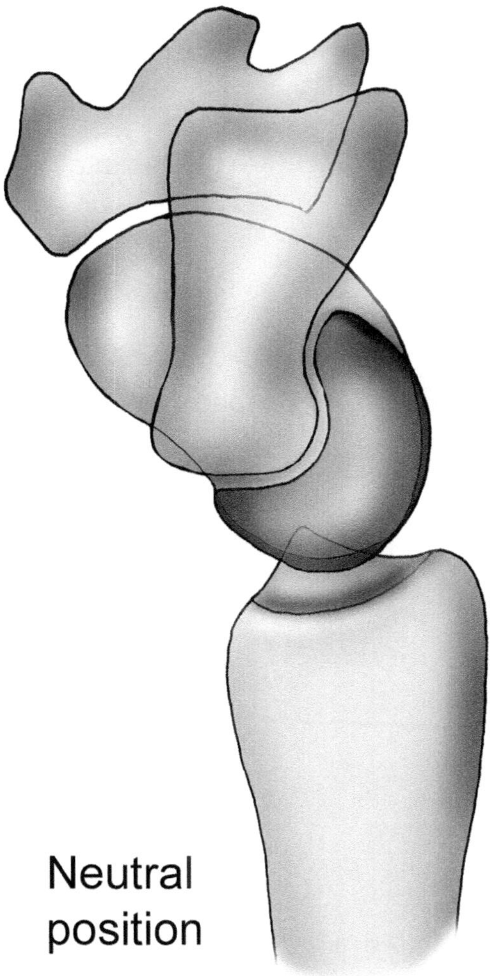

Fig. 5.36 Palmar non-dissociative instability

Secondly, the dorsal radiocarpal ligament, which avoids the flexion of the first row, loosens and lets the first carpal row tilt in flexion.

Dorsal Instability

The dorsal instability corresponds to a dorsal subluxation of the capitate in wrist ulnar inclination and is much rarer than the palmar instability.

It can be shown by Louis' test (Louis et al. 1984) in which the therapist presses on the scaph-

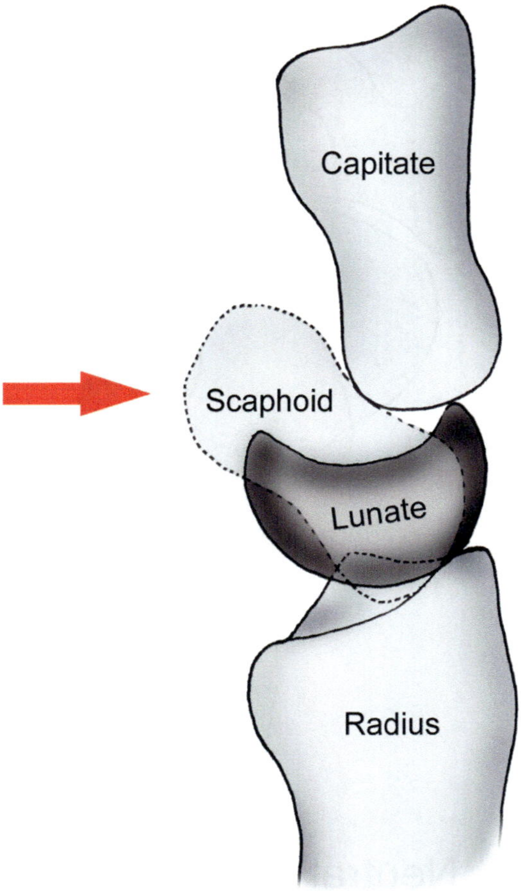

Fig. 5.37 Louis' test

oid's tubercle, with a slight traction and the wrist in slight flexion and ulnar inclination. If this maneuver creates a painful dorsal subluxation of the capitate relative to the lunate, it is positive (Fig. 5.37).

Combined Instability

It corresponds to a palmar instability with a positive Louis' test. It is very rare but can happen in hypermobile people, especially if they practice sports with repetitive movements such as volleyball, tennis, or gymnastics.

Adaptive Instability

The adaptive form appears secondarily to an extrinsic cause, mainly a forearm fracture with a vicious callus. This forearm deformity can provoke an "adaptive" deformation of the carpus to make daily activities easier.

Treatment Guidelines

Palmar Instabilities

The initial treatment for palmar instabilities is conservative with a corrective immobilization (Lichtman and Wroten 2006; Wolfe et al. 2012).

For palmar instabilities, the orthosis will be realized in slight ulnar inclination (after the jump showing that the first row has moved from flexion to extension), with a corrective press on the pisiform and the ulnar head. The orthosis must be always worn during 6–8 weeks (Harwood and Turner 2015), with a weekly control of the pressure points to avoid cutaneous complications. During these controls, the wrist must stay in ulnar inclination to prevent the first row from going in flexion.

This immobilization is followed by an adapted proprioceptive rehabilitation where the therapist works with the muscles preventing the flexion of the first carpal row—mainly the hypothenar muscles and the flexor carpi ulnaris. These exercises should be done in closed chain for greater efficiency at the midcarpal level (Fig. 5.38).

If the conservative treatment does not work, surgical techniques can be considered such as capsule-ligamentous interventions or arthrodeses.

Dorsal Instabilities

For dorsal instabilities, the literature is divided regarding the results of the initial treatment (Lichtman and Wroten 2006). In any case, whether it is after surgery or in a conservative treatment, the orthosis will be realized in a neutral wrist position or in slight radial inclination, to prevent the first row from going in extension. In conservative treatments, the orthosis will be worn always for 6–8 weeks.

The proprioceptive rehabilitation will be focused on the extensor carpi radialis and the extensor carpi ulnaris that prevent the extension of the first carpal row (Fig. 5.22(2)).

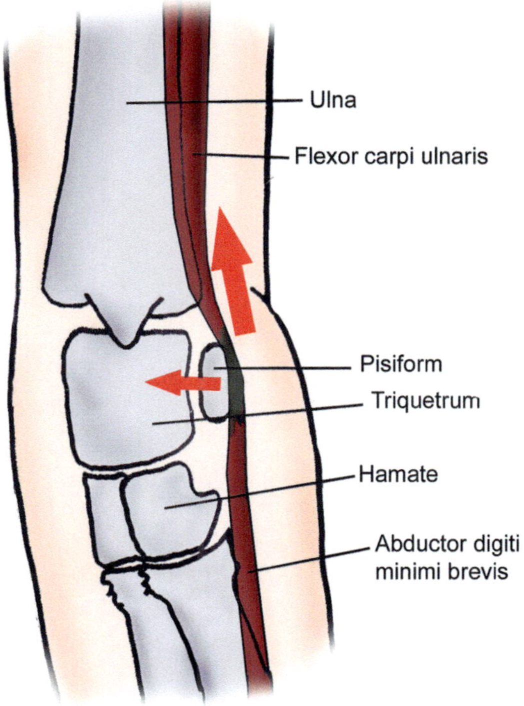

Fig. 5.38 The contraction of the flexor carpi ulnaris in a closed chain creates a palmo-dorsal push opposing the tilt in flexion of the first carpal row

Combined and Adaptive Instabilities

The recommended treatment is surgery, with techniques on the carpus in combined instabilities and techniques on the extrinsic cause in adaptive instabilities (Wolfe et al. 2012).

Bibliography

Athlani L, et al. La ligamentoplastie SLIC dans le traitement de la dissociation scapholunaire : résultats cliniques au recul minimum de 12 mois. Revue de Chirurgie Orthopédique et Traumatologique. 2017;103(7):S59–60.

Athlani L, et al. Treatment of chronic scapholunate dissociation with tenodesis: a systematic review. Hand Surg Rehabil. 2018;37(2):65–76.

Badia A, Khanchandani P. The floating lunate: arthroscopic treatment of simultaneous complete tears of the scapholunate and lunotriquetral ligaments. Hand. 2009;4:250–5.

Christodoulou L, Bainbridge L. Clinical diagnosis of trique-trolunate ligament injuries. J Hand Surg Br. 1999;24(5):598e600.

Ennaciri B, Beaudouin E. Open surgery for lunotriquetral instability. Pan Afr Med J. 2016;24:273.

Esplugas M, et al. The scapholunate gap increases with forearm supination. A laboratory study. FESSH. 2018;

Garcia-Elias M. Carpal instability, in Green's operative hand surgery. Editor: Elsevier; 2011.

Garcia-Elias M, Cantero-Tellez R. Classification and management of carpal instability. In: Rehabilitation of the hand and upper extremity. Elsevier; 2021.

Garcia-Elias M, Lluch AL, Stanley JK. Three-ligament tenodesis for the treatment of scapholunate dissociation: indications and surgical technique. J Hand Surg Am. 2006;31(1):125–34.

Hagert E. Proprioception of the wrist joint: a review of current concepts and possible implications on the rehabilitation of the wrist. J Hand Ther. 2010;23(1): 2–16. quiz 17

Harvey EJ, et al. Bone-tissue-bone repairs for scapholunate dissociation. J Hand Surg Am. 2007;32(2): 256–64.

Harwood C, Turner L. Conservative management of midcarpal instability. J Hand Surg Eur. 2015;41E(1): 102–9.

Karagiannopoulos C, et al. Responsiveness of the active wrist joint position sense test after distal radius fracture intervention. J Hand Ther. 2016;29(4): 474–82.

Lichtman DM, Wroten ES. Understanding midcarpal instability. J Hand Surg Am. 2006;31(3):491–8.

Louis D, et al. Central carpal instability-capitate lunate instability pattern: diagnosis by dynamic displacement. Orthopaedics. 1984;7:1693–6.

Overstraeten LV, et al. Anatomical description of the dorsal capsulo-scapholunate septum (DCSS)-arthroscopic staging of scapholunate instability after DCSS sectioning. J Wrist Surg. 2013;2(2):149–54.

Raja S, et al. New concepts in carpal instability. In: Wrist and elbow arthroscopy with selected open procedures; 2022. p. 173–85.

Rhee PC, et al. Examination of the wrist: ulnarsided wrist pain due to ligamentous injury. J Hand Surg Am. 2014;39(9):1859–62.

Roll R, et al. Illusory movements prevent cortical disruption caused by immobilization. NeuroImage. 2012;62(1):510–9.

Short WH, et al. Biomechanical evaluation of the ligamentous stabilizers of the scaphoid and lunate: part II. J Hand Surg Am. 2005;30(1):24–34.

van de Grift TC, Ritt MJ. Management of lunotriquetral instability: a review of the literature. J Hand Surg Eur. 2016;41(1):72–85.

Wolfe SW, Garcia-Elias M, Kitay A. Carpal instability nondissociative. J Am Acad Orthop Surg. 2012;2012(20):575–85.

Common Tendinopathies in the Wrist

6

Thomas Everaere, Cédric Le Petit, and Grégory Mesplié

De Quervain Tenosynovitis

Description

De Quervain's tenosynovitis (DQ) corresponds to damage to the tendons and synovial sheaths (tenosynovitis) (Dictionnaire médical de l'Académie de Médecine - Définition ténosynovite 2022) of the extensor pollicis brevis (EPB) and abductor pollicis longus (APL) muscles (Bouillot 2011) (Fig. 6.1).

The tendons of these muscles run in an inextensible osteofibrous tunnel, located in the first dorsal compartment of the wrist (Nguyen et al. 2012). This compartment consists of the radial gutter and the extensor retinaculum. If there is a mismatch between the content (tendons) and the container (osteofibrous tunnel), the tendons' ability to slide within their sheaths is impaired, resulting in the classic DQ pain on the outside of the wrist.

This characteristic pain is located opposite the radial styloid, in the path of the two tendons of the APL and EPB muscles. It is provoked by the palpation of the area, the contraction and/or stretching of these muscles, and may be accentuated by movements of the thumb and wrist (Nguyen et al. 2012).

The De Quervain tenosynovitis is a common condition (Wolf et al. 2009) that can occur at any age, although it classically affects people over 40 years (Nguyen et al. 2012) and women (Shen et al. 2019). It also seems more likely to occur in pregnant women and young mothers (Avci et al. 2002). It can also be found in people who have suffered injury or trauma, or who overuse their thumb or wrist. This is the case, for example, in certain sports and activities (volleyball, golf, racket sports), or in certain professions: manual workers (housekeepers, carpenters, gardeners), office workers (computer keyboarding), sign language interpreters and musicians (Calvo-Cerrada et al. 2012; Rodineau 1991; Hassan et al. 2013).

De Quervain's tenosynovitis is one of the most common musculoskeletal disorders (MSD) of the upper limb (INRS 2022a) and is recognized as an occupational disease according to table 57C (INRS 2022b). DQ represents around 8% of hand and wrist MSDs compensated each year in France (Petit Le Manac'h et al. 2011). It should also be noted that the number of MSDs has increased by 60% since 2003 (Ameli 2022).

Tenosynovitis

Etymologically speaking, tenosynovitis is an inflammation of the synovial sheath surrounding a tendon (Dictionnaire médical de l'Académie de

T. Everaere · C. Le Petit
Institut Sud Aquitain de la Main et du Membre Supérieur, Biarritz, France

G. Mesplié (✉)
ISAMMS, Biarritz, France

G. Mesplié (ed.), *Wrist Functional Anatomy and Therapy*,
https://doi.org/10.1007/978-3-031-42879-1_6

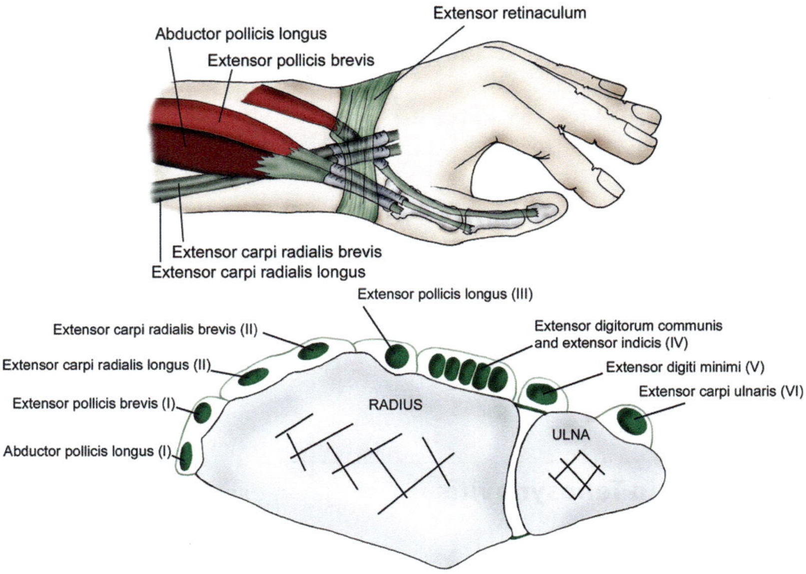

Fig. 6.1 (**a**) EPB and APL under the extensor retinaculum on the radial side of the wrist. (**b**) Axial sectional view showing the six dorsal compartments

Médecine - Définition ténosynovite 2022). Two forms of tenosynovitis can be distinguished: exudative and stenosing (Artru 1999).

- *Exudative tenosynovitis*

In this type of tenosynovitis, the synovial sheath is thickened, and edema and hypervascularization are present, together with an effusion of variable importance (Revue médicale suisse 2022). Clinically, it is characterized by swelling along the tendon (sometimes erythematous), and by a limited mobility—often of algesic origin. Pain is also present when the tendon is palpated or tensioned (passive thumb flexion or resisted thumb extension). In the case of chronic exudative tenosynovitis, crepitations linked to fibrin deposition may be felt during passive mobilization.

- *Stenosing tenosynovitis*

This type of tenosynovitis is what characterizes De Quervain's tenosynovitis. Stenosing tenosynovitis is the result of a disproportion between the fibrous structures under which the tendons slide, and the size of the tendons. The result is a thickening of the structures and a constriction that limits tendon sliding and increases friction (Revue médicale suisse 2022) (Fig. 6.2).

For many years, this condition was considered an inflammatory response. It was only recently in the last century, thanks to the development of more sophisticated research techniques, that studies demonstrated the absence of systematic inflammatory cells in DQ and confirmed the presence of tendon degeneration (Read et al. 2000; Meachim and Roberts 1969; Clarke et al. 1998). This reflects a degenerative or reactive pathology, linked to mechanical stress, rather than a disease of inflammatory origin (McAuliffe 2010).

Epidemiology

Tenosynovitis of the extensor sheaths is most common in the first compartment (INRS 2022b). The reported prevalence in the population varies from 0.5 to 0.7% in men and from 1.3% to 2.1% in women (Petit Le Manac'h et al. 2011; Walker-Bone et al. 2004; Roquelaure et al. 2006).

The condition affects women in 72.7% of cases, versus 27.3% in men (Shen et al. 2019). Various case series also suggest that DQ affects women 3–7 times more than men (De Quervain 2005; Beutel et al. 2020; Monaco 1996; De Keating-Hart et al. 2016).

The predominance of the female gender is classic (Nguyen et al. 2012), particularly in meno-

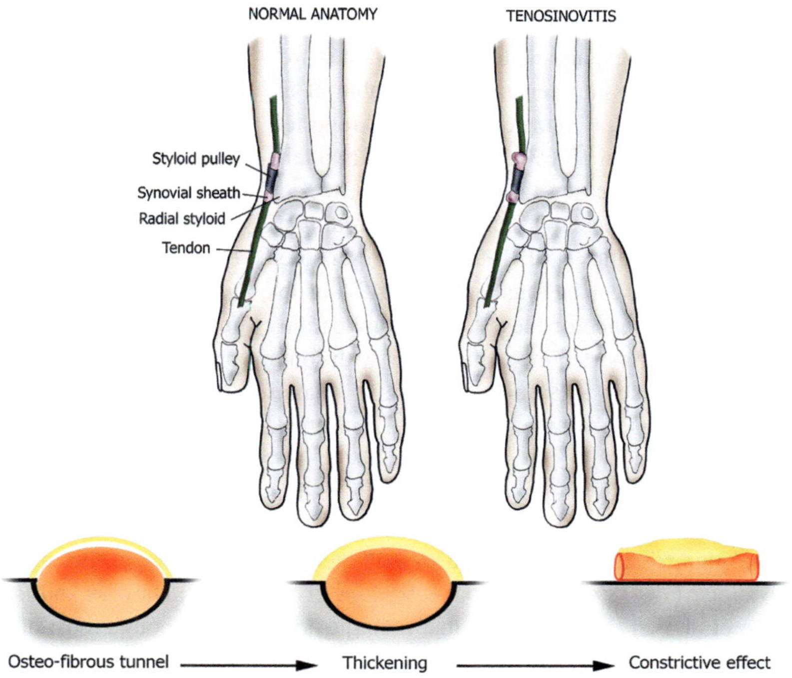

Fig. 6.2 (**a**) Mismatch content/container. (**b**) The osteofibrous tunnel. The thickened slide has a constrictive effect on the tendon

pausal women (Moore 1997; Muckart 1964). DQ has also been reported in pregnant women, particularly in the last trimester, but also in nursing mothers and women with young children (Avci et al. 2002; Monaco 1996; De Keating-Hart et al. 2016). The condition is most often unilateral, but can sometimes be bilateral (Nguyen et al. 2012), especially in new mothers or childminders (Laoopugsin and Laoopugsin 2012; Stahl et al. 2015).

Etiologies

Mechanical Causes

The development of the pathology, which is more frequent in the first compartment than in the other compartments of the wrist, suggests a mechanical origin. Different anatomic variations and biomechanical constraints could play a role in the onset of the pathology, as well as in the response to treatment, although this is still a matter of debate (De Keating-Hart et al. 2016; Lee et al. 2017).

Anatomical Variations

The literature lists numerous anatomical variations of the first extensor compartment. These include the presence of one or more total or partial sub-compartments in the first compartment, the variability of the tendons' distal insertions, and the possibility of tendon duplication—especially the APL. These anatomical variations within the first extensor compartment are frequent. In a study on 300 cadaver wrists by Jackson et al. (Jackson et al. 1986), the number of tendons in the first extensor compartment differed from the standard anatomical description in 75% of cases.

The study by Beutel et al. (2020) showed that 79.4% of subjects had a sub-compartment separate from the EPB. Numerous case series (Lee et al. 2017; Kulthanan and Chareonwat 2007; Nayak et al. 2009; Shiraishi and Matsumura 2005; Alemohammad et al. 2009) report similar data: in cadavers, the prevalence of a septum ranges from 20 to 43.7%, while in patients with DQ, the prevalence ranges from 58 to 76%. Hajder et al. (2013) conclude that the prevalence of a septate first dorsal compartment in subjects with DQ is significantly higher than in subjects without DQ. Kutsumi et al. (2005) showed that the presence of an additional septum increased the sliding resistance of the EPB tendon.

The APL muscle is sometimes subdivided into two fleshy bodies, and its terminal tendon is frequently divided into several strips (Bahm et al. 1995). One study (Gonzalez et al. 1995) reported a single tendon in 13.6% of APL cases, two tendons in 69.7% of cases, three tendons in 13.6% of cases and 4 tendons in 3% of cases. According to Bahm et al. (Bahm et al. 1995), the presence of several tendons can be found in 56 to 94% of subjects. The presence of these tendon duplications is commonly reported in the literature, with some relating as many as 9 tendon divisions (Bahm et al. 1995; Gonzalez et al. 1995; Lane et al. 2001).

Interestingly, while several case series (Bahm et al. 1995; Matzon et al. 2019; Choi et al. 2011) have reported a very high rate of APL tendon divisions (74–78%) in DQ patients, Lee et al. (Lee et al. 2017) have shown that a single APL tendon was more common in this same population, compared to cadaveric studies. This could imply that the pathological process of DQ is not necessarily related to the presence of multiple APL tendons, but rather to the specific distal insertion site of this tendon, which may vary between individuals.

The distal insertion of the APL presents several possible anatomical configurations. A study (Loomis 1951) showed that only 10.2% of subjects had an APL that was inserted only on the lateral tubercle of the base of the first metacarpal. In the remaining 89.8% of cases, the APL had several insertions: on the abductor pollicis brevis (59%), on the trapezium (58%), on the opponens pollicis (15.7%), on the first phalanx of the thumb (7.1%), and at the level of the thumb's carpometacarpal joint (2.3%). One study (Dos Remédios et al. 2005) demonstrated that the various possible variations in APL tendon insertion increase the friction generated in the first extensor compartment and may contribute to DQ symptoms. However, Chang et al. (Chang et al. 2017) did not confirm an association between the site of insertion and DQ in their recent MRI study, and further studies are therefore required.

About the EPB muscle, if we refer to evolutionary processes, we can see that it is a relatively young structure. This muscle used to be mixed with the APL, and only individualized in humans and gorillas. The EPB is often thinner than the APL and is absent in 2–7% of human subjects (Gonzalez et al. 1995; Wolfe et al. 2010). Most often with a single tendon, in rare cases (<5%) it may have two or more tendons (Nayak et al. 2009; Shiraishi and Matsumura 2005; Bahm et al. 1995; Gonzalez et al. 1995). The EPB may also have various insertions. One study showed insertions on the first phalanx (72%), on both phalanges (21.2%) and on the distal phalanx (6.8%) (Loomis 1951). When the EPB has an additional accessory tendon, it may have different attachment points, including the trapezium, the base of the first metacarpal, the interosseous membrane, and the base of the proximal or distal phalanx of the thumb (Brunelli and Brunelli 1992; Dawson and Barton 1986).

Although most of these data come from retrospective studies, a prospective study (Matzon et al. 2019) of 130 DQ patients corroborates these findings with comparable rates of under-sheaths (63%), multiple APL tendons (78%), and a single EPB (92%).

Significant anatomical variability therefore exists in the first extensor compartment. People with DQ seem more likely to have a septum dividing the first extensor compartment between the two tendons of the APL and EPB. Although multiple tendon divisions may also represent a risk factor, current studies seem to give a more important role to the presence of a septum in the occurence of DQ. It should be noted that most surgical series concerning patients with DQ are carried out on a selected population unresponsive to non-surgical therapies. As such, the presence of these variations could, in addition to being a potential risk factor, be associated with a poor response to non-surgical therapies and represent a poor prognosis factor.

These anatomical features are clinically relevant to the pathophysiology and treatment of DQ. They may explain the presence of tenosynovitis in this anatomical zone. A clear understanding of anatomical variations will guide both the conservative and surgical management of this condition and contribute to a better chance of successful treatment.

Human Evolution

According to Bouillot (2011), the two APL and EPB muscles form an integral part of a global dorsal stabilizing muscle chain. This chain starts with the posterior spinal chain, which ensures uprightness, and continues with the scapula stabilizer muscles, the lateral shoulder rotator muscles and the lateral epicondylar muscles. As man evolved from a quadruped to a biped, the purpose of the upper limb evolved from a closed kinetic chain of support to an open kinetic chain of grip. This evolution has transformed the physiological properties of the upper limb muscles. From a functional point of view, this predominantly tonic, posterior stabilizing chain counterbalances the anterior muscular chain (medial shoulder rotators and elbow, wrist, and finger flexors), which mainly plays a phasic role, oriented toward grasping objects. During these grasping activities, the anterior chain works mainly by shortening, while the posterior chain works mainly by lengthening. The APL and EPB muscles work mainly isometrically or eccentrically, and act as a brake on movements of the thumb column, on ulnar inclination, and on pronation, with their muscular bodies in an extended position. In the elongated position, the muscles make greater demands on their aponeurotic and collagenous tissue than on their contractile muscle fibers. In this configuration, the APL and EPB muscles promote wear on the fascial and collagenous structures. This elongation is favored during pronation: while most of the movement takes place within the forearm, the final degrees of movement are made possible by a torsion of the carpus. When stretched, the APL and EPB muscles act as brakes on carpal movements. The constraints on these tendon structures can contribute to the presence of DQ.

Radial Ascension

Gerlac (Gerlac and Gerlac 2015) reports that if the radius is ascended relative to the ulna, the angle of penetration into the first dorsal compartment by both the APL and the EPB tendons is increased (Fig. 6.3). This increases friction

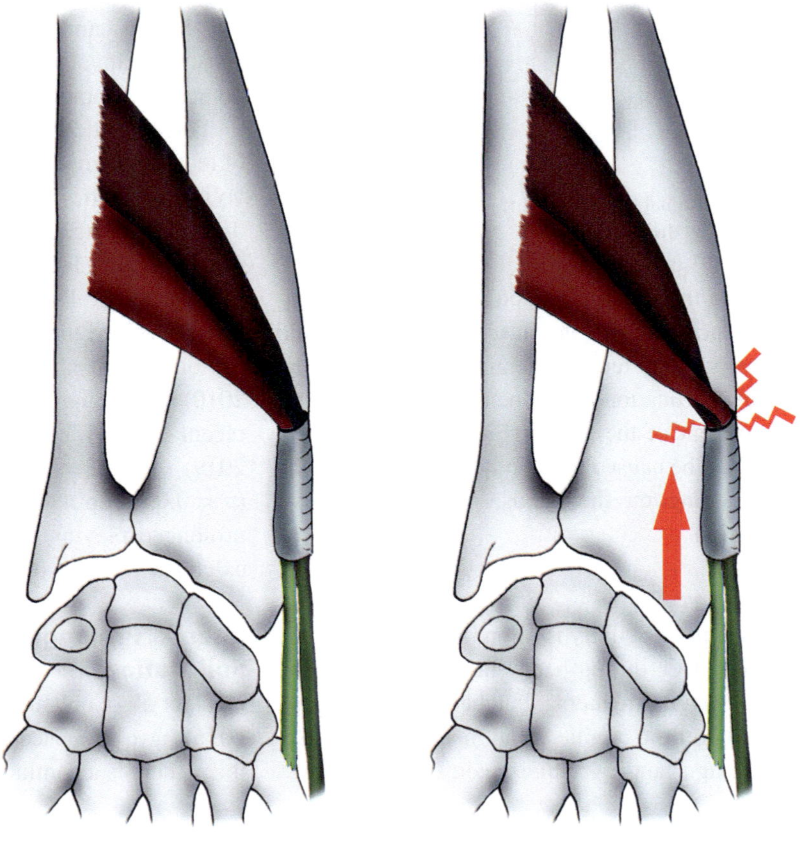

Fig. 6.3 Conflict between the tendon at the level of the entrance of the first compartment, when the radius is ascended

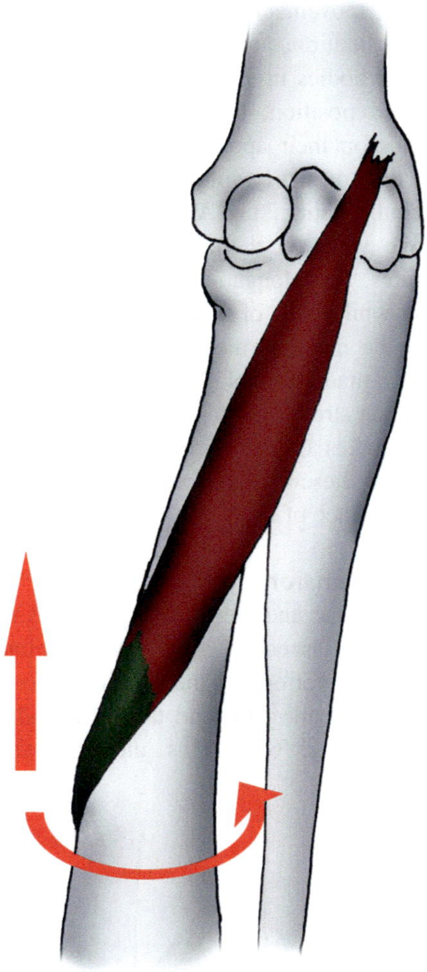

Fig. 6.4 Radial pronation and ascension components produced by the pronator teres

between the different structures of the first compartment. One possible cause of this ascent could be the pronator teres, which in addition to having a major pronation component, has an ascending component of the radius (Fig. 6.4). This ascent may also be caused by repetitive movements or a fall landing on the hands, resulting in radial ascension.

Activities

Occupational activity is often incriminated in the onset of DQ: during heavy tasks (housekeepers, carpenters, gardeners, butchers, fishmongers, cooks), during applied and fine but repetitive tasks (sign language interpreter, dactylographer, office workers, seamstress), as well as in certain artistic occupations (pianist) (Calvo-Cerrada et al. 2012; Rodineau 1991; Kutsumi et al. 2005). The repetitive movements incriminated mainly concern thumb abduction and ulnar inclination of the wrist (Redvers-Chubb 2016). According to Petit le Manac'h (Petit Le Manac'h et al. 2011), a higher prevalence of DQ has been observed in manual workers. Ranney et al. (1995) showed that DQ was the most prevalent wrist tendinous disorder in their study group of female manual workers performing highly repetitive tasks. In office workers, the incidence can reach 3.6% after 1 month's work and 14.7% after 1 year's work (Gerr et al. 2002).

Although many studies suggest that DQ may be work related, no large case series has demonstrated this. A systematic review and meta-analysis (Stahl et al. 2013) of manual occupations involving repetitive work, heavy labor, or ergonomically "stressful" work (inappropriate posture, prolonged movement) found no relationship between occupational risk factors and DQ. There is little evidence that this condition is caused directly by occupational activities, but the symptomatology can certainly be aggravated by the constraints involved in using the hand at work, at home, or in sports (Burge 2022).

This condition has also been reported in cases of tendon overuse during sports activities such as volleyball, golf, racket sports, rowing, canoeing, discus throwing, javelin throwing, cycling, and motorcycling (Jeyapalan and Choudhary 2009; Le Viet 1997; Rossi et al. 2005). Two studies have described the possible involvement of overuse of the cell phone for texting (Ashurst et al. 2010) or playing games (Ma et al. 2019). In their recent study of 500 patients, Ma et al. (Ma et al. 2019) identified three factors significantly ($p < 0.05$) correlated with a higher risk of DQ: prolonged playing time, playing frequency, and extended wrist posture during playing.

Intense, Prolonged, or Repeated Solicitations

Cook et al. (Cook and Purdam 2009; Cook et al. 2016) have proposed that in overuse tendinopathies, there is a continuum of tendon pathologies,

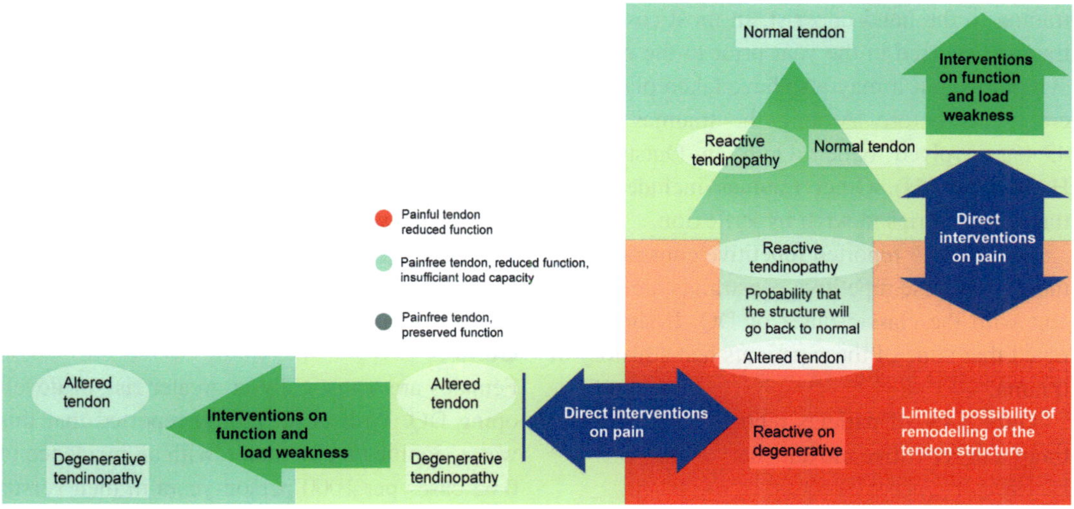

Fig. 6.5 Pathological continuum of the tendinopathies according to Cook et al.

with three main stages: reactive tendinopathy, reactive over-degenerative tendinopathy, and degenerative tendinopathy (Fig. 6.5).

The stages are described in different ways, but there is continuity between them. This model indicates that the addition or removal of load is the principal stimulus for the tendon to evolve along the continuum. Load appears to be a determining factor in the onset, improvement, or worsening of the pathology. Managing tendon stress is therefore the key to treating tendinopathies.

The various anatomical constraints associated with a varied combination of wrist and thumb movements over a prolonged period could be enough to trigger DQ. This condition is recognized in sign language interpreters (Bouillot 2011). This profession does not require any particular effort of strength, but rather a high degree of dexterity and mobility in both thumb and wrist, over prolonged durations. DQ is not systematically associated with a notion of force or load, it can also be linked to a notion of prolonged movement, in a constrained gliding space. Repetitive movements are also incriminated. This is shown by a higher prevalence among people in occupations or activities requiring repetitive wrist and thumb movements (Bystrom et al. 1995; Kurppa et al. 1991). Frictions within the first compartment are increased by repetitive glidings of the tendons in their sheaths. Ilyas et al. (2007) hypothesize that DQ may be secondary to sustained or repetitive tension on the tendons contained in the first dorsal compartment. This state of tension, generated by a fibroblastic response, would lead to swelling and thickening of the first compartment, resulting in discomfort when using the wrist and hand.

The thumb is the most used finger and the one with the greatest freedom of movement. Nguyen et al. (Nguyen et al. 2012) describe several gestures that could be incriminating in DQ: repeated flexion/extension movements of the wrist and fingers, prolonged maintenance of static postures when carrying heavy loads, and pronosupination, ulnar tilt, and wrist extension movements. Adams et al. (Adams and Habbu 2015) reported that activities involving repeated radioulnar deviations, such as hammering, could promote the onset of DQ. The Occupational Health and Safety Research Institute (IRSST) has highlighted various movements that most frequently stress the APL and EPB tendons (Patry et al. 1997). It is indicated that these different stresses may constitute risk factors for the onset of DQ. They include flexion/extension of the thumb with effort, and abduction or extension of the thumb under stress.

Trauma

A 2016 study (Redvers-Chubb 2016) found that 73.2% of patients with DQ had had a previous trauma to the hand or wrist. In most cases, this trauma occurred in the year prior to the onset of symptoms, but it may also have taken place several years before. Among the traumas found, 43.4% involved Fallen Onto an Outstretched Hand (FOOSH). Other traumas included fractures and injuries in wrist hyperflexion.

Only 24.4% reported repetitive constraints on the wrist. These repetitive constraints are consistent with the classic onset of DQ. It should be noted that none of these patients had a history of trauma.

Only 2.4% of patients reported no history of trauma or repetitive movements.

Muscle Weakness and Ligament Instability

The Redvers-Chubb study (Redvers-Chubb 2016) showed extensor carpi ulnaris (ECU) muscle weakness in 82.9% of patients with DQ. Ligament instability was also noted in 46.3% of patients. Among those with ligament instability, 84.7% reported the occurrence of a traumatic event in the three previous years, versus 54.5% in those without ligament instability, which is statistically significant ($p = 0.005$).

This chapter supports the idea that DQ is not always an isolated pathology but may be secondary to an underlying concomitant wrist condition. This condition may arise because of trauma, such as a sprain or ligament damage, and/or muscular weakness in the forearm, particularly in the ECU. The close collaboration between the ECU on the one hand and the APL and EPB on the other, as collateral stabilizers of the wrist, has been described by Van Oudenaarde et al. (1997) and Johanson et al. (1998). Weakness of the ECU may lead to over-solicitation of the APL and EPB muscles in order to compensate for the lack of stability and function. This over-solicitation could lead to the development of DQ.

Individual Factors

Age

DQ can affect all age groups, but epidemiological data from Wolf et al. (2009) indicate that age over 40 years is a significant risk factor. In their large study, the incidence was 0.6 cases per 1000 person-years in people under 20, compared with 2.0 cases per 1000 person-years in people over 40 years.

Petit le Manac'h et al. (2011) point out that these data are consistent with the physiological degeneration of tendons that occurs with advancing age.

Gender

Females are statistically at greater risk of developing DQ. Wolf et al. (2009) reported that this was a significant risk factor, with an incidence of 0.62 cases per 1000 person-years in men versus 2.81 cases per 1000 person-years in women ($p < 0.0001$).

It is difficult to determine the exact reason for this female predominance. Various hypotheses have been put forward, such as the impact of hormones, discussed below. On the other hand, anatomical variations according to gender have been ruled out by several studies: Beutel et al. (2020) found that men and women had a similar rate of double compartment (80% and 82.4%, respectively), and two cadaveric studies found no statistically significant difference between the genders regarding the presence of tendon variations or a septum (Shiraishi and Matsumura 2005; Mahakkanukrauh and Mahakkanukrauh 2000).

Pregnancy and Hormones

DQ is nicknamed "baby wrist" or "mother's thumb" (Vuillemin et al. 2012; Patel et al. 2013). These names suggest a possible close link between pregnancy and the onset of DQ. Young mothers seem to be particularly prone to it. In these cases, the age of onset is much lower (33 years old on average), and the involvement is often bilateral (Skoff 2001). We do not know whether this is due to hormonal changes during and after pregnancy, or to repeated child-raising movements (Burge 2022) that combine wrist flexion and ulnar tilt with thumb extension (Anderson et al. 2004). The condition occurs not only in young mothers but also in childminders. The clinical presentation is similar to that classically described in DQ, but resolution is often spontaneous and occurs once the child's lifting movements are less frequent (Avci et al. 2002; Laoopugsin and Laoopugsin 2012; Stahl et al. 2015).

Hormones also appear to play an important role. Vuillemin et al. (2012) have suggested that estrogen deficiency or excess may be a potential risk factor. This hypothesis seems to be confirmed by histological findings of hormonal receptors in the intermediate layer of the retinacula. Some hormonal treatments for breast cancer in post-menopausal women (aromatase inhibitors) have side-effects involving aggravation of musculoskeletal symptoms. Belkhir (2010) notes that this treatment leads to periarticular changes in 93% of cases, with DQ in 50%. Shen et al. (2015) reported that estrogen receptor (ER-β) expression was higher in patients with DQ, and that the degree of expression was related to disease severity. However, it is difficult to distinguish between the roles played by the mechanical constraints involved in caring for a newborn and the hormonal factors associated with pregnancy.

Other Factors

Tenosynovitis of the upper limb can be linked to a variety of comorbidities. These include hypothyroidism, gout, diabetes, ankylosing spondylitis, rheumatoid arthritis, and microbial or tuberculosis infections (Patry et al. 1997; Rosen and Weiland 1998; Lopes et al. 2008; Rettig 2004).

Laterality may also play a role in the onset of this condition. Unilateral involvement is most common, but bilateral involvement is also possible (Nguyen et al. 2012), particularly after pregnancy (Skoff 2001). According to Kay et al. (Kay 2000), hand dominance does not appear to influence the onset of DQ symptoms.

Genetic predisposition may also be linked to the onset of DQ. Kim et al. (2017) identified a genetic marker (rs35360670) on chromosome 8 that was significantly associated with DQ ($p = 1.9 \times 10^{-8}$). This study is the first to suggest genome-based screening for DQ. The presence of this DNA marker could be used to inform people, particularly at risk of developing DQ, to better prevent the onset of this condition.

Other factors have been identified as increasing the risk of DQ, notably psychosocial factors (anxiety, depression) (Stahl et al. 2013; Beleckas et al. 2018). The IRSST cites other factors such as cold, vibration, and glove wearing as possible contributors to the onset of this condition (Patry et al. 1997).

Clinical and Paraclinical Signs

Clinical Signs

The initial diagnosis of DQ is usually made based on clinical symptoms, in combination with a physical examination (Huisstede et al. 2014). Occasionally, further investigations may be required to confirm or refute the diagnosis.

Clinically, tenosynovitis will manifest itself in particular as a "symptomatic triad" (Artru 1999), which is to say the presence, in addition to pain on palpation, of pain on passive tensioning and resisted contraction of the tendon. The pain described by the patient will be increased by certain passive or active mobilizations of the thumb and wrist (de Quervain 1997; Batteson et al. 2008; Drossos et al. 2009). Pain-increasing movements include thumb abduction, wrist extension, and ulnar or radial deviation (De Quervain 2005; Ilyas et al. 2007; Adams and Habbu 2015; Patry et al. 1997).

Pain may also be exacerbated during resisted contractions of the APL and EPB muscles, particularly during resisted isometric extension and abduction movements of the thumb column (Bouillot 2011; Batteson et al. 2008; Harrington et al. 1998). In some advanced cases, pain may be always present (Bouillot 2011).

It is also pertinent to test the muscular strength of the wrist stabilizing muscles (particularly the ECU) in relation to the contralateral side and to report any ligament instability that may be related to previous trauma. This helps to shed light on any underlying pathology. These tests are not part of the usual assessment of a patient with DQ. They can highlight muscles or ligaments that may be affected, and thus guide treatment or indicate certain complementary tests (Redvers-Chubb 2016).

- *Provocation tests*

Since De Quervain (1997) described the clinical entity of DQ in 1895, much has been written about the diagnosis, etiology, pathology, and treatment of this condition. Various tests have also been proposed: the Finkelstein test, the Brunelli test, the Eichhoff test, and the WHAT test.

Here, we describe the Finkelstein test (the most widely used) and the WHAT test (offering the best sensitivity and specificity). These tests must be performed bilaterally by a qualified healthcare professional, with adequate knowledge of the anatomy of the wrist compartments, and an understanding of the clinical significance of the test results.

– *Finkelstein's test*

As discussed by Finkelstein in his paper (Finkelstein 1930), the maneuver results in intense pain. This seems to be in line with the biomechanical study by Kutsumi et al. (2005), which indicates that the test position generates significantly ($p < 0.05$) greater stress in terms of resistance and structural tension. It therefore seems important for practitioners to take this high pain threshold into consideration when performing the test. Thus, when carrying out the test, it seems logical to try to reach the diagnosis without causing intense pain to the patient.

Given the multitude of different descriptions of the Finkelstein test in the literature, and the errors that can be found in the execution of this maneuver, other authors have subsequently described this test more precisely. Dawson et al. (Dawson and Mudgal 2010), for example, recommend a progressive, well-tolerated three-step procedure for the accurate diagnosis of DQ, the last of which corresponds to the original maneuver described by Finkelstein.

As mentioned by Finkelstein (1930), the test that bears his name can result in severe pain. The multi-stage progression described by Dawson et al. (Dawson and Mudgal 2010) is designed to limit the induction of severe pain. In fact, these different stages put progressive constraints on the concerned structures. As soon as pain is felt, the test is stopped, allowing a precise diagnosis to be made, without necessarily doing the final maneuver which is likely to be very painful.

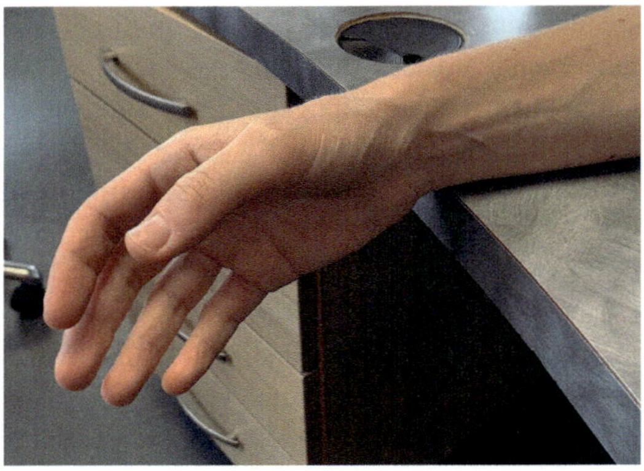

Fig. 6.6 The hand is placed at the edge of the table, with the forearm in a neutral rotation and the ulnar side of the wrist in contact with the table

The test is performed as follows (Dawson and Mudgal 2010): the patient sits in front of the examination table, facing the therapist. The tested upper limb is relaxed, with the ulnar part of the forearm resting on the table and the wrist outside the table, on the therapist's side. The forearm is held in neutral rotation (Fig. 6.6) (Bouillot 2011; Rosen and Weiland 1998; Rettig 2004). At first, the patient's pain is assessed without any external force being applied by the therapist. The aim here is to assess the patient's active ulnar deviation, helped by gravity. Patients in the acute phase may experience pain with this simple maneuver. The test is positive if the patient reports increased pain at the tip of the radial styloid (Dawson and Mudgal 2010) (Fig. 6.7). If this step does not cause pain, the therapist can apply a slight force to bring the hand into ulnar deviation, resulting in increased passive stretching of the structures of the first dorsal compartment (Fig. 6.8). The test is positive if the patient reports increased pain in the radial styloid process. If this does not cause pain either, the therapist can then perform the third stage of the test, which corresponds to the original maneuver described by Finkelstein (Finkelstein 1930). This last stage is suitable for patients with chronic pain who are unlikely to experience significant pain during the first two stages. In this last stage, the therapist grasps the thumb and gently moves it

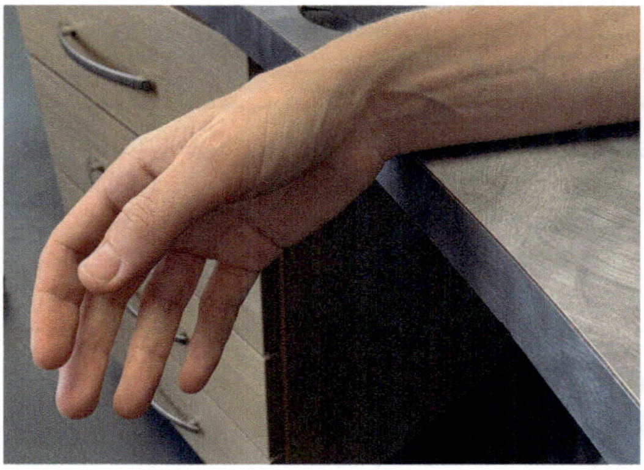

Fig. 6.7 The patient actively brings the wrist in ulnar inclination

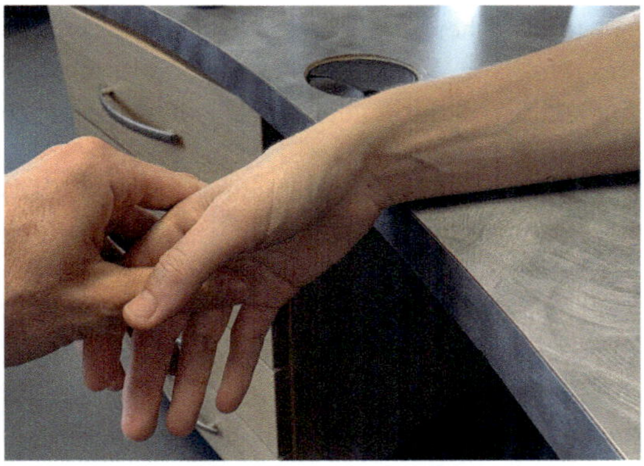

Fig. 6.8 The therapist increases the ulnar inclination

into passive flexion (Fig. 6.9). The test is positive when the patient feels increased pain at the tip of the radial styloid.

It should be noted that, although the Finkelstein test has long been regarded as a pathognomonic sign of DQ (Le Viet 2002), most clinicians and textbooks describe what is actually the Eichhoff test (Darowish and Sharma 2014; Elliott 1992; Waseem et al. 2005), where the thumb is placed in the fist and tightly gripped by the patient's long fingers.

– *WHAT test*

The WHAT test (Wrist Hyperflexion and Abduction of the Thumb test) was developed in response to the following constraints: make the patient as active as possible during the test, to control pain better and specifically target the tendons of the first dorsal compartment of the wrist

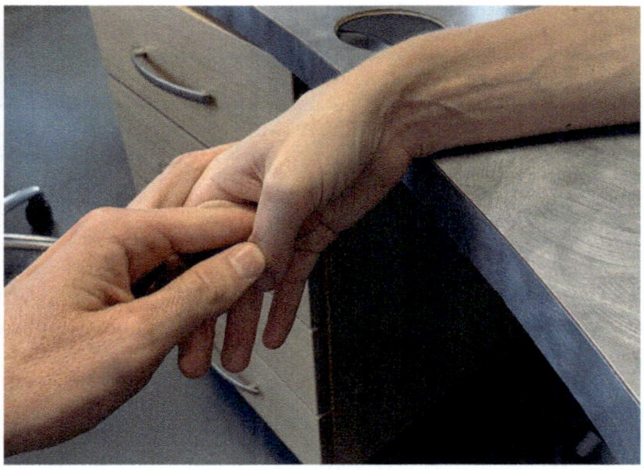

Fig. 6.9 In the final step, the therapist takes the patient's thumb and brings it in a passive flexion toward the palm. This last step corresponds to the maneuver originally described by Finkelstein

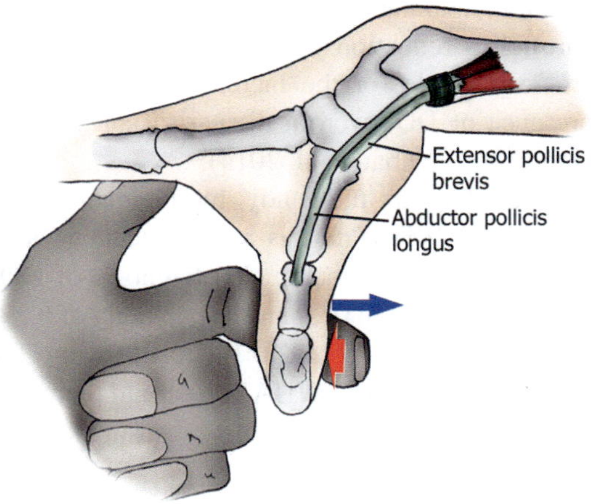

Fig. 6.10 What Test mechanism: the black arrow shows the place where the shearing mechanisms occur

(Goubau et al. 2014). The test is based on active mobilization by the patient, allowing him or her to interrupt the test at any time. Indeed, unlike a test performed passively by the therapist, it is the patient's own pain threshold that ends the test immediately, with a positive result.

The WHAT test is performed as follows: the patient is asked to flex the wrist as far as possible. The wrist is then held by the therapist in this position. The thumb is placed in abduction, with full extension of the metacarpophalangeal and interphalangeal joints. The therapist then applies an increasing resistance to thumb abduction (Fig. 6.10). When the patient is unable to main-

5 severity subgroups		5 duration subgroups
Symptoms	Pain	Duration (steps)
1 – Very light	Very light pain/other symptoms	1 – < 1 month (acute)
2 – Light	↓	2 – 1 < 2 months (subacute)
3 – Mild		3 – 2 < 3 months (subacute)
4 – Severe		4 – 3 < 6 months (chronic)
5 – Very severe	Unbearable pain/other symptoms	5 – > 6 months (chronic)

Fig. 6.11 De Quervain tenosynovitis classification depending on symptomatology

tain the force against the therapist, he or she is free to release the pressure and the test ends. Pain on resisted pressure against the therapist indicates a positive test result. In this configuration, the APL and EPB muscles are actively contracted, producing tension and shear on the distal end of the palmar surface of the first dorsal compartment's reflection pulley. These mechanisms are responsible for the increase of pain in the presence of DQ, even in the early stages of the pathology (Goubau et al. 2014).

According to the study by Goubau et al. (2014), the WHAT test is a more accurate tool than the Eichhoff test for the diagnosis of DQ, with a sensitivity of 0.99 and a specificity of 0.29, compared with 0.89 and 0.14, respectively, for the Eichhoff test. The WHAT test could therefore be adopted to guide clinical diagnosis in the early stages of this pathology.

- *Summary of the assessment*

Batteson et al. (2008) have proposed a seven-point diagnosis screening tool, known as the De Quervain Screening Tool (DQST), which considers various diagnosis criteria. The seven criteria are radial styloid pain, pain on movement, tenderness in the first extensor compartment, positive Finkelstein test, pain on extension of the thumb against resistance, swelling/edema in the first extensor compartment, and thickening of the APL and EPB tendon sheaths. It was developed by a panel of experts in the management of hand pathologies. The test has excellent inter-rater reliability and high test-retest reliability, with a high level of agreement on the seven criteria included (Rosen and Weiland 1998). It allows DQ to be distinguished from two other wrist disorders (carpal tunnel syndrome and osteoarthritis of the base of the thumb) with a sensitivity of 1 and a specificity of 1. However, the authors point out that further research is needed to determine the relevance of two criteria: the swelling and thickening of the tendon sheath, their presence being less frequent.

A European study (Huisstede et al. 2014) brought together experts in the management of hand pathologies to reach a consensus on the management of DQ. Five levels were created to highlight the relationship between severity and duration of the disease so that therapies could subsequently be adapted. The experts described the severity of DQ in terms of the amount of pain or severity of symptoms (from very mild to very severe). The duration of DQ was expressed in terms of the phase: acute, sub-acute or chronic, and the number of weeks or months required for recovery. The combination of these expressions made it possible to identify five sub-groups in terms of both severity and duration (Fig. 6.11) (Harrington et al. 1998).

- *Differential diagnosis*

Various pathologies can lead to localized pain in the radial styloid, looking like the symptoms of DQ. It is important to consider and diagnose these conditions, as they can lead to inappropriate and therefore ineffective therapies. The presence of these pathologies may be isolated or associated with DQ. Differential diagnosis includes cheiralgia paresthetica or Wartenberg syndrome (damage to the sensitive branch of the radial nerve), intersection syndrome (conflict between the first and second extensor compartments), scaphoid fracture, or rhizarthrosis.

Paraclinical Signs

Clinical findings alone can diagnose the presence of DQ. Imaging may be necessary in cases of uncertainty or if there are associated lesions. The literature describes several types of complementary exams to support the diagnosis. However, when the clinical symptoms are clear, the systematic use of such exams is not necessary (Ilyas et al. 2007).

- *X-rays*

In DQ, X-rays are usually normal. This examination will rule out any pathology with a bony origin, especially a fracture of the scaphoid or the lower extremity of the radius, as well as the presence of osteoarthritis of the base of the thumb. On the lateral side of the radius' cortex, we look for changes such as bone erosion, periosteal apposition, or focal bone condensation. These phenomena, sometimes perceptible at the level of the radial styloid, can directly irritate the first dorsal compartment (Ilyas et al. 2007; Darowish and Sharma 2014). The presence of such abnormalities is significantly ($p < 0.05$) correlated with the presence of DQ, but their assessment remains difficult. Periosteal appositions should not be confused with the physiological bone spur that can be observed on the lateral side of the radius' cortex, at the level of the fusion of the growth plate. It should be noted that the possible presence of a small radial bone ridge, indirectly showing the presence of a fibrous septum partitioning the first compartment, is not visible on X-rays (Chien et al. 2001).

- *Ultrasound*

Ultrasound is an excellent modality for exploring the anatomy of the first dorsal compartment. It has the advantage of being unexpensive, non-invasive, and does not expose patients or practitioners to radiation. It allows a precise assessment of local damage and anatomical variations.

Ultrasound can be used to see the presence of a septum (complete, partial, or absent) in the first extensor compartment, allowing us to define the type of tenosynovitis (type I: affecting the APL and EPB without signs of septum, or II: affecting the EPB alone). The presence of a bony ridge on which the septum inserts has also been described (Choi et al. 2011; Vuillemin et al. 2012; Rousset et al. 2010; Lee et al. 2014a). According to Kwon et al. (2010), ultrasound has been shown to be 100% sensitive and 96% specific in detecting a persistent intra-compartmental septum after treatment. It is very useful for detecting a septum and ensuring that the drug injected during infiltration diffuses throughout the sub-compartments (Hajder et al. 2013). However, despite its high sensitivity and specificity, a thin or incomplete septum may not be detected, as reported by Nagaoka et al. (2000) and Kwon et al. (2010). A thickening of the retinaculum can also be observed on ultrasounds (Bouillot 2011; Revue médicale suisse 2022).

Ultrasound can also detect a hyperintense Doppler signal in the retinaculum or sheath, reflecting possible secondary inflammatory phenomena (Revue médicale suisse 2022; Vuillemin et al. 2012; Volpe et al. 2010). It may also reveal thickening of the tendons (Bouillot 2011; Jeyapalan and Choudhary 2009) or of the synovial sheath surrounding the APL and EPB tendons (Rousset et al. 2010; Volpe et al. 2010). Dynamic ultrasonography may reveal impaired tendon movement due to fibrous adhesions in chronic diseases (Jeyapalan and Choudhary 2009).

Different anatomical variations of the tendons can also be identified by ultrasound, such as the presence of tendon divisions (Rousset et al. 2010; Daenen et al. 2004). The transversal appearance of these multiple tendons in a sub-compartment looks like a lotus root and has therefore been described as the "lotus root" sign (Fig. 6.12) (Choi et al. 2011).

Several studies have demonstrated the utility of ultrasound in the diagnosis and treatment of DQ. It appears to be a reference exam in the presence of this pathology, making it possible to complete the clinical diagnosis (Bouillot 2011) and to provide precise data essential to the proposed treatment (infiltration, surgery) (Revue médicale suisse 2022).

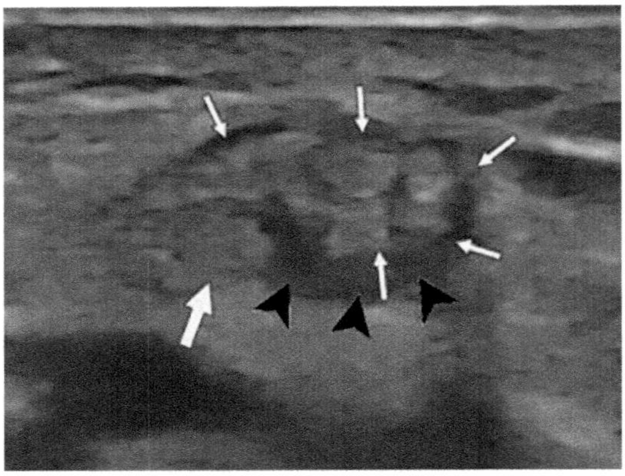

Fig. 6.12 Echography showing the tendon divisions of the APL (thin white arrows) corresponding to the "lotus root" sign, with a synovial thickening around (black arrow). The EPB tendon seems distinct (thick white arrow)

- *Magnetic Resonance Imaging*

Although highly effective, Magnetic Resonance Imaging (MRI) is of limited diagnostic value, given the data provided by ultrasound. It can reveal the presence of an effusion or thickening of the synovial sheath, a multiplicity of tendons or an increase in tendinous volumes, possible infiltration of subcutaneous tissue, and/or signal abnormalities within the tendons themselves (tendinosis) (Nguyen et al. 2012; Goyal et al. 2018). The study by Hadidy et al. (2009) showed that ultrasound was more accurate in identifying a septum or the thickening of the tendon or synovium.

Therapeutic Process

Conservative Treatment

While DQ can sometimes disappear spontaneously within a few weeks, the majority of cases require treatment to ensure a cure and avoid chronicity (Nguyen et al. 2012). Initial treatment is generally conservative and should be carried out as early as possible (Patry et al. 1997; Huisstede et al. 2014; Ilyas 2009).

- *Rest and stress management*

Rest corresponds to a total or partial cessation of the offending activities. It is often recommended for several weeks (Nguyen et al. 2012; Ilyas et al. 2007; Patry et al. 1997; Fichez 2006). The Cook et al. model (Cook and Purdam 2009; Cook et al. 2016) mentioned earlier (Fig. 6.5) indicates that the management of the stress applied to the tendon appears to be a key factor in improving the pathology. However, there is no real evidence of its effectiveness in improving symptoms (Moore 1997; Hadianfard et al. 2014; Richie and Briner 2003; Menendez and Ring 2014).

- *Non-Steroidal Anti-Inflammatory drugs*

Many DQ patients are prescribed non-steroidal anti-inflammatory drugs (NSAIDs) on their first visit to the physician, to manage their pain (Ilyas et al. 2007; Ilyas 2009; Jaworski et al. 2010). Although they are frequently used, they do not appear to bring improvement in most cases (Nguyen et al. 2012).

However, determining the efficiency of NSAIDs is not easy as they are often combined with other treatment modalities in most studies about their use in DQ (Lane et al. 2001; Jirarattanaphochai et al. 2004). The prospective study by Jirarattanaphochai et al. (Jirarattanaphochai et al. 2004) demonstrated no additional benefit from adding nimesulide (a NSAID) to corticosteroid injection in a prospective randomized double-blind study of 160 patients.

- *Orthosis*

Although some studies have indicated an inefficiency of the orthosis (Richie and Briner Jr 2003; Menendez et al. 2015), many authors recommend resting orthoses (Nguyen et al. 2012; Ilyas et al. 2007; Adams and Habbu 2015; Mardani-Kivi et al. 2014; Mehdinasab and Alemohammad 2010).

A 2016 literature review and meta-analysis (Cavaleri et al. 2016) indicates that combining orthosis and corticosteroid injection is more effective than the injection alone in the treatment of DQ. Significantly more participants ($p < 0.05$)

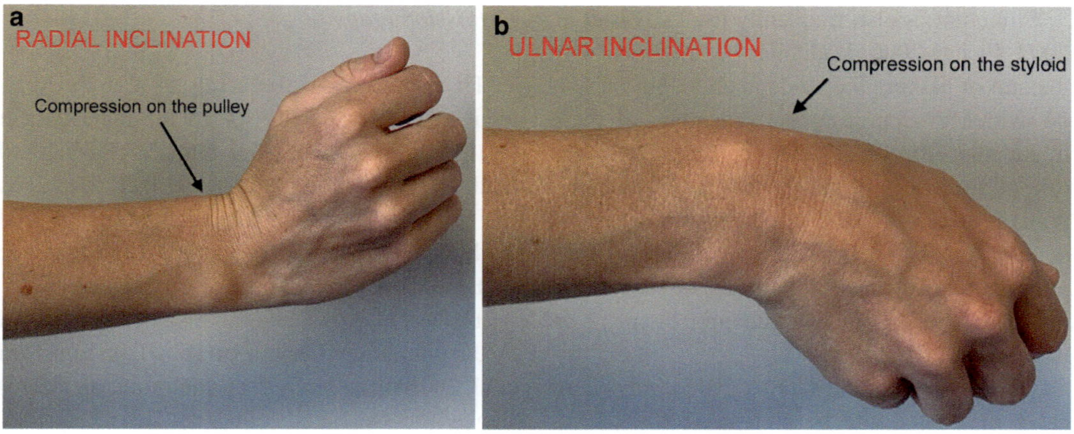

Fig. 6.13 Compression forces in radial (**a**) and ulnar (**b**) wrist inclinations

were successfully treated with a combined orthosis/corticosteroid injection approach than with the orthosis alone and the injections alone.

A European consensus (Huisstede et al. 2014) has been adopted, recommending wearing an orthosis for 3–8 weeks, 24 h a day. Wearing an orthosis is meant to reduce the load exerted on the tenons by relieving them of all mechanical constraints. This eliminates friction and reduces damage to the synovial sheath and tendons, reducing symptomatology (Ashe et al. 2004). The orthosis is designed so that the thumb and hand are aligned with the radius. This limits the tension on the reflection pulley (when the thumb is abducted) or the compression against the radial styloid (when the wrist is in ulnar inclination or the thumb in adduction) (Bouillot 2011) (Fig. 6.13) (Gonzalez et al. 1995; Bystrom et al. 1995; Finkelstein 1930; Dawson and Mudgal 2010).

The interphalangeal joint of the thumb is free, as its mobilization is ensured by the EPL muscle which is not involved in DQ. To limit compression, the orthosis is hollowed at the level of the painful area. The patient must be told how to position the orthosis in the correct position: the straps must be tight to avoid any leverage at the level of the wrist. The straps at the level of the painful area can be looser. When putting on and removing the orthosis, the patient must respect the axis of the thumb column. Once in place, the patient is told to "relax" (Bouillot 2011).

- *Rehabilitation and "gestures" education*
  - *"Gestures" education*
  - It may be necessary, to adapt activities or equipment to get a neutral position of the wrist in various situations. Carrying a load, for example, places the wrist in ulnar deviation with flexion of the metacarpophalangeal joint of the thumb, reproducing the painful kinematics. Depending on the patient, the use of an ergonomic keyboard, or adapting tools so that the wrist is in a neutral position, are examples of possible equipment adaptations that can be added to their daily activities (Robinson 2003).
  - *Rehabilitation*

- *Manual Modalities*

In the presence of edema (reactive phase), massages from distal to proximal can be used to facilitate the reintegration of fluids into the lymphatic circulation. As the effects are temporary, it will be useful to educate the patient on how to perform these techniques. The use of compression garments may also be considered (Goel and Abzug 2015).

After the reactive phase, deep transversal massage (DTM) on the APL and EPB tendons is one of the treatment modalities indicated in several articles (Ilyas et al. 2007; Fichez 2006). Nguyen et al. (2012) recommend 15 minutes of DTM, 3 times a week.

Stretching is also frequently used (Ilyas et al. 2007; Fichez 2006; Hadianfard et al. 2014) with the aim of making the tendons glide, but there is no evidence supporting the efficiency of these treatments. According to Ashe et al. (2004), the role of stretching in the treatment of tendinosis remains uncertain. The effects of stretching on degenerated tendon tissue are poorly understood, and many questions remain to be answered, including the impact of stretching intensity on therapeutic efficiency.

Gerlac (Gerlac and Gerlac 2015), who indicated that DQ could be associated with radius ascension possibly linked to the ascending component of the pronator teres, proposes a three-stage rehabilitation. The first step consists of stretching the pronator teres, thought to be responsible for this ascension. In the second stage, it is suggested to pull the radius distally to reduce friction when the tendons penetrate the sheath, the angle of attack being less aggressive (Fig. 6.14). The third and final stage involves concentric muscle strengthening of the muscles antagonistic to the pronator teres (the muscles doing the ulnar inclination) (Fig. 6.15). The aim is to stabilize the radius in a position that places less stress on the APL and EPB tendons, and to recreate a balance of muscular force moments. It should also be noted that, according to the same study, maintained traction on the radius during the Finkelstein test in patients with DQ makes the test negative in 98% of tested subjects.

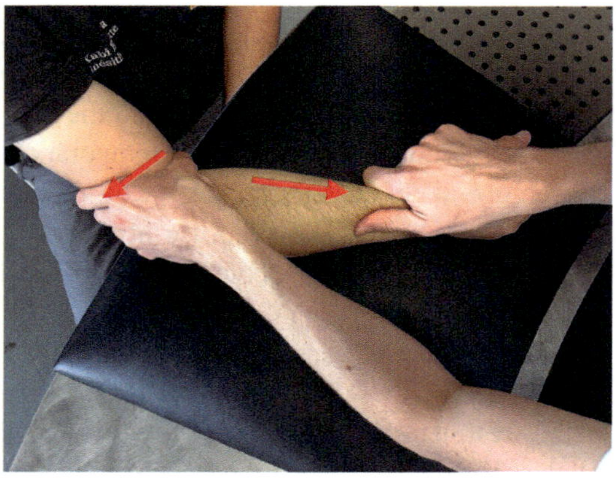

Fig. 6.14 Grip and counter-grip for a distal traction of the radius

- *Physiotherapy*

Thermotherapy is frequently used in the treatment of DQ, especially for edema management (De Quervain 2005; de Quervain 1997; Hadianfard et al. 2014; Goel and Abzug 2015). It is used as ice application, hot pad, or alternating hot and cold (Nguyen et al. 2012), but there is no evidence of its efficiency in the management of DQ.

The use of ultrasound has also been described in the literature (Ferrara et al. 2020; Lunsford et al. 2016). The study by Lunsford et al. (2016) showed a beneficial effect of low-frequency pulsed ultrasound in the treatment of DQ, with a statistically significant improvement in the numerical pain score ($p = 0.046$). Hassan et al. (2013) compared two groups, one with ultrasound use, and the other without, to determine the efficiency of ultrasound. They showed a statistically significant improvement in pain ($p < 0.05$) in the ultrasound group compared with the no-ultrasound group. 96% of patients in the ultrasound group had a VAS (Visual Analog Scale) pain score between 0 and 4, compared with 52% in the no-ultrasound group. The post-treatment pain score showed a significant improvement ($p < 0.01$) in patients in the ultrasound group (72%) compared to the non-ultrasound group (24%). In the non-ultrasound group, 16% of subjects were completely healed (no pain, tenderness, and swelling), compared with 32% in the ultrasound group.

Laser therapy also appears to be effective in the management of DQ (Ferrara et al. 2020), as is iontophoresis, a therapeutic modality used to control pain (Goel and Abzug 2015). According to Lunsford et al. (Lunsford et al. 2016), iontophoresis with dexamethasone, an anti-inflammatory agent, has a statistically significant effect in the treatment of DQ, with an improvement in the Quick-DASH functional score ($p = 0.028$).

- *Corticosteroid injections*

Corticosteroid injection into the first dorsal compartment is perhaps the most common and effective treatment for DQ. A 2015 systematic

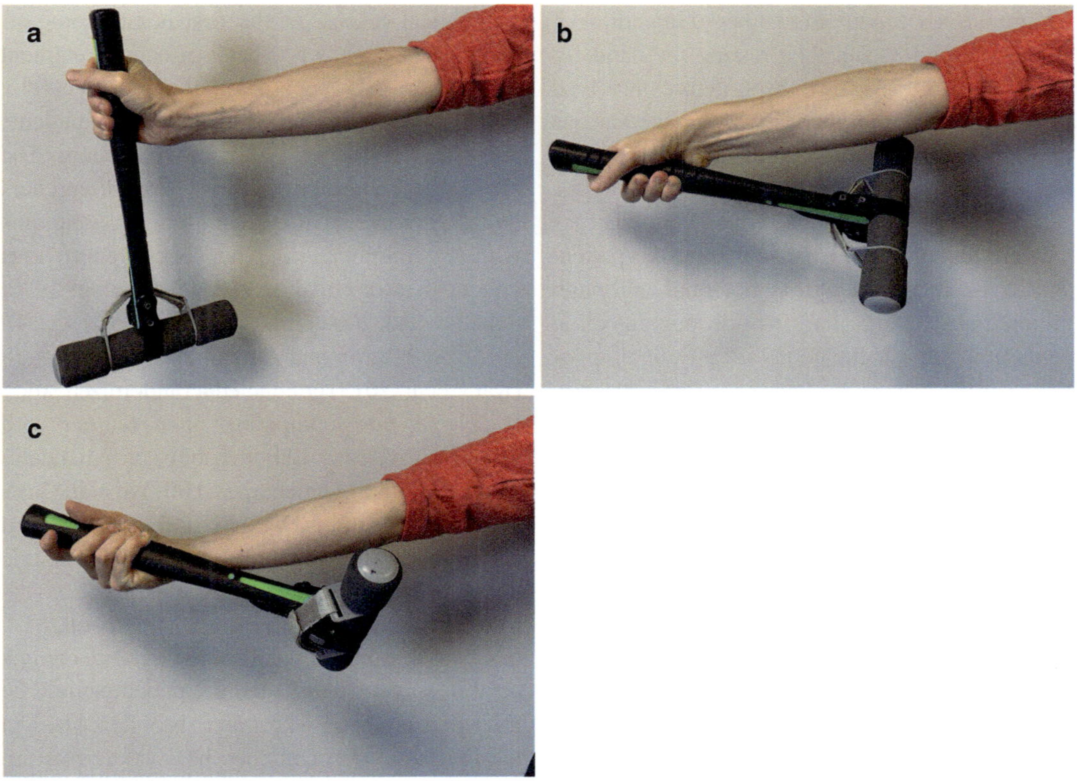

Fig. 6.15 (**a**, **b**, **c**) Concentric exercise for the muscle's antagonist to the APL and EPB

review and meta-analysis (Rowland et al. 2015) of 165 patients found that corticosteroid injection resulted in a statistically significant ($p < 0.05$) improvement in symptom resolution, pain, and hand function. A quantitative literature review by Richie et al. (Richie and Briner Jr 2003) reported a healing rate of 83% in 226 wrists from seven experimental studies. Various success rates have been reported in the literature, ranging from 58 to 100% (Avci et al. 2002; Lane et al. 2001; Zingas et al. 1998; Witt et al. 1991).

Corticosteroids are injected into the first dorsal compartment (Rettig 2004; Jaworski et al. 2010; Harvey et al. 1990). Poor response to corticosteroid injection has been correlated with poor technique (injection outside the sheath) and anatomical variations in the first dorsal compartment, especially the presence of a septum (Hajder et al. 2013; Ilyas et al. 2007; Richie and Briner Jr 2003; Harvey et al. 1990; Mirzanli et al. 2012). Plotkin et al. (Plotkin et al. 2016) recommend using an injection technique adapted to the ultrasound results, as a steroid injection in the first extensor compartment may not disperse around the two tendons if there is an intermediate septum. Two separate injections may be necessary if a septum is discovered. Ultrasound can also be used during infiltration to guide the injection into the tendon sheath with greater precision, and to select the pathological compartment (one compartment alone can be concerned) to avoid failures that could be explained by infiltration into the healthy compartment (Volpe et al. 2010). A recent randomized study demonstrated the superiority of ultrasound-guided injections over injections performed with an anatomical landmark when an intra-compartmental septum is present (Kume et al. 2012).

A second injection can be performed after a delay of 5 to 8 weeks in a patient who has experienced an improvement in symptoms following the first injection but continues to report discomfort (Ilyas et al. 2007; Patel et al. 2013). A European consensus (Huisstede et al. 2014) recommends a maximum number of injections of between 1 and 3, and then resting the hand for 7 days to avoid stressing the structures involved in DQ. If symptoms persist after these various infiltrations, and other pathologies have been ruled out, surgery may be considered.

After an infiltration, various complications may be found. Before the injection, the patient should be informed of the potential, although minor, risks, which may include post-injection pain, infection, subcutaneous atrophy, depigmentation of the skin at the injection site (especially in dark-skinned subjects), and neuritis of the sensitive branch of the radial nerve (Richie and Briner Jr 2003; Jirarattanaphochai et al. 2004; Anderson et al. 1991; Neustadt 1991; Sampson et al. 1994). Hajder et al. (Hajder et al. 2013), in their study of 71 wrists, reported a complication rate of 8%, the most frequent complication being local depigmentation of the skin. Injection directly into the tendon should be avoided, as it may weaken it. Tendon rupture, although unusual, may occur (Ilyas et al. 2007; Nguyen and Jones 2012; Wharton et al. 2015).

Although the latter therapeutic modality is the most effective, there is no clear consensus as to which conservative treatment protocols confer the best results (Abi-Rafeh et al. 2020).

Surgery

- *Description, results, and complications*

In the event of persistent pain or recurrence despite conservative measures, surgery is indicated (Nguyen et al. 2012; Huisstede et al. 2014). The surgical intervention consists of releasing the first dorsal compartment by longitudinally transecting the extensor retinaculum. Once the sheath has been released, the entire first compartment needs to be explored to identify the presence of a septum. If one or more sub-compartments are present, they will also be freed. The presence of a sub-compartment has been identified as a factor increasing the risk of surgical failure if not identified, with a risk of recurrence or residual symptoms (Matzon et al. 2019; Ilyas et al. 2007).

Surgical release of the first dorsal compartment has been shown to be an effective treatment for DQ. A 10-year study of 91 patients by Scheller et al. (2009) found that 100% of patients achieved long-term symptom resolution. The "cure rate," as described by several researchers (corresponding to the resolution of symptoms without complications), has been reported as greater than or equal to 91% (Finkelstein 1930; Scheller et al. 2009; Lapidus and Fenton 1952; Ta et al. 1999; Zarin and Ahmad 2003). Kang et al. (Kang et al. 2013) conducted a randomized study of 52 patients, comparing open release with endoscopic release. In both groups, a statistically significant improvement ($p < 0.001$) in pain (VAS score) and function (DASH score) was measured at 12 and 24 weeks post-surgery. They conclude that this less invasive surgical method delivers results as satisfactory as the open approach.

Although rare, several surgical complications need to be considered, and the patient should be informed of them. The main risks described in the literature are mentioned here (Matzon et al. 2019; Adams and Habbu 2015; Sampson et al. 1994; Belsole 1981; White and Weiland 1984). As said earlier, there is a risk of recurrence or residual symptoms in the event of incomplete release of the first compartment. There also is a risk of skin adhesions or scarring, which early mobilization will attempt to fight. Nerve damage to the superficial branch of the radial nerve may also occur, and intraoperative precautions should be taken to limit this risk. In some cases, section of the extensor retinaculum, which acts as a pulley, may be accompanied by tendon protrusion due to an anterior subluxation of the tendons during thumb retropulsion and wrist flexion movements. Some authors suggest reconstruction of part or all of the radial styloid pulley to avoid this protrusion, although this brings a risk of recurrence (Nguyen et al. 2012). Risks of scar complications (infection, hypertrophy, hypersensitivity) and the secondary development of complex regional pain syndrome (CRPS) have also been described.

- *Post-operative care*

The bandage is kept on for around 10 to 15 days, and an analgesic treatment is administered. The hand should be elevated above the level of the heart as much as possible to limit the development of edema. It will be necessary to mobilize the patient's fingers the day after the operation to limit joint stiffness (Huisstede et al. 2014).

As soon as the stitches have been removed, the scar should be cleaned frequently and massaged to limit adhesions and promote gliding (Bouillot 2011). DTM can be performed to limit the development of scar tissue, which could create adhesions and restrict thumb and wrist mobility (Goel and Abzug 2015).

Desensitization of the scar and nerves can be performed if the patient reports scar hypersensitivity (Ilyas et al. 2007; Goel and Abzug 2015). This desensitization can be achieved using Transcutaneous Vibratory Stimulation (TVS) devices (Watson et al. 2010). Initiated at the periphery of the painful area, they are progressively applied at the level of the painful point. Other forms of desensitization include exposure of the scar or skin to a variety of textures, including soft, rough, dull, and moist objects for sensory rehabilitation (Goel and Abzug 2015). Painful sensitivity may persist for several months, but this should not limit the use of the hand.

Ilyas et al. (2007) report that an orthosis immobilizing the thumb and wrist for 1–2 weeks is recommended following release surgery to restrict thumb activity and promote the healing of the structures. They add that the orthosis is usually taken off when the stitches are removed (10–14 days after surgery).

- *Prevention and patient education*

Daily and professional activities will be analyzed and discussed with the patient to identify possible risk factors and prevent recurrences (Patry et al. 1997). Information on risk factors and minor adjustments can help to reduce the risk of pain in the upper limbs, and thus help to avoid the onset of the resulting MSDs (Calvo-Cerrada et al. 2012).

A European study (Huisstede et al. 2014) involving experts in the management of hand pathologies reported a consensus regarding the instructions to be given to patients in the presence of DQ. This same study also indicated that these recommendations should always be given to the patients, whatever treatment is used. These instructions are divided into three levels: activity instructions, function instructions, and pain management instructions. Activity instructions focus on patient-specific activities that may increase symptoms. Function instructions refer to specific movements or gestures to be avoided, such as repetitive movements of the thumb and wrist, significant flexion of the thumb, or ulnar deviation of the wrist. Pain management instructions will focus on avoiding painful hand movements and powerful manual movements whenever possible, and on recognizing signs of overuse.

In the event of surgery, certain recommendations should also be given to the patient, such as raising the hand above the heart to limit edema or mobilizing the fingers several times a day to avoid scar adhesions and joint stiffness. Carrying heavy loads and intensive activities should be avoided for 2–6 weeks after the surgery, and the hand should be rested. All these recommendations on the preventive measures to be taken play an essential role in preventing symptoms from worsening or recurring (Patry et al. 1997).

It is also important to inform the patient about the pathology and the duration of the healing process, and to indicate a realistic and appropriate recovery timetable. Ashe et al. (2004) suggest that clinicians prepare their patients for a recovery period of several months rather than weeks. Information can help patients take a calmer approach to their condition and empower them to take an active role in its management (Bouillot 2011).

- *Therapy hierarchy*

A European consensus (Huisstede et al. 2014) has been reached on a therapeutic hierarchy. Treatment options have been classified hierarchically (Fig. 6.16), according to the sequence in

	THERAPEUTIC HIERARCHY
1	IN (instructions + NSAI)
2	IO (Instructions + orthosis)
3	INO (Instructions + NSAI + orthosis)
4	IC (Instructions + corticoid injection)
5	ICO (Instructions + corticoid injection + orthosis)
6	IS (Instructions + surgery)

Fig. 6.16 Proposition of therapeutic hierarchy

Table 6.1 Potential therapeutic options depending on the severity and duration of the De Quervain tenosynovitis

DURATION ↑	1 Very benign symptoms			2 Begnin syptoms			3 Mild symptoms			4 Severe symptoms			5 Very severe symptoms		
5 Chonic stage ≥ 6 months									IS			IS			IS
			ICO			ICO									
4 Chronic stage 3 ≤ 6 months		IC			IC			IC	IS		IC	IS			IS
			ICO			ICO			ICO			ICO			
3 Subacute stage 2 ≤ 3 months	IO			IO	IC		IO	IC	IS		IC	IS		IC	IS
		INO			INO	ICO		INO	ICO			ICO			ICO
2 Subacute stage 1 ≤ 2 months	IO			IO	IC		IO	IC			IC			IC	
	IN	INO		IN	INO	ICO		INO	ICO			ICO			ICO
1 Acute stage ≤ 1 months	IO			IO	IC		IO	IC			IC			IC	
	IN	INO		IN	INO			INO							

Very light pain / other symptoms → Unbearable pain / other symptoms

→ SEVERITY

IN: Instructions + no steroidal anti-inflammatory drugs
IO: Instructions + orthosis
INO: Instructions + no steroidal anti-inflammatory drugs + orthosis
IC: Instructions + corticoid injection
ICO: Instructions + corticoid injection + orthosis
ICh: Instructions + surgery

which they are logically prescribed, to guide physicians and therapists. This approach can, of course, be adapted to suit each patient and his or her history. Each proposed treatment is combined with patient instructions. Therapies include NSAIDs, orthosis, corticosteroid injection, and surgery.

Experts have suggested that the main factors in choosing a treatment option are the severity of the disease, the duration of the disease, and previously given treatments (Huisstede et al. 2014). Depending on duration and severity, a summary table of possible treatment options has been proposed (Table 6.1).

Conclusion

De Quervain's tenosynovitis, although common (INRS 2022b), is a complex and poorly understood condition. It affects the tendons of the APL and EPB muscles, which run in the first dorsal compartment of the extensors (Ilyas et al. 2007). A mismatch between container and content leads to stenosis and thickening of this fibrous corridor, increasing friction between the various structures (Nguyen et al. 2012). The exact mechanisms and causes of this pathology are still unclear but appear to be linked to a variety of intertwined risk factors, making it difficult to identify any of them with certainty.

The complexity of this condition is also reflected in the difficulties found in making the diagnosis. This diagnosis is usually based on a combination of clinical signs and detailed questioning. Various provocation tests have been developed, but the most used are not necessarily the most reliable, and their reproduction by therapists remains uncertain (Waseem et al. 2005). Complementary exams, especially ultrasound, can support the diagnosis (Kwon et al. 2010), but their use is not systematic.

Treatment is conservative at first, with corticosteroid injections giving very good results (Rowland et al. 2015). The use of n orthosis, combined with infiltration, is also a recommended treatment modality (Cavaleri et al. 2016). Other therapeutic modalities, such as physiotherapy techniques, are generally implemented as part of the patient's care pathway, despite the limited level of evidence of their efficiency. These techniques are poorly documented in the literature, and the few studies that do exist have no conclusions with a high level of evidence. Surgery can be used as a second-line treatment when non-surgical therapies fail, with very good results and a high level of evidence.

Tendinopathies of the Extensor Carpi Ulnaris

Physiopathology

During pronation and supination movements of the forearm, the tendons in the first five extensor compartments follow the movements of the radius. This behavior is explained by a system of partitions linking the extensor retinaculum to the radius. However, the tendon of the extensor carpi ulnaris (ECU), which runs in the sixth extensor compartment, does not belong to the radius, and is therefore not constrained by the extensor retinaculum, but by the tendon sheath of the EUC (Fig. 6.17) (Garcia-Elias 2015).

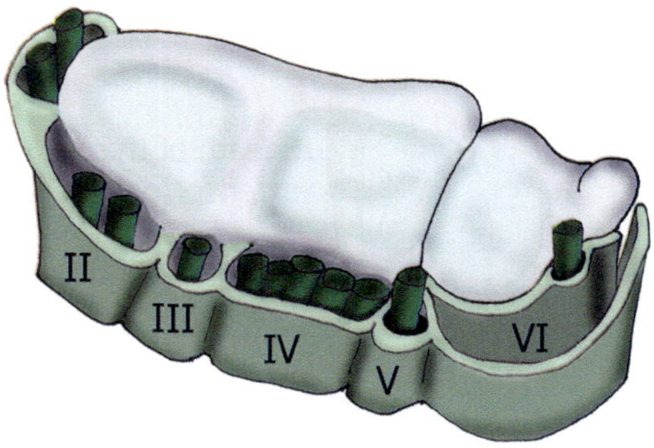

Fig. 6.17 Dorsal compartments of the wrist: extensor compartments (I–VI), extensor retinaculum (light green), ECU tendon, under-sheath of the ECU (dark green)

When activated, the ECU tendon contributes to reducing the dorsal translation of the ulna by almost 30%. However, this attenuating force is neutralized when the under-sheath of the ECU is severed. Spinner and Kaplan (Spinner and Kaplan 1970) have highlighted the role of the ECU and its sheath as secondary stabilizers of the distal radioulnar joint. Moreover, as the position of the ECU relative to other wrist structures changes with forearm pronosupination, its tendon must be both mobile and stable.

Under normal conditions, the under-sheath of the ECU can neutralize the dislocating force of the ECU. This neutralization must allow the tendon to slide freely and ensure a sufficient tendon stability. If it is excessively constrained, the tendon may eventually develop lesions. If, on the other hand, the tendon is excessively loose, it loses its effectiveness. In both cases, the wrist eventually becomes dysfunctional and symptomatic (Garcia-Elias 2015).

The unique anatomical configuration of the ECU tendon and its osteofibrous tunnel may predispose it to pathologies. During the forearm rotation, the ECU tendon remains fixed proxi-

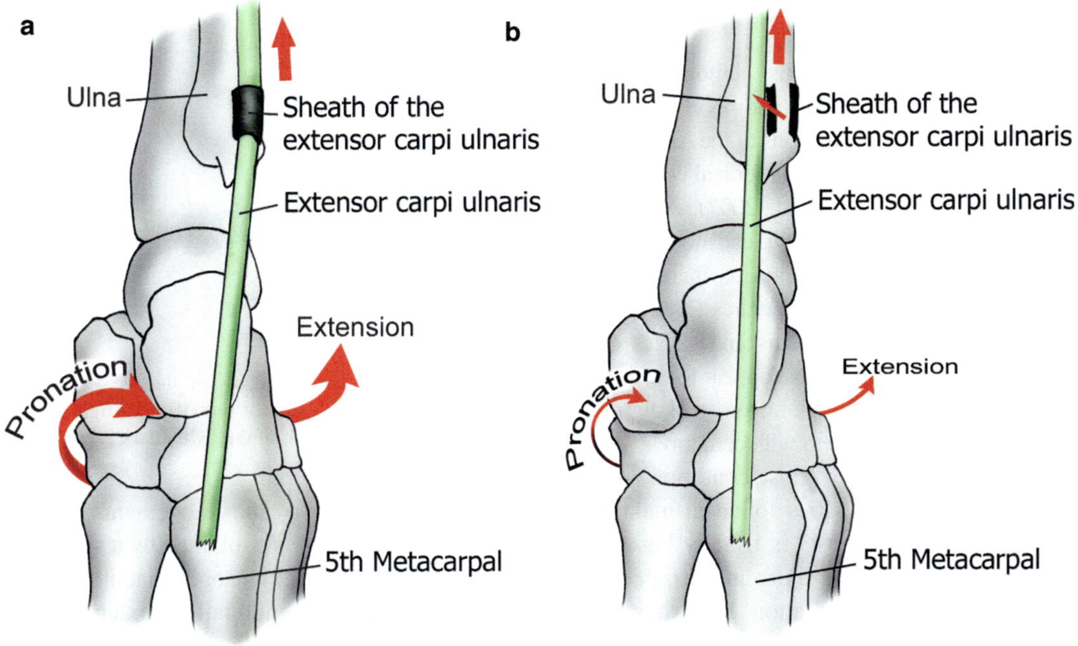

Fig. 6.18 (**a**) Location of the ECU tendon, with its insertion of the basis of the fifth metacarpal. (**b**) Palmar subluxation of the ECU after section of its sheath, causing the loss of its mechanical advantage on the distal part of the ulna

mally along the ulnar groove in the sixth dorsal compartment but must slide more distally over the ulnar styloid to allow full rotation. In the event of trauma, depending on the force involved, the ECU and sixth compartment may be damaged. In the most extreme cases, the medial wall of the compartment is torn, and the tendon may subluxate in palmar, exiting the ulnar groove (Crimmins and Jones 1995).

When the sheath of the ECU is ruptured, the pronation of the scaphoid and capitate decreases significantly, by up to 40% and 50%, respectively. This is because the ECU moves toward palmar and loses its mechanical advantage (Fig. 6.18). This fact may be relevant in cases of partially incompetent ligaments, especially those located on the ulnar side of the wrist, where the carpus could be dynamically destabilized, revealing a previously asymptomatic ligament injury (Salva-Coll et al. 2012).

The structures that stabilize the tendon of the ECU can be damaged in various sports activities, such as tennis, golf, or rugby (Campbell et al. 2013); or sports practiced with an object such as a racket, club, bat, or ball (Graham 2012a).

At abnormally high loads, the constraints generated by this type of activity can cause permanent damage to the concerned structures (Shaaban et al. 2006). The tendon of the ECU is a frequent target of this type of stress, especially when the wrist is in flexion, ulnar inclination, and full supination (Allende and Le Viet 2005; Inoue and Tamura 1998; Yamabe et al. 2012) (Fig. 6.19).

This combination of movements places maximum stress on the ECU's under-sheath and is explained from a biomechanical point of view: in pronation, the ECU rests in the center of the groove and adopts a direct path toward its distal insertion. Therefore, in pronation, there is minimal force on the under-sheath and the ECU serves as a pure ulnar deviator of the wrist. In supination, the ECU translates radially. There is maximum stress on the under-sheath because the ECU now takes an oblique path toward its insertion (Ruchelsman and Vitale 2016). When the wrist is in this position, not only is the tendon of

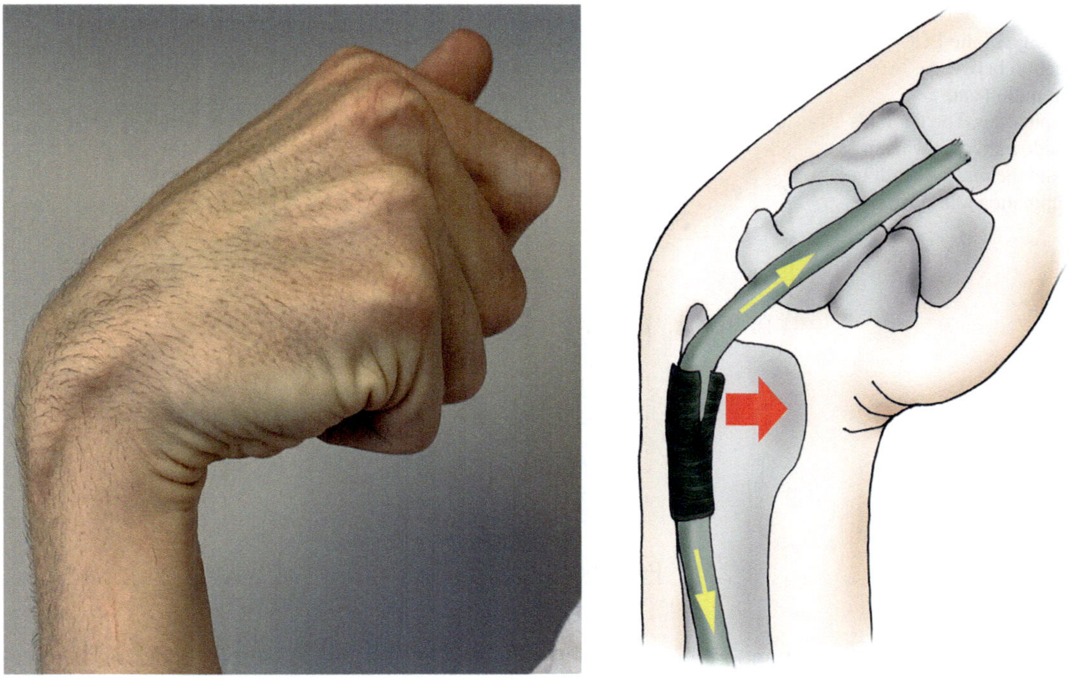

Fig. 6.19 Position in which the ECU tendon (light green) is in maximal tension (yellow arrows). This position combines flexion, ulnar inclination, and supination. It is in this position that the risk of injury of the under-sheath (dark green) by a violent ECU contraction is highest: palmar subluxation (red arrow)

the ECU extremely tight, but there is also a maximum risk of it dislocating out of its compartment (Spinner and Kaplan 1970; Kauer 1992). The tendon lies in the deepest part of the groove of the ECU in maximum pronation and tends to subluxate in maximum supination (Singh et al. 2016).

There is an angulation between the axis of the tendon in its proximal part and the axis of the tendon at its insertion on the base of the fifth metacarpal, even in a neutral wrist position. This angle increases when the wrist is in supination and ulnar deviation. If there is an inadequate containment, the contraction forces of the ECU muscle result in a medial force vector that favors tendon subluxation (Graham 2012a; Wolfe 2011; Montalvan et al. 2006; Hosteins 2015).

As the forearm moves from a neutral position toward supination, the ECU emerges from the under-sheath at an increasingly acute angle, reaching its maximum at around 30° supination (Fig. 6.20). An ulnar deviation accentuates this angle, as does the resulting ulnar translational force applied by the tendon to the under-sheath of the ECU (Campbell et al. 2013; Graham 2012a).

Tension on the retinaculum and under-sheath of the ECU is therefore greater during activities involving forearm supination, especially when this position is associated with wrist flexion and ulnar deviation. This combination of positions occurs especially when a person holds an object firmly and close to the chest (a rugby ball for example) (Campbell et al. 2013).

The risk of a violent contraction of the ECU disrupting the under-sheath of the ECU is greatest in the flexion, ulnar tilt, and supination positions mentioned above. In this configuration, the angle imposed by the under-sheath on the tendon is maximal, and so is tendon tension. It is in this position that acute ECU dislocations occur, most often in athletes using bats or handles, which increase the lever arm as well as the disruptive energy of the tendon against the under-sheath (Graham 2012a; Melone Jr et al. 2010).

The only structure that prevents the tendon of the ECU from dislocating is its under-sheath. It

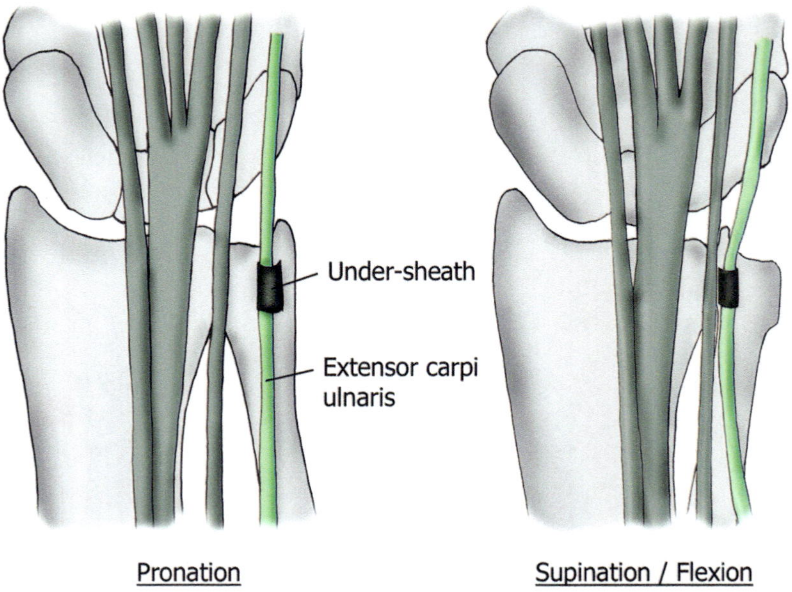

Fig. 6.20 Position change of the ECU tendon between pronation and supination. The tendon's angle increases when it exits the under-sheath in supination and flexion

allows the tendon to remain moored in the dorsal groove of the ECU. The absence of elastic fibers within this under-sheath suggests an unusual resistance to rupture, a key feature for a tissue expected to play a major stabilizing role (Spinner and Kaplan 1970; Kauer 1992; Iwamoto et al. 2006).

The structural integrity of the tendon and osteofibrous tunnel is essential for normal wrist mechanics and function (Campbell et al. 2013). Disruption or insufficiency of these structures can lead to an anteromedial subluxation of the tendon of the ECU and subsequent destabilization of the distal radioulnar and radiocarpal joints.

Sometimes, the problem is not the sheath itself, but an excessive friction between the sheath and the tendon, leading to painful degeneration of the tendon (tendinopathy) and/or its sheath (tenosynovitis), which may or may not be accompanied by tendon blockage. Some everyday activities, such as using a screwdriver or opening a jar, are examples of weight-bearing pronosupination tasks that can trigger this condition (Garcia-Elias 2015; Shaaban et al. 2006).

Pathologies of the tendon of the ECU include tenosynovitis of the tendon sheath, tendinopathy, and tendon instability or rupture. These conditions may occur on their own or simultaneously.

It should be noted that rupture of a normal tendon is unusual, and is mainly observed in lacerating, penetrating, or high-force injuries (Campbell et al. 2013).

Tendinopathy

Generally speaking, the stress induced in the ECU by the majority of the weight-bearing activities in pronosupination is well tolerated by the tendon. However, if the same stress is applied repeatedly over a long period of time, an overuse tendinopathy may develop. This repetitive stress generates an adaptive response in the tendon that thickens and becomes disorganized, accompanied by alterations to its internal vascularization with zones of deterioration and zones of remodeling, surrounded by reactive tenosynovitis. In advanced tendinopathies, the degeneration of the collagen matrix may evolve in a disorganized way. If poorly managed, tendon rupture is possible (Campbell et al. 2013; Melone Jr et al. 2010).

In certain circumstances, it is not excessive stress but a chronic inflammatory disease (chondrocalcinosis, gout, or tuberculosis) that may be the cause of the symptomatic tendon degeneration, which usually progresses macroscopically in a similar way to overused tendons (Garcia-Elias 2015).

Tendinopathy appears to be an adaptive response of the tendon to repetitive stress and/or trauma and may progress through stages of increasing severity (Campbell et al. 2013). Cook's model (Cook and Purdam 2009; Cook et al. 2016) describes three different stages of tendinopathy: reactive tendinopathy, over-degenerative reactive tendinopathy, and degenerative tendinopathy. These three stages occur as a continuum rather than as three completely distinct phases.

Reactive tendinopathy usually involves the tendon responding to a rapid increase in load or direct trauma. The tendon remains structurally intact and there is minimal change in the collagen integrity. This short-term adaptation to overload thickens the tendon and increases its rigidity.

An over-degenerative reactive tendinopathy occurs with continuous excessive loading. The structure of the tendon begins to change, with greater degradation of the matrix. There may be an increased vascularization and neuronal growth.

A degenerative tendinopathy is more common in older athletes due to chronic overload. The tendon becomes less efficient at adapting to load. The collagen becomes progressively disorganized, with advanced degradation of the matrix, which can lead to partial tearing or even rupture (Campbell et al. 2013).

Tendinopathy leads to metabolic changes, especially an abnormal neovascularization combined with the emergence of small nerve endings (Fedorczyk 2012).

- *Tenosynovitis*

Sometimes, it is not the tendon itself, but the tendon sheath that thickens, progressively restricting movement of the ECU. It can be induced by a recent trauma but occurs more often for unknown reasons. ECU tenosynovitis is the second most common tenosynovitis after De Quervain's (Garcia-Elias 2015; Salva-Coll et al. 2012).

ECU tenosynovitis is a pathology that can occur at any age, with a higher prevalence from the age of 40 years onward, probably linked to tissue aging. It mainly affects an active, sporting population. Recovery must therefore be optimal, to enable a return to previous activities, and especially to the movements that caused this tenosynovitis (Hosteins 2015). This condition has also been described in office professions (Singh et al. 2016).

The notion of "over-use" more often (Giffin and Stanish 1993) is often found. These repetitive movements are said to subtly damage the synovium, leading to tenosynovitis in patients with no history of traumatic events. The history may include a new activity or a change in an existing activity in which the mechanical use of the hand and wrist has been altered (Sato et al. 2016).

Repetitive sports activity can lead to the development of ECU tenosynovitis. Tendon instability may be a contributing factor. The tendon sheath of the ECU may be irritated by repetitive flexion/extension of the wrist, especially in supination, at the point of angulation of the tendon at the exit of the osteofibrous tunnel (Campbell et al. 2013). Cases of stenosing tenositis of the ECU have been reported, but these are rare and do not appear to be related to sports activities. The site of sheath stenosis is unclear and has not been documented. Inflammatory conditions such as rheumatoid arthritis should be considered in patients with ECU tenosynovitis who do not engage in typically predisposing sports activities. This may be due to its coexistence with other inflammatory processes, where tenosynovitis may be directly involved in the physiopathology leading to the erosive disease (Campbell et al. 2013; Lillegraven et al. 2011).

- *Instability*

An acute injury and chronic insufficiency of the ECU under-sheath can lead to a symptomatic instability of the ECU at the level of the distal bone groove of the ulna (Ruchelsman and Vitale 2016).

The spectrum of tendon instability ranges from minor subluxation of the ECU during pronosupination movements to frank dislocation and forearm locking. In addition, instability may be

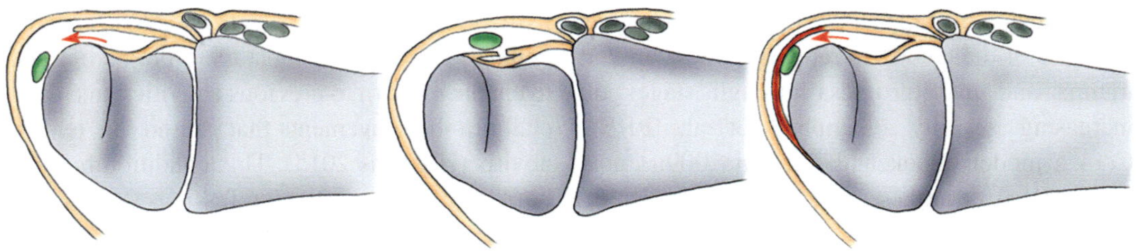

Fig. 6.21 Inoue and Tamara's classification of the most common clinical forms of ECU luxations

increased by the presence of one or more associated local lesions, the most common of which is a lesion of the triangular ligament, with tearing of the peripheral insertion. It goes without saying that the consequences of partial or total dislocation of the tendon will be different: total dislocation makes the ECU tendon ineffective in its role as a stabilizer of the distal radioulnar joint (Campbell et al. 2013; Allende and Le Viet 2005).

Partial or complete ruptures of the ECU under-sheath are rare in the normal population. On the other hand, they are frequently found in athletes practicing sports using a bat or handle, for example.

A complete tear of the ECU under-sheath can happen when a violent contraction of the muscle occurs while the forearm is in a fully supinated position and the wrist in ulnar flexion and tilt. Such circumstances are not uncommon in bat/racket sports. In tennis, for example, a two-handed backhand combines these parameters. Under such conditions, a violent contraction of the muscle can lead to an increase in tension in the under-sheath, which may be enough to cause a rupture. When this phenomenon occurs, the ECU tendon will have a tendency to dislocate in the anteromedial direction (Garcia-Elias 2015; Shaaban et al. 2006; Melone Jr et al. 2010).

Instability is the result of a rupture or dysfunction of the ECU under-sheath. These acute ruptures usually occur as a single traumatic event. Retaining structures are particularly at risk of acute injury when the wrist moves from pronation to supination, while fixed in flexion and ulnar deviation. Less frequently, the under-sheath may break because of repetitive stress (Campbell et al. 2013).

According to the classification of Inoue and Tamura (Inoue and Tamura 1998) (Fig. 6.21) (Kang et al. 2013; Hosteins 2015), the most common forms of ECU dislocation are:

- *Type A (ulnar rupture of the sheath)*: The ulnar edge of the ECU under-sheath has broken, or the medial ridge of the ulnar groove has been avulsed. Usually, injured structures retract rapidly, making the repair almost impossible unless approached immediately after the accident. According to Allende and Le Viet (2005), this is the most common type of under-sheath injury.
- *Type B (middle or radial rupture of the sheath)*: The ECU under-sheath has suffered a tear on its middle part, or more often on its radial edge. This leaves part of the sheath (ulnar side) interposed between the subluxated tendon and the ulnar groove. For this type of injury, surgery to remove the incarcerated tissue is always necessary.
- *Type C (subperiosteal tear of the under-sheath's ulnar insertion)*: A strong shearing of the ECU tendon against the ulnar edge of the sixth compartment may not disrupt the ECU under-sheath but detach the periosteum from the medial part of the ulna, allowing the ECU tendon to leave the sixth compartment and enter the enlarged subperiosteal pocket thus created.

A pathological subluxation can also occur. Similar in appearance, it is diametrically different in terms of prognosis. It may occur when the ECU tendon luxates in palmar after a progressive weakening of the under-sheath due to a rheumatoid tenosynovitis of the ECU (Garcia-Elias 2015).

Etiology

Trauma Related to Sports Practice

ECU pathologies have been most frequently reported in tennis and golf, although injuries of the stabilizing structures of the ECU also happen in some contact sports such as rugby. Sports with a risk of ECU injury share common characteristics: either a load applied to the wrist when the ECU is in a vulnerable position (flexion, ulnar deviation, and supination), or a sudden lateral force applied to the wrist when the tendon is in a strong isometric contraction. In tennis, the incriminating movement is the two-handed backhand.

In golf, it is the impact at the end of the swing that can lead to ECU injuries on the wrist facing the target. At this exact moment in the swing, the ECU muscle is in isometric contraction to fight the impact of the club with the ball. If the club hits a hard object on the ground at impact, or in the case of hard ground play, the swing is suddenly interrupted. The upper body and limbs keep moving forward, while the club (and hands) do not.

In rugby, injuries can occur when the ball is held in the tackle. The ball is held firmly against the chest. The forearm is maximally supinated, the wrist in flexion and ulnar inclination. The ECU contracts isometrically. A sudden increase in the isometric force within the ECU, as the player attempts to grip the ball more firmly on contact, can lead to a tear of the under-sheath with acute subluxation of the ECU tendon. This can be felt as a painful snapping sensation on impact (Campbell et al. 2013; Montalvan et al. 2006).

Repetitive Movements

Repetitive movements can also subtly damage the synovium, leading to tenosynovitis. This is more likely to be the cause in patients with no known history of traumatic events. In cases of displaced ulnar styloid fracture, osteophyte, or ulnar head dislocation, an irregularity of the sixth compartment's floor can fasten damage to the tendon's synovial sheath. Erosion of the compartment's floor will expose the tendon to the abrasive effects of the bone during glidings. The bone, in turn, may show signs of chronic damage, including sclerosis, osteolysis, and osteophyte formation, all of which can be detected on X-ray (Crimmins and Jones 1995).

Anatomical Variation

The presence of an accessory tendon of the ECU tendon or the extensor digiti minimi traveling through the ECU under-sheath has been documented in 5.6%–34.2% of patients. It has been suggested that this accessory tendon may contribute to stenosing tenosynovitis, as it may increase the size of the bundle that has to go through the ECU under-sheath (Kollitz et al. 2015).

Negative Ulnar Variance

The study by Chang et al. shows a significant correlation between a negative ulnar variance and the presence of ECU tendon pathologies and/or ECU subluxation. Their study also indicates that patients with ECU pathologies had a shorter and shallower ECU groove, but not significantly so.

Although these results cannot establish causality, the anatomical relationship between the ECU tendon and the distal ulna supports a plausible connection between tendon pathology and distal ulnar morphology.

A shallower bone groove may impose a greater stabilizing load on the ECU tendon's fibrous under-sheath and imply greater susceptibility to injury of these structures (Cooney 2011; Chang et al. 2014).

Morphology of the Extensor Carpi Ulnaris' Ulnar Groove

Kohyama et al. (2017) hypothesized that the ECU groove morphology, especially its shape, is related to ECU injuries. They developed a brief classification to enable a better understanding of the pathologies. Grooves with the deepest point oriented toward the radial slope (type R) could be more prone to ECU injuries, compared to other groove types (orientation of the deepest point of the groove toward the ulnar slope (type U) or in the middle of the groove (type M)), especially because there is no medial bone buttress (Fig. 6.22).

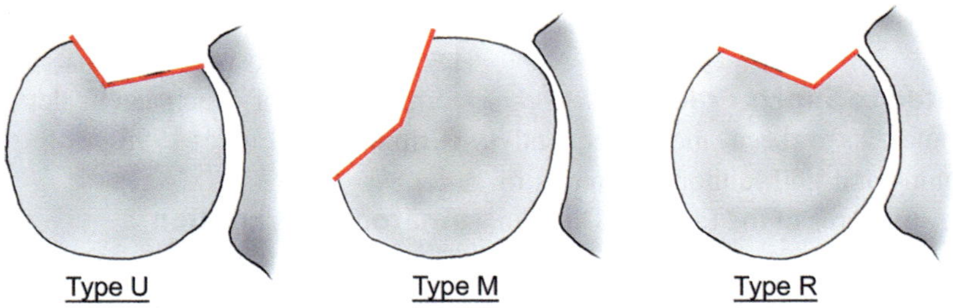

Fig. 6.22 Three main types of ECU groove depending on the position of the deepest point in the groove. Type U: the deepest point is on the ulnar side. Type M: the deepest point is in the middle. Type R: the deepest point is on the radial side

Other studies have hypothesized that a shallow groove of the ECU may represent an anatomical variation that could predispose affected patients to subsequent ECU instability and symptomatic subluxations, despite a stable under-sheath and absence of previous trauma. The presence of a relatively flat groove appears to be a risk factor for the development of tendon subluxations. It would be easier for the tendon to dislocate with a "smooth" morphology as opposed to a hollowed groove with a sharp edge. However, a recent study seems to show that this risk factor is not as important as previous studies seemed to suggest (Allende and Le Viet 2005; Singh et al. 2016; Iorio et al. 2014; Oka and Handa 2001; MacLennan et al. 2008).

Clinical and Paraclinical Signs

Clinical Signs

Tendinopathy, tenosynovitis, or instability of the ECU tendon present clear results on physical examination that can be observed or evoked (Graham 2012a).

A thorough history and clinical evaluation are essential for the diagnosis of ECU tendon disorders. There are many other causes of pain on the ulnar side of the wrist, and the area or site of discomfort requires accurate localization by both patient and therapist (Campbell et al. 2013).

- *Tendinopathy and tenosynovitis*

Pain on the dorso-ulnar side of the wrist, opposite the sheath, and a burning sensation are the most frequently reported complaints. In stable ECU tendinopathies, it is more common to describe a "zone" of discomfort or pain, rather than a specific precise "point" of pain. In these circumstances, other causes of pain on the ulnar side of the wrist should be considered (Campbell et al. 2013; Graham 2012a; Kollitz et al. 2015).

The pain has two components: a constant dull aching sensation on the dorso-ulnar side of the wrist, and a sudden burning longitudinal pain felt along the path of the ECU tendon during active contraction of the muscle (Campbell et al. 2013).

In contrast to an under-sheath injury, patients with ECU tendinopathy or tenosynovitis usually report a gradual, insidious onset of their pain over the past weeks or months. In most cases of tendinopathy and tenosynovitis, there is no history of trauma. Pain is usually increased by activity and may be provoked or aggravated by certain movements. In tendinopathy, stretching or resisted contraction of the muscle will cause increased pain (Garcia-Elias 2015; Kollitz et al. 2015).

It is common for a person with stable ECU tendinopathy to describe a growing awareness of functional disorders and pain. Loss of muscle strength is also common (Garcia-Elias 2015; Campbell et al. 2013).

Patients with reactive tendinopathy and ECU tenosynovitis will often have an imprecise, subtle swelling along the sixth extensor compartment. A stenosing tenosynovitis with grinding, may also occur (Campbell et al. 2013).

A test called the "ECU synergy test" has been developed to help the examiner distinguish between ulnar intra-articular pain and pain of tendinous origin (Ruland and Hogan 2008). The test

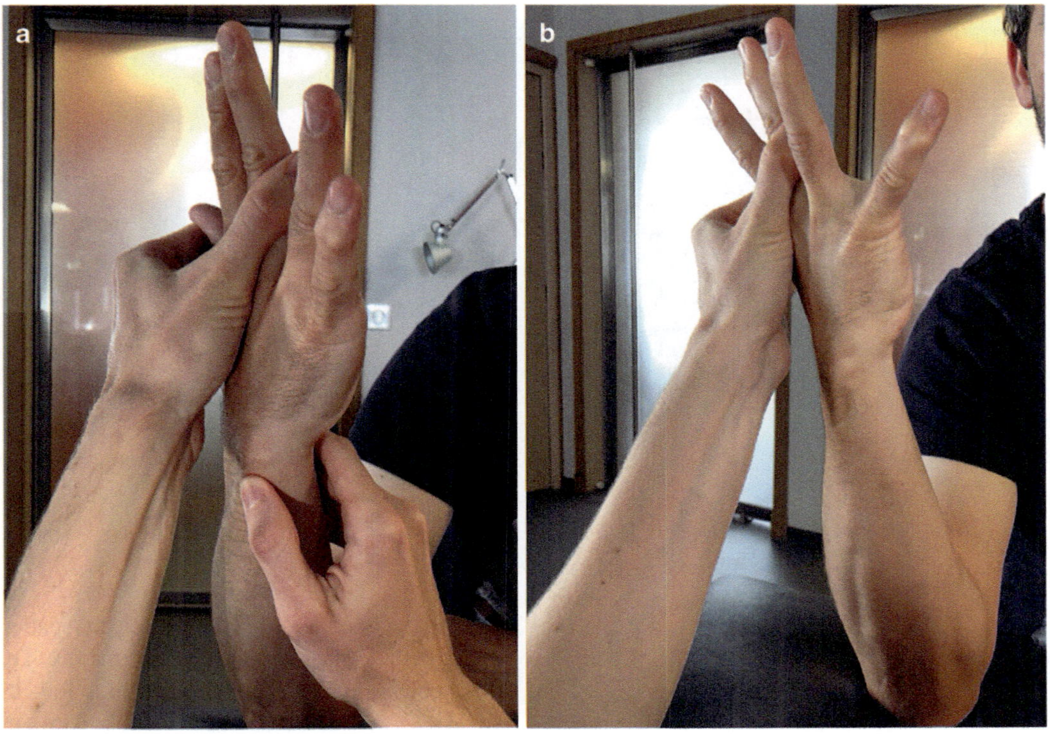

Fig. 6.23 The synergic test for the ECU is performed by asking for a resisted radial deviation of the thumb (extension) (**a**). The bowstring of the ECU tendon can be seen under the skin (**b**)

consists in applying an isolated tension to the ECU, without overstressing other structures. This test has been shown to have good sensitivity (73.3%) and specificity (85.7%) in the diagnosis of ECU tendinopathy (Sato et al. 2016; Ruland and Hogan 2008). This test is performed by exploiting an isometric contraction of the ECU during a resisted radial deviation of the thumb. The test is performed by resting the patient's arm on the examination table with the elbow bent at 90° and the forearm fully supinated. The wrist is held in a neutral position, with the fingers fully extended (Fig. 6.23). Facing the patient, the examiner grasps the patient's thumb and middle finger with one hand and palpates the ECU tendon with the other. The patient then extends the thumb ("radial abduction") against resistance, isometrically activating the ECU (Ruland and Hogan 2008). The presence of both FCU and ECU muscle contraction is confirmed by direct palpation. Reproduction of pain along the dorso-ulnar side of the wrist is considered to be a positive result of this ECU tendinopathy test (Campbell et al. 2013).

Another test, the carpal supination test (Fig. 6.24), appears to be more sensitive (86% sensitivity and 67% specificity) for the detection of ECU tendinopathy (Yoshida 2010). This test is performed by holding the patient's hand and passively supinating both hand and forearm and is considered positive if it reproduces the patient's pain. One study seems to confirm that this test is not only the most sensitive but also the most specific; however, it was not performed in vivo, which may constitute a significant bias (Kataoka et al. 2015).

Considerable pain on passive flexion and radial deviation of the wrist (reverse Finkelstein test) is the most characteristic feature of tenosynovitis (Garcia-Elias 2015).

- *Instability*

ECU disorders are fairly rare in the general population but are unusually prevalent in one particular population: athletes who play racquet sports, or who need to manipulate a handle. Most

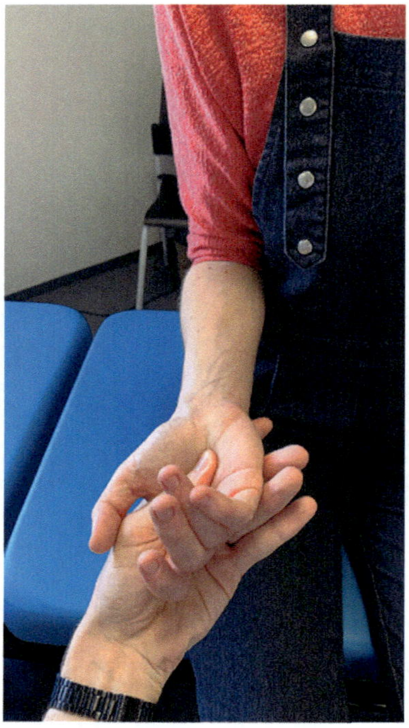

Fig. 6.24 The carpal supination test is performed by doing a passive supination of the hand and forearm

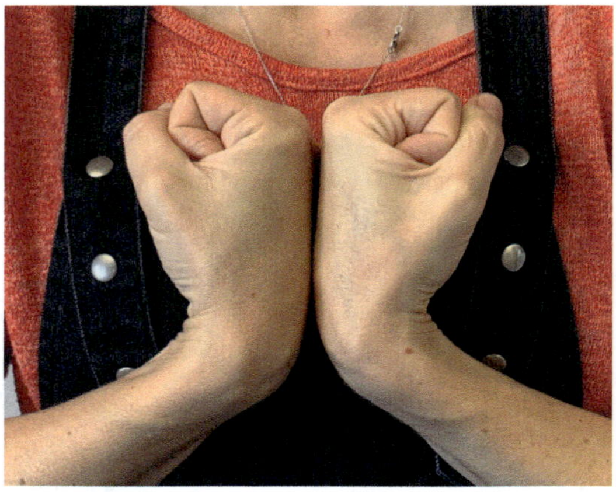

Fig. 6.25 Heart-shaped test, made to create a dislocation of the tendon, highlighting an instability of the ECU tendon

patients have a history of sudden pain due to injury, usually resulting from sports activities, a fall, or a twist (Graham 2012a; Montalvan et al. 2006; Inoue and Tamura 2001).

Acute dislocation of the ECU, especially affects adult males aged 18–40 years, who are professional athletes practicing bat or racket sports. The traumatic mechanism is often identified as the result of combined supination, flexion, and ulnar tilt movements of the wrist, associated with a slow, violent contraction of the ECU. In the acute phase, the most typical clinical presentation consists of pain and slight swelling on the dorso-ulnar side of the wrist (Garcia-Elias 2015; Ruchelsman and Vitale 2016; Hosteins 2015).

In cases of untreated chronic dislocation, the wrist will tend to give way, usually with pain, when the patient attempts to perform a loaded pronosupination. Tendon dislocation can be demonstrated by a test known as the "heart test," which involves reproducing all the movement components that facilitate the tendon dislocation: flexion, ulnar inclination, and supination. This test is performed by asking the patient to hold the two wrists flexed, hands back-to-back, while the forearm is supinated and the ulnar side of the hand is pressed against the chest (Fig. 6.25).

The majority of the instabilities are sensitive to this test, and a "pop" is often perceptible, sometimes audible, indicating dislocation of the tendon out of its compartment. The test appears to have good sensitivity and specificity (Garcia-Elias 2015).

The moment of the onset of symptoms helps to distinguish between acute and chronic causes. The mechanical symptoms at the time of onset are also common descriptors of this condition. Patients will use words such as "snap," "tear," and "jump" in the case of acute sheath rupture.

In some cases, episodes of tendon subluxation can be very painful. In other cases, the subluxation may be entirely asymptomatic and can be easily reproduced by the patient. The subluxating "protrusion" of the tendon as it leaves its groove on the dorsal surface of the ulna can only be produced by an active contraction of the ECU. Passive movements will not produce this characteristic sign, as the tendon is not tensed enough to produce a subluxation. Active supination with the affected wrist held firmly in maximum flexion and ulnar tilt will produce an often-visible subluxation of the tendon (Campbell et al. 2013). A demonstrable subluxation that is clear and unambiguous is one of the major elements in the clinical assessment of this condition. Other signs may be much more subtle and require careful clinical examination. Palpation along the ECU tendon may reveal tenderness located precisely on this structure. The causal movement (especially sports movement) can also reproduce this pain (Reddy and Compson 2005). Pain on resisted active extension with ulnar tilt is pathognomonic of an ECU disorder. Muscle weakness, often associated with pain, may be present. Painless muscle weakness is likely to represent a complete rupture of the ECU tendon (Campbell et al. 2013).

- *Differential diagnosis*

Tendinopathy, tenosynovitis, or instability of the ECU may coexist with other conditions of the ulnar side of the wrist, so the diagnosis should not be taken as an exclusion of all other possible diagnoses. Clinical evaluation and further investigation of other important structures of the ulnar side of the wrist are essential to exclude coexisting pathologies involving the TFCC complex, the lunotriquetral ligament, the distal radioulnar joint, or the ulnar styloid (Campbell et al. 2013).

Possible pathological anatomical structures that may cause ulnar wrist pain involve intra or extra-articular tissues. The first ones include the triangular fibrocartilaginous complex (TFCC), the lunotriquetral ligament, the ulnar styloid, and the distal radioulnar joint. The other includes the wrist's extrinsic ulnocarpal ligament and the ECU tendon (Sato et al. 2016).

The complex relationships between the ECU, its under-sheath, the TFCC, and the ulnar carpus explain the frequent discovery of concomitant ulnar wrist injuries found alongside ECU lesions (Ruchelsman and Vitale 2016).

Tenosynovitis of the ECU should not be confused with Barfred's syndrome, in which there is a juncta between the tendon of the ECU and that of the extensor digiti minimi. This condition is characterized by pain in supination of the wrist, with impaired extension of the fifth finger (Hosteins 2015).

Since a variety of painful conditions at the lower end of the ulna may coexist with lesions of the ECU, a full clinical screening is required, with further investigations if necessary (Garcia-Elias 2015).

Paraclinical Signs

Conventional X-rays are not always necessary and are usually normal in ECU pathologies, however, some authors have noted an erosion of the ulnar styloid in the presence of ECU tenosynovitis. Crimmins and Jones have also stressed the importance of X-rays in detecting bony abnormalities that would cause or be caused by an ECU tendinopathy, such as pseudarthrosis of an ulnar styloid fracture with erosive or osteolytic changes to the styloid (Crimmins and Jones 1995; Campbell et al. 2013).

In equivocal or difficult cases, ultrasound or MRI are the imaging modalities of choice to complete the clinical diagnosis of tendinopathy and instability of the ECU. The ECU tendon is subcutaneous, easily palpable, and visible on ultrasound, enabling early diagnosis and management of these conditions (Campbell et al. 2013; Ruchelsman and Vitale 2016).

Ultrasound and MRI can be used to better assess the relationship of the tendon and under-sheath with the distal ulna (Kollitz et al. 2015).

Ultrasound has several advantages, including low cost, non-invasive technique, and harmless soft tissue evaluation. The examination is fast, inflammatory changes can be assessed by Doppler imaging without the need for intravenous contrast agents, the contralateral limb can be used for comparison, and a dynamic assessment can be performed between pronation and supination. MRI can assess other structures such as the TFCC, which is not easily accessible with ultrasound (Campbell et al. 2013).

These examinations can be useful in confirming the presence or absence of dislocation and/or injury of the ECU strap (Hosteins 2015).

A systematic clinical examination using the contralateral side as a reference, together with a careful study of the patient's anamnesis, will reveal most ECU injuries. Further investigations are not systematic and may be necessary to confirm uncertainties in misleading cases, as well as to provide additional information to guide the treatment. In the case of equivocal pathology, MRI would appear to be the most appropriate option. On the other hand, if the aim is merely to confirm suspicions and get additional information to guide the treatment, ultrasound would appear to be the best option (Campbell et al. 2013). As this pathology is superficial, and current equipment has excellent resolution, the exact location and extent of tendon and sheath lesions can be correctly assessed and anticipated. Ultrasound appears to have a major role to play in the future diagnosis of ECU injuries (Garcia-Elias 2015).

Therapeutic Process

As in most client situations, treatment must be individualized for each patient. In most cases, a conservative treatment will relieve the pathology (Campbell et al. 2013). If this fails, surgical treatment may be considered.

Tendinopathy

In all cases, it is necessary to identify and treat the underlying etiology of the problem (Garcia-Elias 2015).

- *Conservative treatments*

The main goal of the treatment is to prevent further degeneration and subsequent rupture of the affected tendon. Conservative treatments are usually effective in the management of overuse tendinopathy (Garcia-Elias 2015; Spinner and Kaplan 1970; Graham 2012a).

Acute ECU tendinopathies usually respond to non-surgical measures of rest, immobilization, rehabilitation, and activity modification, administration of anti-inflammatory drugs, and one or more infiltrations of local corticosteroids (Campbell et al. 2013).

- *Immobilization*

Wearing a short resting orthosis (wrist in ulnar tilt and 30° extension) allows the muscle to be positioned in the shortening position (Campbell et al. 2013; Hosteins 2015). Some authors recommend a long resting orthosis, with the forearm pronated, so that the ECU tendon is comfortably located in the dorsal ulnar groove. There is no evidence to support one type of orthosis over another.

Continuous wear for 3–6 weeks (Garcia-Elias 2015; Hosteins 2015), together with anti-inflammatory treatment, and muscle rehabilitation in a controlled program, tends to resolve most of these pathologies.

- *Rehabilitation*

The origin of the tendinopathy should be identified, and postural and/or gestural adaptation proposed to avoid exposing the arm to the same repeated stresses that contributed to the appearance of the lesion (Garcia-Elias 2015).

Rehabilitation strategies are based on the severity of the tendinopathy (Cook and Purdam 2009; Cook et al. 2016). Treatment of the early reactive phase consists of load management and isometric exercises until the pain stabilizes (generally over 5–10 days). The load can then be increased in stages. The use of NSAIDs (ibuprofen type) can be a useful complement during this phase. Analgesic techniques can also be used, such as massage, Transcutaneous Vibratory Stimulation (TVS) at a frequency of 100 Hz (for analgesic purposes), cryotherapy, or TENS-type electrotherapy. At the same time, passive and active mobilizations can be performed to maintain/restore optimal mobility of the wrist and hand, which may have been diminished by immobilization.

In chronic tendinopathies, without a sudden increase in pain, a combination of load management, eccentric work, isometrics, and strength exercises is likely to help. Some of the changes within the tendon may be reversible, but it is likely to be a condition that will need long-term management (Campbell et al. 2013).

Eccentric muscle exercises play an important role. They involve three parameters (Hosteins 2015):

- Tendon length: The resting length is increased, generating less tension on the tendon during movements.
- Progressive increase in load, increasing the tendon's intrinsic resistance.
- Increasing the speed at which the exercise is performed, which in turn increases the developed force.

Eccentric muscular training in tendinopathy helps reduce neovascularization by capillary flow without reducing oxygen saturation. Physical activity also promotes the active metabolism of the tendinous tissue, due to the plasticity of tendons in response to variations in mechanical solicitations. Eccentric muscle work stimulates type 1 collagen synthesis, without altering its rate of degradation (Hosteins 2015).

Eccentric training also reduces the tendon's volume in the thickened zone associated with tendinopathy (Ohberg and Alfredson 2004). Repetition of an eccentric-type protocol over time will also have a prophylactic effect on tendon and muscle lesions.

This anisometric mode of contraction helps to improve muscle mass and develop the vascularization of the epitendon, making the tendon more resistant to longitudinal traction (Middleton and Montero 2004).

On the other hand, it should be borne in mind that eccentric work can lead to muscle soreness, known as Delayed Onset Muscle Soreness (DOMS), especially when performed in internal race. Work through the entire joint amplitude should therefore be favored (Hosteins 2015). A study of DOMS (Bakhtiary et al. 2007) in the lower limb showed that the application of vibrations (frequency 50 Hz) for a short period before eccentric work reduced the loss of strength induced by eccentric work, lowered the production of serum creatine kinase, and reduced the pain felt. The rehabilitation session could therefore be preceded by a session of vibrotherapy at this frequency, by applying the vibration at the myotendinous junction, increasing the proprioceptive effect and preparation for effort.

Alfredson (Alfredson et al. 1998) proposes a protocol based on the principle that it is necessary to rehabilitate the injured tendon with the goal of approaching the most traumatic position—that of the causal movement. This is achieved by varying the speed and load, depending on the position, and always using eccentric training. He suggests performing three series of 15 movements, indicating that the first 10 movements of each series should be performed without difficulty or pain, and that the last 5 should be more irritating.

It will therefore be necessary to increase the speed of execution from slow to fast, and then the load, starting in the pronation position and ending in the supination position. The protocol evolves according to the patient's pain level: the next stage will only be reached if the exercise is pain-free. The workload is calculated using 30% of the maximum load of the contralateral side. Sessions are spaced 48–72 hours apart, to allow energy reserves (especially glycogen) to recover.

The position of the wrist during eccentric exercises is designed to induce progressive stresses on the tendon and ECU strap at the level of the sixth extensor compartment, but also to progressively increase tendon excursion (Hosteins 2015).

As the eccentric exercises progress, the wrist will be placed in increasingly demanding positions for the tendon and ECU strap, namely (in chronological order):

- Pronation
- Radial inclination and extension
- Ulnar tilt and extension
- Radial inclination and flexion
- Ulnar inclination and flexion
- Supination
- Radial inclination and 15° extension
- Ulnar inclination and 15° extension
- Ulnar inclination and flexion or extension

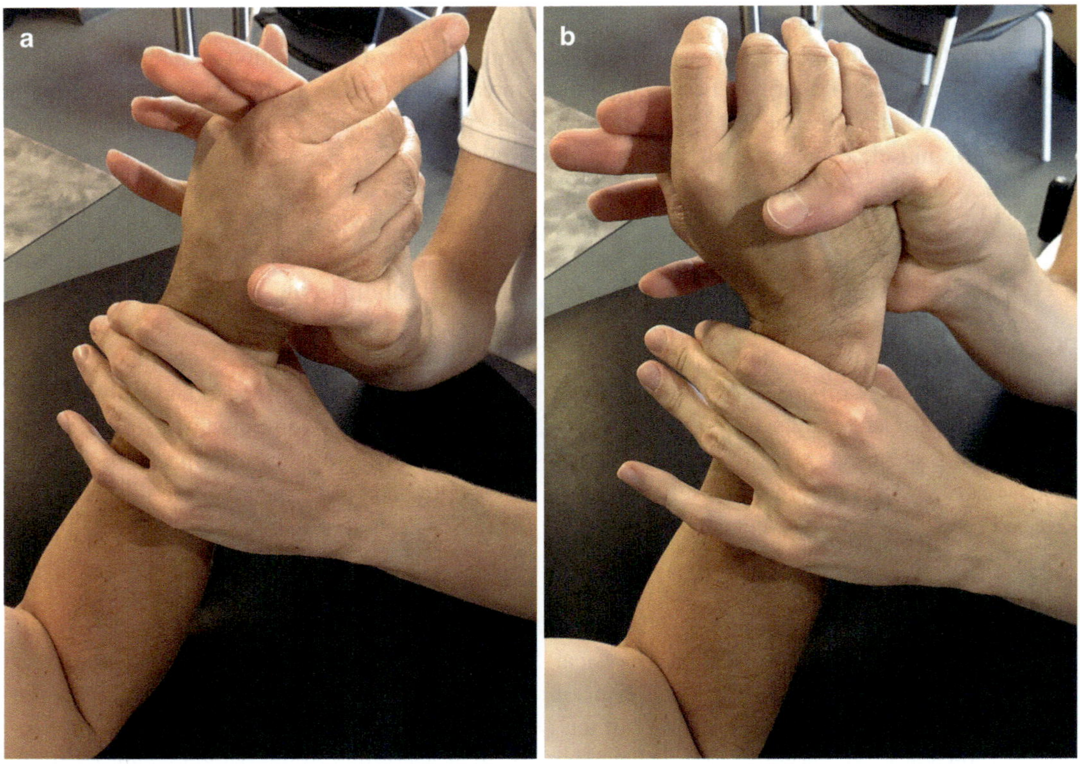

Fig. 6.26 Eccentric exercise for ulnar inclination; start (**a**) and end (**b**) positions

The speed will be modulated when the exercise is performed without pain, as follows:

- D1 and D2: slow speed
- D3 and D4: moderate speed
- D5 and D6: fast speed

At D7, the load is increased, and the patient resumes the next series at a slow speed.

Eccentric exercises are designed to enable the patient to oppose radial flexion and inclination. The goal is to slow the movement down, not stop it. It may be appropriate to make the patient feel what is being asked of him/her, to ensure that the exercise is performed correctly. Initially, resistance is applied manually by the therapist, and it may be useful to work on one component of movement at a time at first (e.g., ulnar tilt against resistance), so that the stimulus is as progressive as possible (Hosteins 2015).

- *Example*

The exercise is initiated with the patient's wrist in pronation, extension, and ulnar tilt. The goal is to reach the final position of pronation, extension, and radial inclination (Fig. 6.26) (Ruchelsman and Vitale 2016).

Subsequently, work can be carried out with an object (such as a club or hammer) to increase the lever arm and get closer to the patient's sports activity.

- *Example* (Hosteins 2015)

Request an eccentric work by slowing down the movement of flexion and radial inclination of the wrist in the pronation position. The starting position is therefore pronation, extension, and ulnar inclination, with the elbow resting on the table. The club is vertically oriented, with the weight above the hand. The patient is asked to control the fall of the club in radial flexion and inclination (Fig. 6.27). Subsequently, the same exercise can be performed in the supination position (Fig. 6.28).

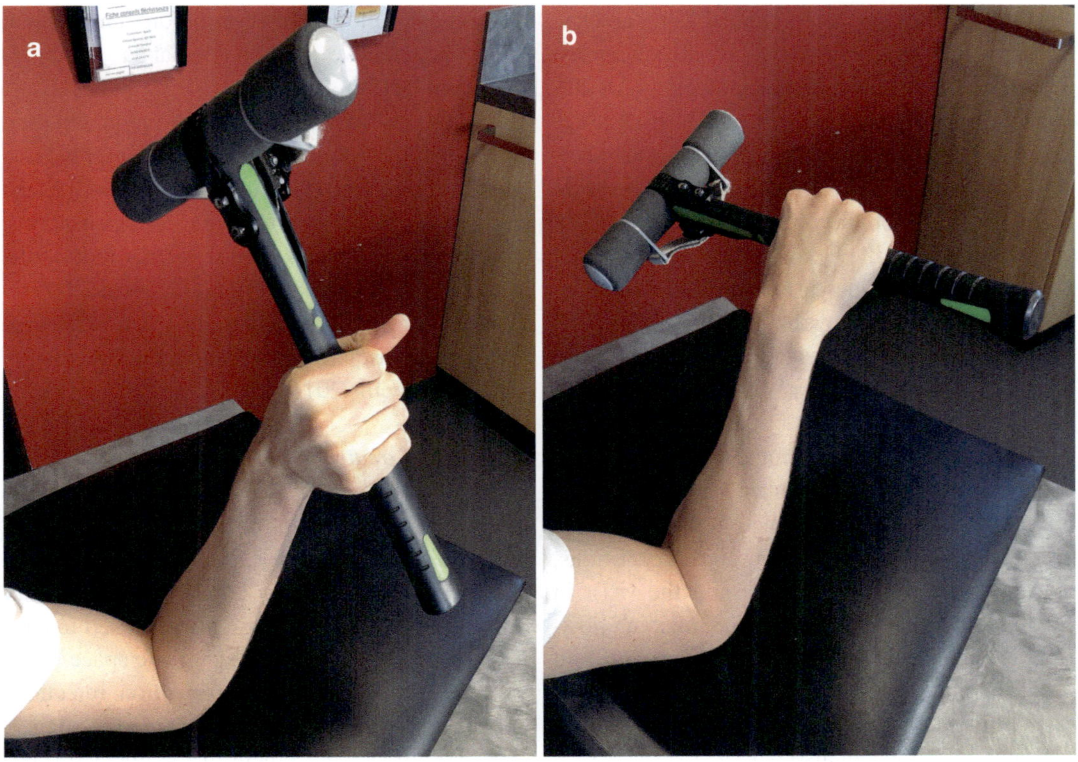

Fig. 6.27 Eccentric exercise for extension and ulnar inclination in pronation; start (**a**) and end (**b**) positions

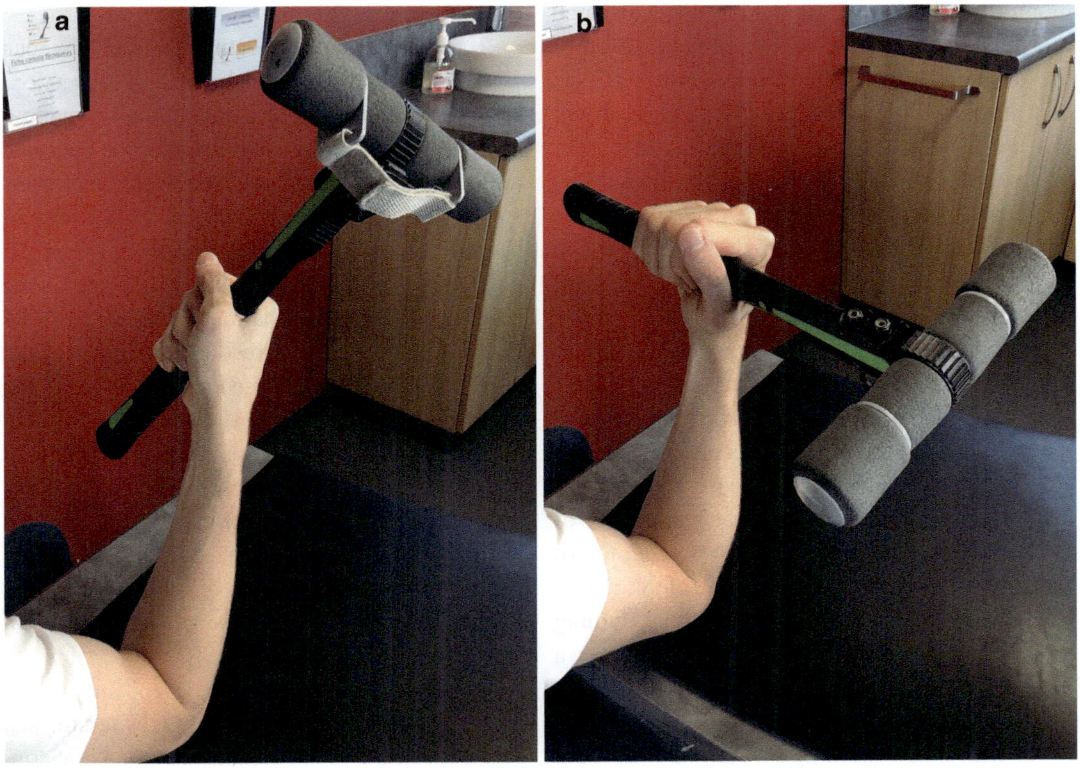

Fig. 6.28 Eccentric exercise for extension and ulnar inclination in supination; start (**a**) and end (**b**) positions

The exercise can be reproduced using an elastic strap, to provide a more global solicitation involving the muscular chains, especially for athletes in training. The patient stands in a lunge position, with the shoulder girdles firmly in place. At first, the elbow is bent during the exercise to work selectively on the wrist. The intensity of the force developed will be progressive, as the tension of the elastic band increases due to its stretching as the movement progresses (Fig. 6.29).

As the end of the treatment approaches, the same type of eccentric load can be applied using Kabat's diagonals.

With the aim of reducing DOMS following eccentric exercises, concentric wrist extension, and ulnar tilt can be performed at the end of the session. This can consist of eight repetitions, starting with the elbow flexed and the wrist in flexion and radial inclination. The finishing position is elbow straight, wrist in extension, and ulnar inclination.

A short period of 50 Hz vibrotherapy at the end of the session can also help recovery.

The main goal of these exercises is to challenge the ECU in its role as a wrist stabilizer and mobility enhancer (e.g., tennis lift), through movements requiring control and modulation of the developed force. Eccentric work will also help improve concentric strength. The goal will also be to improve the agonist/antagonist ratio between the ECU and the FCU in the ulnar stabilization of the wrist and, more generally, in the overall work of the wrist during the acceleration and accompaniment phases of the movement (movement braking).

In wrist rehabilitation, it is always better to aim for a stable wrist rather than a mobile one. Exercises designed to control and brake movement can help improve proprioception.

The goal is to achieve a decrease in pain and a level of strength equal to or greater than 80% of the contralateral strength before a gradual return to sport (Graham 2012a; Topper et al. 1998; Croisier et al. 2001). Static muscular training may be initiated if the assessment indicates a deficiency in this area.

The sport-specific preparation phase should begin with empty training or training with light equipment, followed by resumption of movement with progressive power demands (striking) (Graham 2012a).

An analysis of the gesture and equipment used in sports practice is also relevant to improve and correct the gesture (fine and global) as well as the posture if necessary to avoid compensations. Improving equipment can also help reduce the onset of ECU disorders (Tagliafico et al. 2009).

Appropriate muscular training can be carried out in pre-season to prevent and reduce the risk of injury (Hosteins 2015).

- *Medical treatments*

If symptoms are not relieved, a steroid injection into the osteofibrous sheath may be considered (Campbell et al. 2013). A preliminary injection of local anesthetic may be used to confirm the diagnosis and to help create space in the sheath for subsequent steroid injection. Injections are best performed under ultrasound guidance, ensuring precise placement of the injected product, and avoiding intra-tendinous injection (and the risk of precipitating a subsequent rupture) (Campbell et al. 2013).

Tendinosis, or degenerative tendinopathy, can be difficult to distinguish clinically from tendonitis. As tendinosis is a non-inflammatory overuse syndrome, the role of steroidal and non-steroidal anti-inflammatory treatments remains controversial (Khan et al. 2000). NSAIDs and local corticosteroid injections have been shown to inhibit collagen repair in vitro, and their usefulness in the treatment of tendinosis has been questioned (Bass 2012). Campbell et al. recommended that local corticosteroid injections should be considered after at least 3 weeks of rest and immobilization, and a period of rehabilitation with increasing load and isometric exercise (Campbell et al. 2013).

If diagnosed and treated early, most tendons return to normal function with good healing (Heras-Palou 2012).

- *Non-conservative treatments*

In patients with persistent ECU tendinosis, surgical release of the compartment may be con-

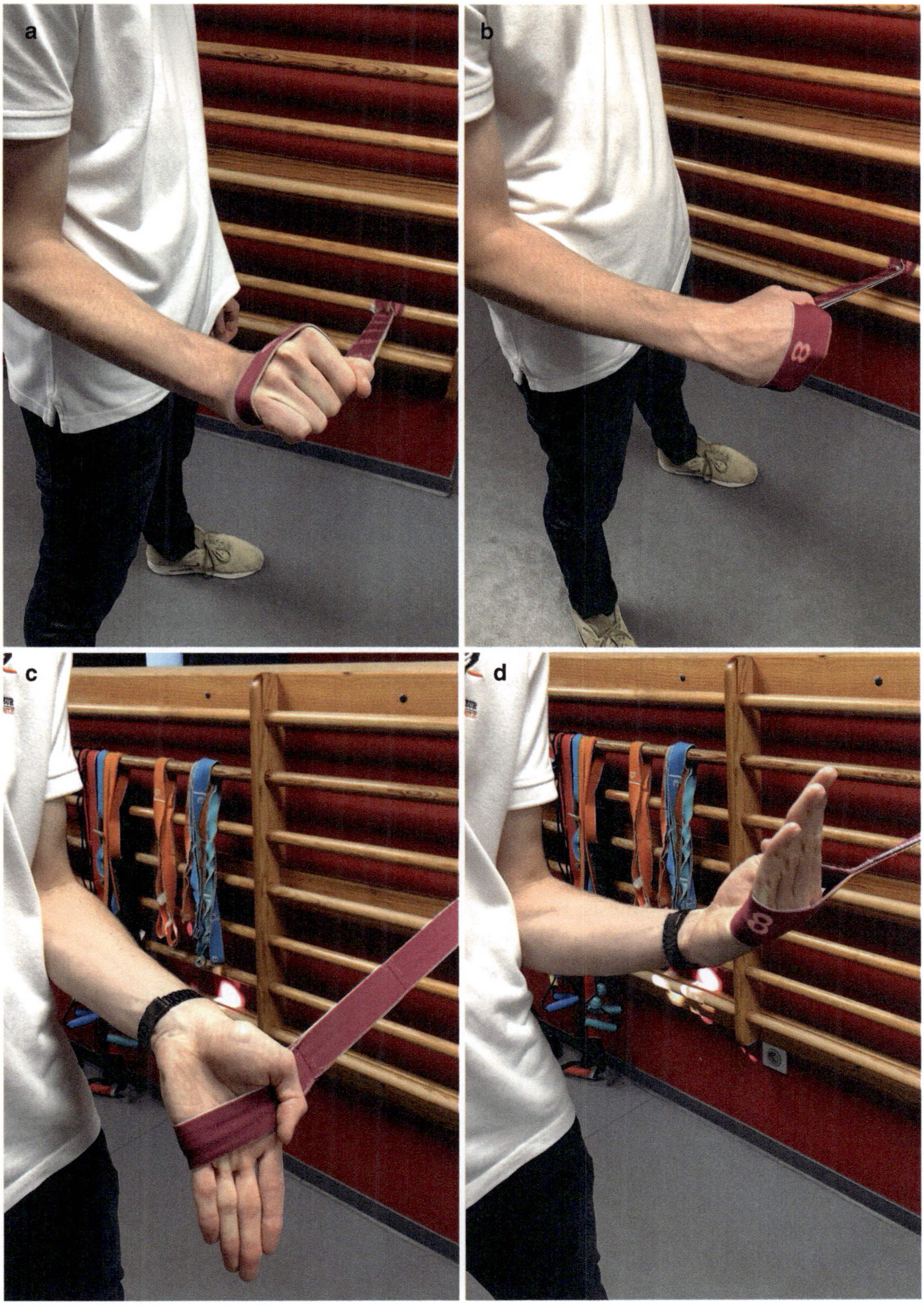

Fig. 6.29 Eccentric exercises in pronation (**a** and **b**) and supination (**c** and **d**)

sidered. This involves division of the intercompartmental septum between the fifth and sixth extensor compartments, thereby increasing the compartmental volume without threatening its stabilizing function (Campbell et al. 2013).

Chronic tendinopathy can be treated by longitudinal division of the fibers and debridement of necrotic tissue. Abnormal tendon stubs should be removed, as their bulking effect may contribute to stenosis (Allende and Le Viet 2005).

Tenosynovitis

As mentioned above, this type of pathology appears especially in sportsmen and women as a result of the stresses placed on the wrist. During rehabilitation, it will be important to keep in mind the objective of reducing pain, but also resuming the causal movement (Hosteins 2015).

- *Conservative treatments*

As in other types of stenosing tenosynovitis of the dorsal wrist, rest, splinting, and corticosteroid injections are generally effective in reducing inflammation and pain. Each modality has its own specific indications and recognized results (Crimmins and Jones 1995; Campbell et al. 2013).

- *Orthotic treatments*

It corresponds to a resting orthosis. The goal is to limit friction between the osteofibrous gliding and the tendon. It allows modification of the force vector transmitted to the sixth extensor compartment (Hosteins 2015). A suggested position is:

- 15–20° wrist extension
- Neutral inclination
- Pronation through ovalization of the orthosis
- Free overlying (elbow) and underlying (metacarpophalangeal joints of the five fingers) joints.

This position allows maximum unloading of the ECU strap. A slight wrist extension places the ECU tendon in a centered position. In this position, pronation reduces tension on the tendon, unlike supination where the tendon undergoes greater stretching due to its elongation when rolled up. Pronation reduces tendon excursion. The orthosis is worn continuously for a minimum of 3 weeks (Hosteins 2015; Horii et al. 1993).

- *Rehabilitation*

To reduce pain and trophic disorders, cryotherapy, analgesic and draining massage, and draining pressotherapy can be used. TENS electrotherapy and TVS (100 Hz) are also part of the therapist's toolbox. Passive and active mobilizations can also be used to help the wrist regain optimal mobility, which may have been diminished by immobilization (Hosteins 2015).

Work can then begin on restoring the ECU to its original condition (Hosteins 2015).

This differs from the work carried out for tendinopathies, as it does not focus on muscular work, but on the sliding of the tendon in relation to its sheath.

This rehabilitation should be coupled with wrist proprioception exercises and a gradual return to functional activities adapted to the patient's professional or sports activities.

A gestural and postural analysis will also be an integral part of the treatment so that advice can be given on healthy lifestyle habits to avoid compensation and limit the risk of recurrence.

- *Medical treatments*

Analgesics may also be indicated to reduce pain. If symptoms are slow to improve, an ultrasound-guided steroid injection into the tendon sheath of the ECU at its distal insertion may be considered. Failing this, the ECU under-sheath may have undergone a "contracture" due to insufficient healing of a partial injury, or some other process of under-sheath thickening. In both cases, surgical release may be recommended (Garcia-Elias 2015).

- *Non-conservative treatments*

Surgery may be considered in cases of persistent tenosynovitis unresponsive to conservative treatment. It generally consists of widening the gliding of the sixth extensor compartment (removal of the external septum while preserving the internal septum) (Crimmins and Jones 1995; Roulot 2012).

Surgical options for the treatment of tenosynovitis include release of the ECU under-sheath, with or without under-sheath reconstruction, or synovectomy. Debridement of necrotic tissue or abnormal tendons may also be indicated (Allende and Le Viet 2005; Kollitz et al. 2015).

Erosion of the floor of the sixth dorsal compartment has been identified as a source of pain in some cases of refractory stenosing tenosynovitis. The bone is exposed to the floor of the ECU under-sheath, which is thought to contribute to inflammation of the tendon. In such cases, a portion of the retinaculum can be used to reconstruct the floor of the compartment to protect the tendon from further damage (Crimmins and Jones 1995; Carneiro et al. 2005).

Instability

The main goal is to reestablish normal relationships between the ulna and the ECU, thereby restoring the stabilizing efficiency of the ECU (Garcia-Elias 2015).

Asymptomatic instability of the ECU tendon, especially if it does not cause significant subluxation, does not always require treatment.

- *Conservative treatments*

Early diagnosis of an unstable ECU tendon in association with acute trauma can be managed by the reduction of tendon subluxation and immobilization for a period of 6 weeks. Reduction is achieved by positioning the wrist in radial deviation, with the forearm pronated (Montalvan et al. 2006; Hosteins 2015; Iorio and Huang 2014). The tendon is repositioned in the ulnar groove and must then be maintained in this position by wearing a long orthosis. The goal here is to reattach the under-sheath to the ulnar edge of the ECU groove (Burkhart et al. 1982).

In top-level athletes, this immobilization can last up to 4 months, with positive results at the end of this period. This prolonged immobilization obviously has an impact on physical condition and athletic performance and may not be favored in certain circumstances (Montalvan et al. 2006).

Immobilization is followed by exercises to treat any resulting stiffness (Iorio and Huang 2014).

In cases of persistent painful ECU snapping, in-season management of athletes may include taping and/or the use of cortisone injections to try to get a pain-free snap until repair/reconstruction can be performed (Ruchelsman and Vitale 2016; Graham 2012b).

It should be noted that in cases of tendon instability associated with secondary tendinopathy, conservative management of the tendinopathy alone is unlikely to be successful.

- *Non-conservative treatments*

Surgical treatment is indicated in refractory cases, where there is significant pain, inadequate function, and/or a high risk of developing imminent friction tendinosis. ECU instability can be classified as acute or chronic. In the case of acute dislocation in young, active patients, surgical reconstruction of the damaged ECU sheath promotes stability and is recommended. Surgical treatment gives good results, as non-surgical management of acute lesions is not always effective, especially in athletes wishing to return to sport as soon as possible (Garcia-Elias 2015; Campbell et al. 2013; Melone Jr et al. 2010; Heras-Palou 2012; Kim et al. 2013).

There are several surgical options described in the literature. These will depend on the type of injury and the surgeon's preferred technique. They include direct repair of the under-sheath, repair of the under-sheath with a graft, repositioning of the under-sheath with trans-osseous sutures or suture anchors, or reconstruction of the sheath with the creation of a sling. Some researchers believe that the presence of a flat, convex ECU groove increases the risk of recurrent subluxation, and recommend deepening this groove. The goal of all these techniques is to increase tendon stability in the groove (Singh et al. 2016; Verhiel et al. 2020).

Acute dislocations often require direct repair of the under-sheath. However, very few articles have been published on this subject (Garcia-Elias 2015; Graham 2012a; Kollitz et al. 2015; Verhiel et al. 2020).

Current evidence favors open relocation of the tendon within its compartment, repair of the ECU under-sheath, followed by immobilization with a long orthosis immobilizing the elbow (Graham 2012a; Kollitz et al. 2015).

The orthosis is designed to immobilize the limb in a pronation position, with a radial tilt or even a slight extension of the wrist. The orthosis should be worn continuously for at least 6 weeks (Garcia-Elias 2015; Melone Jr et al. 2010; Heras-Palou 2012).

Some authors recommend switching from a long to a short orthosis when the patient can achieve 45° of pronation and active supination. This change of orthosis is followed by a progressive resumption of movement. In this case, strengthening is initiated around 10 weeks after surgery. Sport-specific activities are allowed between 3 and 4 months after surgery in most cases (Ruchelsman and Vitale 2016).

In the presence of a chronic dislocation, surgical reconstruction of the damaged under-sheath is rarely possible due to necrosis and retraction of the two sides of the torn sheath. In this situation, open reduction of the tendon, supplemented by reconstruction of a new under-sheath using a sling created from the retinaculum of the remaining extensors may be indicated, especially in high-level athletes. These types of reconstruction are called "non-anatomical" because they do not recreate the normal anatomy of the ECU complex. The repair must not be too tight to allow the tendon to glide smoothly. If the reconstruction is too tight, the tendon may not slide optimally in the sheath, resulting in possible ECU tendon stenosis. If repair is not possible without creating this stenosis, a capsuloplasty may be considered (Garcia-Elias 2015; Allende and Le Viet 2005; Inoue and Tamura 1998; Yamabe et al. 2012; MacLennan et al. 2008; Heras-Palou 2012).

Some authors base surgical decision-making on the classification of Inoue and Tamura (Fig. 6.21): direct repair is preferred when the site of rupture of the under-sheath is radial (type b), whereas a graft from the extensor retinaculum is preferred in the case of ulnar rupture (type a). In cases where the periosteum is detached from the ulna (type c) to form a false pocket in which the ECU could dislocate, repair can be performed using suture anchors to fix the periosteum (Inoue and Tamura 1998; Inoue and Tamura 2001).

It is important to inform the patient that, following surgery, the final result is generally characterized by a loss of mobility in axial rotation. This may be due to the formation of adhesions between the reconstructed ECU tendon sheath and the extensor retinaculum (Garcia-Elias 2015).

The study by Chang et al. (2014), which found a significant correlation between negative ulnar variance and the presence of ECU tendon pathologies, is interesting because current surgical evidence is contradictory. Many surgeons consider a shallow ulnar groove of the ECU to be a source of recurrent subluxations and therefore deepen the groove as a component of surgical stabilization of the ECU to improve congruence of the tendon and groove. Meanwhile, others have discovered that over-aggressive deepening of the groove in conjunction with reconstructive surgery (anchors) of the ECU can also lead to adverse consequences, such as a greater propensity for recurrent subluxation (leading to more tendon damage) and fractures in the ulnar part of the ECU groove that is weakened by the procedure (loss of the medial buttress) (Graham 2012a; Wolfe 2011; Cooney 2011; Chang et al. 2014; MacLennan et al. 2008; Verhiel et al. 2020).

ECU tendon rupture appears to be the product of repeated trauma over time. Treatment with local corticosteroid injections may contribute to definitive tendon rupture. Reconstruction with a palmaris longus tendon graft may be possible (Montalvan et al. 2006; Kollitz et al. 2015; Khan et al. 2000).

All the described techniques have variable post-operative immobilization and rehabilitation programs to allow the reconstruction to heal appropriately.

There are several complications to be considered after reconstruction surgery. Injury to the sensory branches of the ulnar dorsal nerve may cause pain and/or paresthesia. The ECU tendon may rupture because of attrition, weakening due to chronic inflammation, or iatrogenic manipulation. The same conditions can lead to ECU tendinopathy. When the repair is too tight, this can lead to stenosing tenosynovitis of the ECU (Verhiel et al. 2020).

Conclusion

Damage to the ECU tendon is common in sports such as golf, tennis, and rugby. Many cases can be managed by conservative and rehabilitative measures. A distinction must be made between stable and unstable conditions. Tendon subluxation is a difficult condition to assess and can occur in asymptomatic patients. Its management remains controversial (Campbell et al. 2013).

The ECU tendon and its sheath are not only important for the stability of the distal radioulnar joint, but also for the dynamic stabilization of the wrist. Hence the importance of preserving and/or reconstructing the ECU sheath in cases of tendon subluxation (Salva-Coll et al. 2012).

Ultrasound or MRI imaging are useful complements to clinical examination when atypical features are present, and in cases resistant to conservative management. Ultrasound-guided injection therapy is a useful addition to the treatment of tendinopathy or tenosynovitis in certain cases. Surgery is not often necessary but may be indicated in cases of acute traumatic lesions of the sheath and in cases of chronic subluxation associated with tendinopathy (Campbell et al. 2013).

It is necessary to maintain a high level of suspicion for ECU pathologies, among other pathologies affecting the ulnar side of the wrist, as well as acute diagnostic competence and a palette of therapeutic alternatives for their treatment (Graham 2012a).

Tendinopathies of the Flexor Carpi Radialis

Physiopathology

FCR tendon disorders can manifest as tenosynovitis, tendinopathy, synovial sheath cysts with or without STT joint pathology, or partial or complete tendon rupture (Luong et al. 2014; Parellada et al. 2006).

Micro-traumatic tendinopathies are closely associated with STT joint osteoarthritis, a frequent problem in the elderly population.

Impingement of the FCR tendon in the region of the STT complex can result in a wide spectrum of tendon injuries, including tenosynovitis with or without tendinopathy, isolated tendinopathy, and partial or complete tendon tears (Luong et al. 2014; Parellada et al. 2006; Bishop et al. 1994).

Inflammatory disorders such as rheumatoid arthritis (RA) can spread to the synovial sheath surrounding the FCR tendon.

Pathologies may also be associated with synovial sheath cysts of the FCR tendon, which may arise and communicate with the STT joint, or with other synovial proliferative diseases such as pigmented villonodular synovitis (PVNS).

Finally, the FCR tendon, like any other tendon, may be subject to overuse, trauma, intratendinous calcification, or iatrogenic lesions (Luong et al. 2014; Parellada et al. 2006; Hepper and Boyer 2011; DiMatteo and Wolf 2007).

Inflammatory Tendinopathies

The FCR tenosynovitis is characterized by thickening and/or effusion of the synovial membrane surrounding the FCR tendon. The tendinopathy manifests as tendon thickening and heterogeneous hypo-echogenicity, with or without tearing. When the tenosynovitis is of mechanical origin, effusion predominates. On the other hand, when tenosynovitis is associated with RA or other chronic inflammatory disorders, thickening of the synovial membrane (pannus) predominates. Doppler ultrasonography can assess the vascularity of the pannus, providing a measure of the disease's activity. In chronic cases, the teno-synovial pannus may erode into the adjacent FCR tendon, leading to a tear (Luong et al. 2014; Naredo et al. 2012; Filippucci et al. 2012).

It is therefore important to always carefully assess the integrity of the tendon to detect even partial tendon damage. Partial ruptures are diagnosed by partial interruption of the tendon fibers, whereas complete tendon ruptures appear as a discontinuity in the tendon structure, with proximal and distal tendon stumps retracted to varying degrees (Martinoli et al. 2002).

In inflammatory conditions, it is particularly important to assess surface erosions of the scaphoid or trapezium, as these bones are near the tendon sheath of the affected FCR. Examination of the other tendons and joints of the wrist then completes the examination (Luong et al. 2014).

Tendinopathies Related to Proliferative Pathologies of the Synovial Membrane

The FCR tendon can also be affected by proliferative synovial disorders such as pigmented villonodular synovitis (PVNS). The ultrasound appearance of the latter is similar to that of a form of RA. In the latter case, imaging may suggest SVNP, but an MRI or a biopsy is required to make the definitive diagnosis (Luong et al. 2014).

Intra-tendinous Calcifications

Calcification of the FCR tendon appears on ultrasound as a hyperechoic lesion with variable posterior acoustic shading. Doppler can be used to detect local hyperemia to detect the presence of local inflammation.

The presence of an osteoid osteoma of the scaphoid may also be associated with calcifying tendinopathy of the FCR tendon (Michaelides et al. 2018; Park et al. 2016).

Traumatic Tendinopathies and Tendinous Tears

Chronic trauma due to irritating bone fragments after fractures of the radius, scaphoid or trapezium, or acute penetrating trauma, can lead to tenosynovitis, tendinopathy and, in the most severe cases, partial or complete ruptures of the FCR tendon.

Ultrasound can detect the presence of a tendinopathy and determine the exact location of the impingement. Ultrasound can also differentiate between partial and complete ruptures and measure the distance between the tendon stumps in the latter case. Color Doppler can show local hyperemia if the tear is recent. Ultrasound can also accurately assess traumatic FCR tendon tears and locate foreign bodies next to the FCR tendon.

Bone avulsions of the distal FCR tendon insertion are rare and mainly observed in high-energy trauma (Luong et al. 2014; DiMatteo and Wolf 2007; Soejima et al. 2002).

Iatrogenic Tendinopathies and Tears

The presence of an osteosynthesis screw or plate can irritate the FCR tendon, causing lesions ranging from tendinopathy or tenosynovitis to partial or complete tears. Ultrasound can be useful in identifying the positioning of hardware (screws, plates, etc.). Sono-palpation and dynamic evaluation in flexion/extension of the wrist can reveal the conflict between the tendon and the hardware, as well as reproducing the symptoms. Color Doppler may show local hyperemia, supporting the presence of local inflammation (Luong et al. 2014; Soejima et al. 2002; Bianchi et al. 2008).

Tendon ruptures after trapezectomy, as well as those due to corticosteroid infiltration, can be evaluated by ultrasound. Risk factors include intra-tendinous steroid infiltration and/or significant tendinosis and partial tear. It should be noted that there may be normal or acquired communication between the STT joint and the synovial sheath of the FCR tendon, either on a congenital or degenerative basis (Parellada et al. 2006). If there is a communication, a steroid injection into the STT joint could diffuse to the FCR tendon sheath.

Cysts

Cysts in the synovial sheath of the FCR tendon can be identified on ultrasound. The presence of a pedicle between the cyst and the synovial sheath confirms its origin. Coupled with color Doppler, ultrasonography can show local hyperemia that indicates local inflammation (Luong et al. 2014).

Injuries of the Adjacent Structures

Ultrasound can easily identify other pathologies that may clinically mimic or occur at the same time as FCR tendon disorders, especially lesions of the palmar cutaneous branch of the median nerve or pseudoaneurysm of the radial artery (Luong et al. 2014).

Etiology

Apart from the idiopathic origin, several causes have been identified and may occur simultaneously (Gabel et al. 1994).

Origin Related to a Probable Repetitive Activity (Wrist Flexion in Particular)

FCR tendinopathy may occur as part of a primary condition linked to an overuse syndrome, or as a secondary condition associated with soft tissue or bone abnormalities adjacent to the tendon (Gabel et al. 1994).

FCR Tendon Disorders Associated with Lesions of Adjacent Structures (Cyst, Callus, Osteophyte, or Another Degenerative Lesion (Luong et al. 2014; Gabel et al. 1994))

It should be noted that the tendon lies close to several carpal bones and joints, especially the lower end of the radius, the scaphoid tubercle, the STT joint, and the carpo-metacarpal joint of the thumb; as well as a vascular structure: the deep palmar arcade (reunion of the radial artery and ulnar artery at the anterior part of the wrist). Less than a millimeter of soft tissue separates the tendon from the tubercle of the scaphoid, the STT joint, the trapezium, and the carpo-metacarpal joints of the second and third fingers (Bishop et al. 1994).

The characteristics of the FCR tunnel and its proximity to adjacent structures may explain a certain vulnerability of the tendon (Fig. 6.30).

Any change in the anatomy at this level, however slight, such as the result of a trauma or a degenerative process within this narrow tunnel, can lead to a constriction of the tendon and increased constraints, potentially resulting in a tendinopathy or a stenosing tenosynovitis (Bishop et al. 1994; Gabel et al. 1994).

Several conditions, such as a (distal) fracture or cyst of the scaphoid, osteoarthritis of the STT complex or of the trapezo-metacarpal joint have been cited as predisposing to a FCR tenosynovitis (Bishop et al. 1994; Gabel et al. 1994).

The fibrous then osteofibrous sheath provides a gliding space of variable dimensions for the tendon. In the osteofibrous tunnel, 90% of the available sheath space is occupied by the tendon, which is in contact with the slightly rough surface of the trapezium. As a result, the FCR tendon is surrounded in this region by a thicker envelope consisting of a true synovial sheath. Proximal to the tunnel, the tendon occupies only 50–60% of the sheath and is less subject to constriction. However, mechanical irritation may occur secondary to osteophytes or to the callus of a carpal fracture for example, as mentioned previously (Bishop et al. 1994; Gabel et al. 1994).

Iatrogenic Origin

Authors (Low and Hales 2014) have demonstrated a high incidence of FCR tendinopathy following total trapezectomy with suspension tendinoplasty of the abductor pollicis longus (APL).

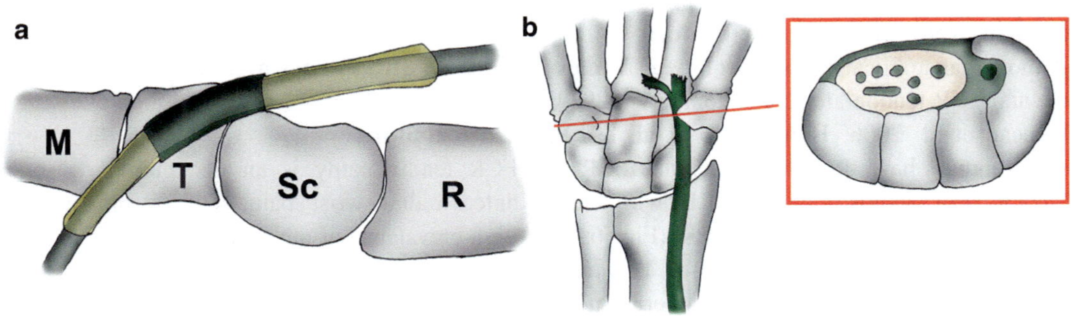

Fig. 6.30 (**a**) Sagittal view showing the FCR tendon in front of the radius (R), the scaphoid (Sc), and the trapezium (T). At the level of the wrist, a synovial sheath surrounds the tendon while it goes under its retinaculum. The tendon then changes direction on the palmar side of the scapho-trapezo-trapezoid joint (STT), before getting deeper just before its insertion. M = first metacarpal. (**b**) Palmar and transversal views of the FCR tendon

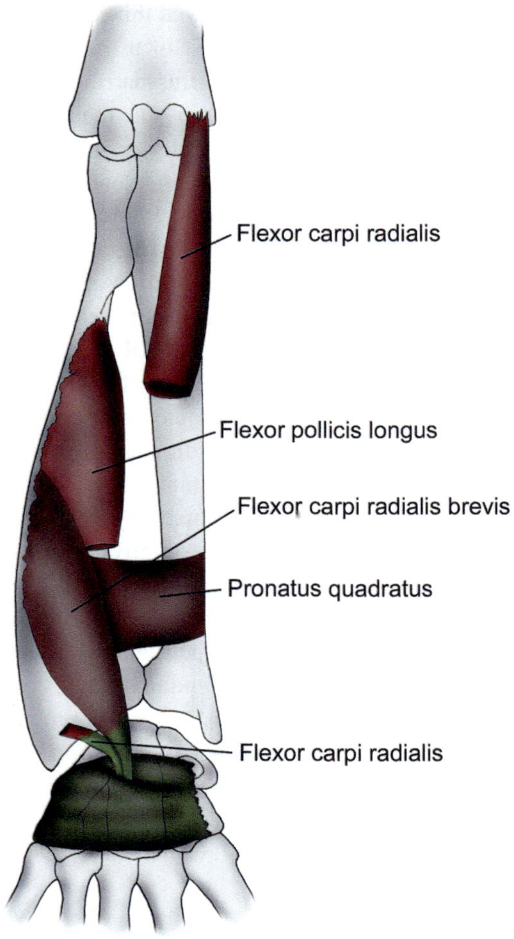

Fig. 6.31 The FCRB starts between the origin of the FPL and the insertion of the pronator quadratus. It then runs superficially next to the pronator quadratus and goes through the osteofibrous tunnel of the FCR

Anatomical Variation (Accessory Muscle or Supernumerary Tendon)

Although anatomical variations of the FCR muscle and FCR tendon are rare (Luong et al. 2014; Duncan et al. 2006; Hongsmatip et al. 2019), some authors have described a doubled FCR or "flexor carpi radialis brevis" (FCRB) with a tendon distinct from that of the FCR (Fig. 6.31) (Bishop et al. 1994; Lee et al. 2014b). This muscle inserts on the distal third of the anterior radial surface of the radius, downwards from the insertion of the flexor pollicis longus (FPL) and upwards from the insertion of the pronator quadratus.

At the level of the radiocarpal joint, it forms a relatively short tendon, parallel and radial to the FCR tendon within the FCR osteofibrous tunnel (Duncan et al. 2006; Hongsmatip et al. 2019). The FCRB tendon can be inserted on the base of the second, third, or fourth metacarpal, on the radial part of the scaphoid, trapezium, trapezoid or capitate, or on the retinacular septum within the osteofibrous tunnel of the FCR (Duncan et al. 2006; Hongsmatip et al. 2019; Lee et al. 2014b). These anatomic variations are often discovered by chance during imaging examinations and surgical procedures. In some cases, however, these accessory muscles may be accompanied by pain (during the compression of a nearby nerve, vessel, or tendon, for example) or by a swelling or mass, simulating a tumor. The prevalence of FCRB muscle has been reported to be 2–8% (Hongsmatip et al. 2019; Lee et al. 2014b), although the presence of this muscle may be higher, as it is often encountered as an incidental intraoperative finding (Lee et al. 2014b; Ho et al. 2011; Mantovani et al. 2010). The presence of this muscle could lead to a tendon intersection syndrome between the FCR and FCRB tendons (Fig. 6.32), which may also be related, at least in part, to irritation by osteophytes of the adjacent STT complex (Parellada et al. 2006). In addition, the presence of the accessory FCRB muscle can lead to compressive neuropathy of the anterior interosseous nerve and denervation of the distal muscles when the FCRB muscle is hypertrophied (Dodds 2006; Andreisek et al. 2006; Dunn et al. 2007).

Clinical and Paraclinical Signs

Clinical Signs

FCR tendinopathy is an uncommon cause of antero-radial wrist pain. The (comparatively) high prevalence of other disorders in this region, combined with a low index of suspicion for FCR tendinopathy, can result in a lack of clinical suspicion, failure to diagnose, and AN inappropriate or delayed treatment. Pain in the antero-radial part of the wrist may be caused by trapezo-metacarpal osteoarthritis, the presence of a cyst

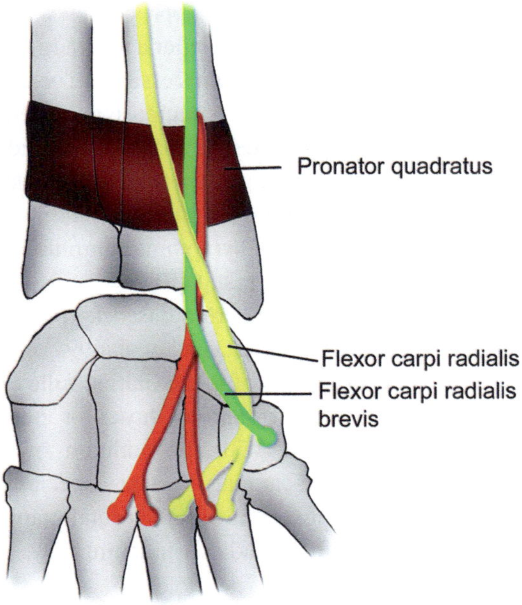

Fig. 6.32 Anterior side of the wrist showing the FCRB tendon's potential pathways and insertions: trapezium or retinacular septum (green spot), capitate (blue spot), or basis of the second and fourth metacarpals (red spot)

or ganglion opposite the scaphoid, De Quervain's tenosynovitis, Linburg syndrome (abnormal inter-tendinous connection between the tendons of the flexor pollicis longus FPL and the second finger's flexor digitorum profundus) or other pathologies. The symptoms of FCR tendinopathy are similar to those of other local conditions, which can make the diagnosis difficult, especially if there is a concomitant local lesion. It will be necessary to consider the patient's history and background (Bishop et al. 1994; Gabel et al. 1994).

Clinically, these conditions come in the form of radial palmar wrist pain accompanied by sensibility to palpation and variable swelling in the area. Symptoms suggestive of FCR tenosynovitis include (Luong et al. 2014; Gabel et al. 1994):

- Pain and/or tenderness over the proximal part of the trapezium, increased by radial flexion and deviation against resistance or by passive extension of the wrist.
- Possible functional limitation in daily, professional, or leisure activities.

Injection of a local anesthetic into the tendon sheath can be used to confirm the diagnosis.

Paraclinical Signs

Since FCR tendon disorders often show non-specific symptoms and a non-diagnostic clinical examination, imaging is often necessary for accurate assessment and therapeutic planning.

Conventional radiography allows good visualization of the surrounding bones and joints, as well as rare intra-tendinous calcifications.

MRI allows the evaluation of the FCR tendon and adjacent anatomical structures with excellent tissue resolution. In comparison, the ultrasound evaluation of the FCR tendon is less frequently described in the literature, despite its affordability, good soft tissue resolution, and the advantages of dynamic, rapid diagnostic imaging. In addition, ultrasound is well tolerated by the patient and facilitates diagnostic and therapeutic injections when they are clinically indicated (Luong et al. 2014; Parellada et al. 2006; McCann et al. 2010).

Ultrasound can accurately guide a diagnostic needle puncture or therapeutic infiltration of the tendon sheath. It allows precise, real-time localization of the needle in the synovial space. It also minimizes the risk of perforating underlying structures such as tendons, nerves, or arteries. Moreover, according to several studies, ultrasound-guided infiltrations are less painful and better tolerated than those guided by anatomical landmarks (Luong et al. 2014; Chavez-Chiang et al. 2012; Sibbitt Jr et al. 2009).

Ultrasound and X-rays are complementary imaging modalities for the evaluation of palmar radial wrist pain with suspected FCR tendon disorders.

X-rays allow a panoramic assessment of the wrist joints and bones and can identify osteoarthritis of the STT complex, the most common cause of FCR tendon injury. Ultrasound allows a precise detection and classification of the FCR tendon pathology.

Dynamic imaging allows direct visualization of the impact of hardware or adjacent structures, and can help differentiate complete and partial tears, or even show the creation of a pseudotendon. Ultrasound evaluation of the FCR tendon should include adjacent structures as indicated to help the differential diagnosis and assess associated lesions (Luong et al. 2014; Low and Hales 2014).

Therapeutic Process

Conservative Treatments

Conservative treatments are usually effective for primary tendinopathies. They include immobilization in a neutral wrist orthosis for 6 weeks, physiotherapy, NSAIDs, and corticosteroid infiltration of the tendon sheath.

However, if there are other local pathological alterations, a conservative treatment is less likely to be successful (Gabel et al. 1994).

Rehabilitation goals include the reduction of trophic disorders and pain. Recovery of full joint amplitudes and proprioceptive abilities of the wrist, as well as total functional recovery, will also be targeted. It will also be necessary to prevent recurrence of primary tendinopathy.

To achieve these goals, the physiotherapist can use several techniques, including draining massage, draining vacuotherapy, and draining pressotherapy. Physiotherapy (cryotherapy, TENS current, Transcutaneous Vibratory Stimulation TVS with a frequency of 100 Hz) may prove beneficial in pain management. Passive and active mobilization and tendon gliding exercises can also be performed. Wrist proprioception exercises and TVS (70–80 Hz) should also be added to the treatment. The therapist's role will also be to provide lifestyle advice on posture and activities (professional and sports) so that the patient can recover optimal wrist functionality adapted to his or her needs, and thus prevent the risk of recurrence. It should be noted that a functional orthosis may be considered for the resumption of some activities.

Non-conservative Treatments

The surgical treatment involves the treatment of any local lesions (such as removal of osteophytes or bone grafting in the case of cysts), as well as the decompression of the tunnel.

Surgical release seems appropriate when symptoms have not improved after a non-surgical treatment. It consists of decompressing the osteofibrous tunnel of the FCR. A decrease in painful symptoms is expected after the surgery, but residual symptoms are common. A history of overuse, work-related compensations, failure of infiltrations, and long-standing symptoms (chronicity) are associated with poor results.

After surgery, patients are advised to wear a splint for around 3 weeks (Gabel et al. 1994).

The goals and means of rehabilitation following surgery will be similar to those for non-surgical management, with the addition of a section dedicated to scar management, especially defibrosing massages and scar vacuotherapy, when the scar is closed and non-inflammatory.

Conclusion

FCR tendon disorders are often overlooked, even though they are a relatively frequent cause of radiopalmar wrist pain. A rigorous clinical examination, possibly supported by complementary tests such as ultrasound, will allow a precise diagnosis and appropriate management. In the case of a primary tendinopathy, a conservative treatment is generally the first choice. In the event of associated lesions or failure of conservative treatment, surgery may be considered.

Tendinopathies of the Flexor Carpi Ulnaris

Physiopathology

In the case of tendons sliding in sheaths, the pathology is most often caused by a stenosing tenosynovitis. However, the tendon of the flexor carpi ulnaris (FCU) muscle has no sheath (Shin et al. 2004).

In this pathology, the histology of the affected tendon is different from that of the normal tendon. The latter normally consists of tightly packed, highly organized collagen bundles oriented along the longitudinal axis of the tendon. It contains a low number of fibroblasts, which are long, thin, flat, fusiform, and longitudinally arranged between the rows of collagen, parallel to the tendon's long axis. The normal tendon is avascular (Budoff et al. 2005).

Tendon lesions are most often the result of excessive mechanical overload. In response to tendon damage, thin, resting fibroblasts become active, multiplying and producing collagen for a normal tendon repair. When the tendon's ability to heal is exceeded, healing fails, and the tendinosis cycle is initiated (Budoff et al. 2005).

Many active fibroblasts persist and must be present to diagnose tendinosis. Tendinosis is defined as a non-inflammatory intra-tendinous degeneration of collagen with the pathological characteristics of angio-fibroblastic hyperplasia. In addition, there may sometimes be areas of local necrosis, calcification, or other elements derived from the mesenchymal cell line, including cartilage and fat.

Tendinosis appears to be painful in itself, but we do not know why. It may be caused by ischemia or chemical irritation, as the degree of tendinosis seems to correlate with the intensity and duration of pain.

The term tendinosis is used rather than tendinitis, as it more accurately defines the histopathological presentation of the degenerative process. The suffix "-osis" implies degeneration, while "-it is" implies inflammation. The term tendinitis has previously been used to describe the theoretical chronic inflammatory changes in the overused tendon. However, histological examination of the tendinopathy has yet to reveal large numbers of macrophages, lymphocytes, or neutrophils (Budoff et al. 2005).

Muscle variations in the forearm flexor compartment, although usually asymptomatic, can also cause FCU pathologies by inducing limb postural deformities or compression neuropathies. The FCU muscle is a pertinent example, with muscle variations shown in anatomical dissections and clinical cases, and an accessory flexor carpi ulnaris muscle has been described. This anatomical variation may be unilateral or bilateral, and there is a wide variation in their characteristics. We can find:

- An abnormal origin or insertion: elbow joint capsule, connection with the insertion of the flexor digitorum superficialis of the flexor's retinaculum, palmar aponeurosis, direct connection to the FCU tendon.
- A partial muscle belly, or additional FCU head, or two FCU bellies.
- Combined insertions with the FCU.
- An abnormal innervation (other than the ulnar nerve).

The presence of a supernumerary muscle belly is rare compared with descriptions of abnormal insertions or small extra-tendinous expansions (Ciftcioglu et al. 2011; Alvin et al. 2011; Vollala and Kumar 2007; Niumsawatt et al. 2013; Pressney et al. 2020).

Furthermore, there are inconsistencies in the literature regarding the nomenclature of supernumerary muscles, which have included digastric FCU, accessory FCU, and palmar FCU (Alvin et al. 2011; Vollala and Kumar 2007). The lack of a universal classification system makes it impossible to precisely list the presence of these anomalies and to determine their technical characteristics and incidence.

Knowledge of these variations is essential to avoid complications in radio-diagnosis and surgical procedures. They are important not only for anatomists, but also for upper limb surgeons, radiologists, and physiotherapists (Niumsawatt et al. 2013).

A study of 5000 cadaveric dissections to assess anatomical variations in the forearm identified an incidence of 0.16% for flexor compartment anomalies and 0.02% for FCU anomalies. The incidence of FCU anomalies varies between studies, ranging from 0.02% to 0.2%. These studies also suggest that the frequency of these abnormalities may be greater than previously thought (Vollala and Kumar 2007; Niumsawatt et al. 2013; Ang et al. 2010).

These anomalies can be classified as follows (Niumsawatt et al. 2013):

- Abnormal origin of FCU
- Abnormal termination of the FCU
- Abnormal size or number of muscle bellies

- Abnormal junction of the FCU with another forearm muscle
- Abnormal innervation

OR (Pressney et al. 2020):

- One muscle with two tendons
- Two muscle bodies with two tendons
- Accessory FCU adjacent to normal FCU

Etiology

Mechanical Overload (Budoff et al. 2005; Waldman 2019)

The FCU tendon can develop tendinopathy after a significant or inappropriate mechanical overload, especially when performing activities requiring repeated flexion and ulnar inclination of the wrist. Acute FCU tendinopathy has been observed in clinical practice with increasing frequency due to the growing popularity of handle sports such as tennis, baseball, and golf. Inadequate stretching of the FCU muscle and tendon before the exercise has also been implicated in the development of tendinopathy of this muscle, as well as acute rupture of the tendon. Injuries ranging from partial to complete tendon damage can occur when the distal tendon undergoes direct trauma while the muscle is fully contracted and under stress.

Anatomical Variation

Most of the forearm accessory muscles described in the literature are located at the level of the radial side of the forearm (variations of the flexor digitorum superficialis, flexor carpi radialis, and palmaris longus are commonly described). On the ulnar side of the wrist, variations of the hypothenar muscles are frequently described, the most common being the presence of an accessory abductor digiti minimi brevis (Sookur et al. 2008).

Clinical and Paraclinical Signs

Clinical Signs

Wrist tendon pain is a frequently encountered complaint. The FCU tendinopathies usually cause pain over the distal part of the tendon, with a particularly marked tenderness 3 cm proximal to its insertion on the pisiform.

Pain may occur spontaneously or may be provoked by movements such as resisted flexion and ulnar deviation of the wrist. Pain may also occur in connection with the patient's professional or personal activities.

The differential diagnosis of ulnar wrist pain should include FCU tendinopathy, piso-triquetral arthritis, lesions of the triangular fibrocartilage complex (TFCC), ulnar impingement, lunotriquetral instability, fracture of the hamulus of the hamate, hypothenar hammer syndrome, and distal radioulnar joint instability (Waldman 2019; Wick et al. 2011).

Paraclinical Signs

X-rays are indicated in all patients with wrist and hand pain (Waldman 2019). Depending on the patient's clinical presentation, further investigations may be indicated. MRI or ultrasound of the wrist and hand is indicated if a tendinopathy or tearing of the FCU is suspected. MRI or ultrasound evaluation of the affected area can also help delineate the presence of calcific tendinopathy or other hand pathology.

Broadly speaking, an angio-fibroblastic hyperplasia (tendinosis) appears characteristically dull, gray, friable, and edematous, compared with the firm, off-white appearance of a normal tendon.

These significant changes seem less evident in the FCU tendon, probably because the relatively smaller size of the tendon implies less tendinosis (Budoff et al. 2005).

Therapeutic Process

Conservative Treatments (Budoff et al. 2005; Waldman 2019)

Distinguishing tendinosis from tendinitis is more than a matter of semantic precision and is important for two reasons. First, it helps explain the cause of tendon pain, which comes from an intrinsic degenerative pathology. Unlike the tendons of the FCR and the flexors and extensors of the fingers that cross the wrist, the FCU tendon has no sheath. As a result, it cannot develop stenosing tenosynovitis, which is the most common pathology affecting these other tendons. Second, an appropriate treatment depends on a correct understanding of the patho-ethiology, which determines the goals of the therapeutic intervention.

The term tendonitis is misleading and can lead the treatment to focus on non-existent inflammation rather than a degenerative process, for which it is better to provide a treatment based on strengthening and stretching exercises, like the recommendations for other upper limb tendinopathies such as tennis elbow and rotator cuff. Any repetitive activity likely to exacerbate the patient's symptoms should be avoided. Although NSAIDs, steroid injections, and other therapeutic modalities may provide temporary comfort, they have no proven long-term curative efficiency. It should be noted that the opposite is true for a traditional treatment of stenosing tenosynovitis, where splints, rest, and steroid injections can potentially be curative.

Over time, if the tendinopathy is left untreated, muscle atrophy and calcific tendinopathy may occur, or the distal musculotendinous unit may suddenly break. Patients who suffer a complete rupture of the FCU tendon will not be able to flex the hand fully and forcefully or perform a full ulnar inclination of the wrist.

Non-conservative Treatments (Budoff et al. 2005)

Surgical debridement of the pathologic tendinosis tissue is an efficient treatment for patients whose non-surgical management has failed.

Conclusion

The distal musculotendinous unit of the flexor carpi ulnaris muscle is subject to a surprisingly wide range of constraints as it performs its function of flexing and ulnar tilting the hand. The relatively poor blood supply to the distal musculotendinous unit limits the ability of the muscle and tendon to heal when traumatized. Over time, muscle damage and tendinopathy can develop, weakening the musculotendinous unit and making it susceptible to further damage and ultimately complete rupture.

Bibliography

Abi-Rafeh J, Kazan R, Safran T, Thibaudeau S. Conservative management of de Quervain stenosing tenosynovitis: review and presentation of treatment algorithm. Plast Reconstr Surg. 2020;146(1):105–26.

Adams JE, Habbu R. Tendinopathies of the hand and wrist. J Am Acad Orthop Surg. 2015;23(12):741–50.

Alemohammad AM, Yazaki N, Morris RP, Buford WL, Viegas SF. Thumb interphalangeal joint extension by the extensor pollicis brevis: association with a subcompartment and de Quervain's disease. J Hand Surg Am. 2009;34:719–23.

Alfredson H, Pietilä T, Jonsson P, Lorentzon R. Heavy-load eccentric calf muscle training for the treatment of chronic Achilles tendinosis. Am J Sports Med. 1998;26(3):360–6.

Allende C, Le Viet D. Extensor carpi ulnaris problems at the wrist. Classification, surgical treatment and results. J Hand Surg Br. 2005;30:265–72.

Alvin M, Alan N, Leone J, Fredieu J. A unilateral accessory flexor carpi ulnaris muscle observed during cadaveric dissection. Clin Anat. 2011;24(8):971–3.

Ameli. Comprendre les troubles musculo-squelettiques - Assuré [En ligne]. Disponible sur: https://www.ameli.fr/flandres-dunkerque-armentieres/assure/sante/themes/tms/comprendre-troubles-musculosquelettiques. Consulté le 22 avr 2022.

Anderson BC, Manthey R, Brouns MC. Treatment of de Quervain's tenosynovitis with corticosteroids. A prospective study of the response to local injection. Arthritis Rheum. 1991;34:793–8.

Anderson SE, Steinbach LS, De Monaco D, et al. "Baby wrist": MRI of an overuse syndrome in mothers. Am J Roentgenol. 2004;182:719–24.

Andreisek G, Crook DW, Burg D, Marincek B, Weishaupt D. Peripheral neuropathies of the median, radial, and ulnar nerves: MR imaging features. Radiographics. 2006;26(5):1267–87.

Ang G, Rozen W, Vally F, Eizenberg N, Grinsell D. Anomalies of the flexor carpi ulnaris: clinical case report and cadaveric study. Clin Anat. 2010;23:427–30.

Artru L. Démarche diagnostique et traitement d'une douleur du poignet. Encycl Méd Chir. Paris: Elsevier; 1999.

Ashe MC, McCauley T, Khan KM. Tendinopathies in the upper extremity: a paradigm shift. J Hand Ther Off J Am Soc Hand Ther sept. 2004;17(3):329–34.

Ashurst JV, Turco DA, Lieb BE. Tenosynovitis caused by texting: an emerging disease. J Am Osteopath Assoc. 2010;110(5):294–6.

Avci S, Yilmaz C, Sayli U. Comparison of nonsurgical treatment measures for de Quervain's dis-

ease of pregnancy and lactation. J Hand Surg Am. 2002;27(2):322–4.
Bahm J, Szabo Z, Foucher G. The anatomy of de Quervain's disease: a study of operative findings. Int Orthop. 1995;19(4):209–11.
Bakhtiary AH, Safavi-Farokhi Z, Aminian-Far A, Rezasoltani A. Influence of vibration on delayed onset of muscle soreness following eccentric exercise * COMMENTARY. Br J Sports Med. 2007;41(3):145–8.
Bass E. Tendinopathy: why the difference between tendinitis and tendinosis matters. Int J Ther Massage Bodywork. 2012;5(1):14–7.
Batteson R, Hammond A, Burke F, Sinha S. The de Quervain's screening tool: validity and reliability of a measure to support clinical diagnosis and management. Musculoskeletal Care. 2008;6(3):168–80.
Beleckas CM, Wright M, Prather H, Chamberlain A, Guattery J, Calfee RP. Relative prevalence of anxiety and depression in patients with upper extremity conditions. J Hand Surg Am. 2018;43(06):571–8.
Belkhir R. Atteinte des mains de patientes traitées par inhibiteurs de l'aromatase: données cliniques et échographiques. Paris: Univeristé Paris V René Descartes; 2010.
Belsole RJ. De Quervain's tenosynovitis diagnostic and operative complications. Orthopedics. 1981;4:899–903.
Beutel BG, Doscher ME, Melone CP. Prevalence of a septated first dorsal compartment among patients with and without De Quervain tenosynovitis: an in vivo anatomical study. Hand. 2020;15(3):348–52.
Bianchi S, van Aaken J, Glauser T, Martinoli C, Beaulieu JY, Della SD. Screw impingement on the extensor tendons in distal radius fractures treated by volar plating: sonographic appearance. AJR Am J Roentgenol. 2008;191(5):199–203.
Bishop AT, Gabel G, Carmichael SW. Flexor carpi radialis tendinitis. Part I: Operative anatomy. J Bone Joint Surg Am. 1994;76(7):1009–14.
Bouillot F. La Ténosynovite de De Quervain. Diplôme inter-universitaire de rééducation et d'appareillage en chirurgie de la main. [Mémoire de Diplôme Inter-Universitaire de Rééducation et d'Appareillage en Chirurgie de la Main]. [Faculté de médecine de Grenoble]: Université Joseph Fournier; 2011.
Brunelli GA, Brunelli GR. Anatomy of the extensor pollicis brevis muscle. J Hand Surg. 1992;17(3):267–9.
Budoff JE, Kraushaar BS, Ayala G. Flexor carpi ulnaris tendinopathy. J Hand Surg janv. 2005;30(1):125–9.
Burge P. The British Society for Surgery of the Hand. De Quervain's syndrome [En ligne]. Disponible sur : https://www.tims.nhs.uk/wp-content/uploads/2018/12/BSSH-de_quervain_leaflet_2016.pdf. Consulté le 03 mai 2022.
Burkhart SS, Wood MB, Linscheid RL. Posttraumatic recurrent subluxation of the extensor carpi ulnaris tendon. J Hand Surg Am. 1982;7(1):1–3.
Bystrom S, Hall C, Welander T, Kilbom A. Clinical disorders and pressure-pain threshold of the forearm and hand among automobile assembly line workers. J Hand Surg. 1995;20(6):782–90.
Calvo-Cerrada B, Martínez JM, Dalmau A. Adoption of preventive measures after returning to work among workers affected by De Quervain's tenosynovitis. J Occup Rehabil. 2012;22(4):579–88.
Campbell D, Campbell R, O'Connor P, Hawkes R. Sports-related extensor carpi ulnaris pathology: a review of functional anatomy, sports injury and management. Br J Sports Med. 2013;47(17):1105–11.
Carneiro RS, Fontana R, Mazzer N. Ulnar wrist pain in athletes caused by erosion of the floor of the sixth dorsal compartment: a case series. Am J Sports Med. 2005;33(12):1910–3.
Cavaleri R, Schabrun SM, Te M, Chipchase LS. Hand therapy versus corticosteroid injections in the treatment of de Quervain's disease: a systematic review and meta-analysis. J Hand Ther. 2016;29(1):3–11.
Chang CY, Huang AJ, Bredella MA, Kattapuram SV, Torriani M. Association between distal ulnar morphology and extensor carpi ulnaris tendon pathology. Skeletal Radiol juin. 2014;43(6):793–800.
Chang CY, Kheterpal AB, Vicentini JRT, Huang AJ. Variations of anatomy on MRI of the first extensor compartment of the wrist and association with DeQuervain tenosynovitis. Skeletal Radiol. 2017;46(8):1047–56.
Chavez-Chiang NR, Sibbitt WL, Band PA, DeLea SL, Park KS, Bankhurst AD. The outcomes and cost-effectiveness of intraarticular injection of the rheumatoid knee. Rheumatol Int. 2012;32(2):513–8.
Chien AJ, Jacobson JA, Martel W, et al. Focal radial styloid abnormality as a manifestation of De Quervain tenosynovitis. AJR. 2001;177:1383–6.
Choi SJ, Ahn JH, Lee YJ, Ryu DS, Lee JH, Jung SM, et al. de Quervain disease: US identification of anatomic variations in the first extensor compartment with an emphasis on subcompartmentalization. Radiology. 2011;260(2):480–6.
Ciftcioglu E, Kopuz C, Corumlu U, Demir M. Accessory muscle in the forearm: a clinical and embryological approach. Anat Cell Biol. 2011;44(2):160–3.
Clarke MT, Lyall HA, Grant JW, Matthewson MH. The histopathology of de Quervain's disease. J Hand Surg (Br). 1998;23:732–4.
Cook JL, Purdam CR. Is tendon pathology a continuum? A pathology model to explain the clinical presentation of load-induced tendinopathy. Br J Sports Med. 2009;43(6):409–16.
Cook JL, Rio E, Purdam CR, Docking SI. Revisiting the continuum model of tendon pathology: what is its merit in clinical practice and research? Br J Sports Med. 2016;50(19):1187–91.
Cooney WP. The wrist: diagnosis and operative treatment. Riverwoods, IL: Lippincott Williams and Wilkins; 2011.
Crimmins CA, Jones NF. Stenosing tenosynovitis of the extensor carpi ulnaris. Ann Plast Surg. 1995;35(1):105–7.

Croisier J-L, Forthomme B, Foidart-Dessalle M. Treatment of recurrent tendinitis by isokinetic eccentric exercises. Isokinet Exerc Sci. 2001;9:133–41.

Daenen B, Houben G, Bauduin E, et al. Sonography in wrist tendon pathology. J Clin Ultrasound JCU. 2004;32:462–9.

Darowish M, Sharma J. Evaluation and treatment of chronic hand conditions. Med Clin North Am. 2014;98(4):801–15.

Dawson S, Barton N. Anatomical variations of the extensor pollicis brevis. J Hand Surg. 1986;11:378–81.

Dawson C, Mudgal CS. Staged description of the Finkelstein test. J Hand Surg. 2010;35(9):1513–5.

De Keating-Hart E, Touchais S, Kerjean Y, Ardouin L, Le Goff B. Presence of an intracompartmental septum detected by ultrasound is associated with the failure of ultrasound-guided steroid injection in de Quervain's syndrome. J Hand Surg Eur. 2016;41(2):212–9.

de Quervain F. On a form of chronic tendovaginitis by Dr. Fritz de Quervain in la Chaux-de-Fonds. 1895. Am J Orthop Belle Mead NJ. 1997;26(9):641–4.

De Quervain F. On the nature and treatment of stenosing tendovaginitis on the styloid process of the radius. J Hand Surg. 2005;30(4):392–4.

Dictionnaire médical de l'Académie de Médecine - Définition ténosynovite [En ligne]. Disponible sur : https://www.academie-medecine.fr/le-dictionnaire/index.php?q=ténosynovite. Consulté le 07 aout 2022.

DiMatteo L, Wolf JM. Flexor carpi radialis tendon rupture as a complication of a closed distal radius fracture: a case report. J Hand Surg [Am]. 2007;32(6):818–20.

Dodds SD. A flexor carpi radialis brevis muscle with an anomalous origin on the distal radius. J Hand Surg. 2006;31(9):1507–10.

Dos Remédios C, Chapnikoff D, Wavreille G, Chantelot C, Migaud H, Fontaine C. The abductor pollicis longus: relation between innervation, muscle bellies and number of tendinous slips. Surg Radiol Anat. 2005;27:243–8.

Drossos K, Remmelink M, Nagy N, de Maertelaer V, Pasteels JL, Schuind F. Correlations between clinical presentations of adult trigger digits and histologic aspects of the A1 pulley. J Hand Surg. 2009;34(8):1429–35.

Duncan SFM, McCormack RR, Roberts CC. Characteristics of the flexor carpi Radialis brevis tendon on magnetic resonance imaging and its use in basal joint arthroplasty. Radiol Case Rep. 2006;1(1):24–6.

Dunn AJ, Salonen DC, Anastakis DJ. MR imaging findings of anterior interosseous nerve lesions. Skelet Radiol. 2007;36(12):1155–62.

Elliott BG. Finkelstein's test: a descriptive error that can produce a false positive. J Hand Surg. 1992;17(4):481–2.

Fedorczyk JM. Tendinopathies of the elbow, wrist, and hand: histopathology and clinical considerations. J Hand Ther Off J Am Soc Hand Ther. 2012;25(2):191–200.

Ferrara PE, Codazza S, Cerulli S, Maccauro G, Ferriero G, Ronconi G. Physical modalities for the conservative treatment of wrist and hand's tenosynovitis: a systematic review. Semin Arthritis Rheum. 2020;50(6):1280–90.

Fichez O. Tendinopathies du poignet dans la pratique sportive. Congrès "Sport et Appareil Locomoteur" Organisé par le Dr Thierry Boyer; 2006; Centre de Rhumatologie et Traumatologie du Sport Le Saint-Louis, Saint Raphael.

Filippucci E, Gabba A, Di Geso L, Girolimetti R, Salaffi F, Grassi W. Hand tendon involvement in rheumatoid arthritis: an ultrasound study. Semin Arthritis Rheum. 2012;41(6):752–60.

Finkelstein H. Stenosing tendovaginitis at the radial styloid process. J Bone Jt Surg. 1930;12(3):509–40.

Gabel G, Bishop AT, Wood MB. Flexor carpi radialis tendinitis. Part II: results of operative treatment. J Bone Joint Surg Am juill. 1994;76(7):1015–8.

Garcia-Elias M. Tendinopathies of the extensor carpi ulnaris. Handchir Mikrochir Plast Chir. 2015;47(5):281–9.

Gerlac D, Gerlac D. Ténosynovite de De Quervain : "replacer" le radius atténue la symptomatologie. Prof Kiné. 2015;49:18–22.

Gerr F, Marcus M, Ensor C, et al. A prospective study of computer users: study design and incidence of musculoskeletal symptoms and disorders. Am J Ind Med. 2002;41:221–35.

Giffin JR, Stanish WD. Overuse tendonitis and rehabilitation. Can Fam Physician Médecin Fam Can. 1993;39:1762–9.

Goel R, Abzug JM. De Quervain's tenosynovitis: a review of the rehabilitative options. HAND. 2015;10(1):1–5.

Gonzalez MH, Sohlberg R, Brown A, Weinzweig N. The first dorsal extensor compartment: an anatomic study. J Hand Surg Am. 1995;20:657–60.

Goubau JF, Goubau L, Van Tongel A, Van Hoonacker P, Kerckhove D, Berghs B. The wrist hyperflexion and abduction of the thumb (WHAT) test: a more specific and sensitive test to diagnose de Quervain tenosynovitis than the Eichhoff's test. J Hand Surg Eur. 2014;39(3):286–92.

Goyal A, Srivastava DN, Ansari T. MRI in De Quervain tenosynovitis: is making the diagnosis sufficient? Am J Roentgenol. 2018;210(3):W133–4.

Graham TJ. Pathologies of the extensor carpi ulnaris (ECU) tendon and its investments in the athlete. Hand Clin. 2012a;28(3):345–56.

Graham TJ. Treatment of ECU injuries in professional baseball players. Hand Clin. 2012b;28(3):357.

Hadianfard M, Ashraf A, Fakheri M, Nasiri A. Efficacy of acupuncture versus local methylprednisolone acetate injection in De Quervain's tenosynovitis: a randomized controlled trial. J Acupunct Meridian Stud. 2014;7(3):115–21.

Hadidy A, Hadidy S, Haroun A, et al. De Quervain's tenosynovitis imaging: ultrasonography versus magnetic resonance imaging. J Bahrain Med Soc. 2009;21:328–31.

Hajder E, de Jonge MC, van der Horst CMAM, Obdeijn MC. The role of ultrasound-guided triamcinolone injection in the treatment of De Quervain's disease: treatment and a diagnostic tool? Chir Main. 2013;32(6):403–7.

Harrington JM, Carter JT, Birrell L, Gompertz D. Surveillance case definitions for work related upper limb pain syndromes. Occup Environ Med. 1998;55:264–71.

Harvey FJ, Harvey PM, Horsley MW. De Quervain's disease: surgical or nonsurgical treatment. J Hand Surg Am. 1990;15(1):83–7.

Hassan MK, Rahman MH, Sobhan F, Shoma FK, Walid CM. Role of ultrasound in the management of De'Quervain's disease. Med Today. 2013;24(1):31–5.

Hepper CT, Boyer M. Repair of flexor carpi radialis tendon laceration at the wrist in a professional ice hockey player. Orthopedics. 2011;34(6):225.

Heras-Palou M. Extra-articular ulnar-sided wrist pain. Arthroscopic management of ulnar pain. Heidelberg: Springer; 2012. p. 335–48.

Ho SY, Yeo CJ, Sebastin SJ, Tan TC, Lim AY. The flexor carpi radialisbrevis muscle—an anomaly in forearm musculature: a review article. Hand Surg. 2011;16(3):245–9.

Hongsmatip P, Smitaman E, Delgado G, Resnick DL. Flexor carpi radialis brevis: a rare accessory muscle presenting as an intersection syndrome of the wrist. Skeletal Radiol mars. 2019;48(3):457–60.

Horii E, An KN, Linscheid RL. Excursion of prime wrist tendons. J Hand Surg [Am]. 1993;18:83–90.

Hosteins E. Prise en charge des ténosynovites de l'extenseur ulnaire du carpe après traitement orhtétique. Mémoire du Diplôme inter universitaire de rééducation et d'appareillage de la main. Université Joseph Fourier Faculté de médecine de Grenoble; 2015, 27 p.

Huisstede BMA, Coert JH, Friden J, Hoogvliet P, for the European HANDGUIDE Group. Consensus on a multidisciplinary treatment guideline for de Quervain disease: results from the European HANDGUIDE study. Phys Ther. 2014;94(8):1095–110.

Ilyas AM. Nonsurgical treatment for de Quervain's tenosynovitis. J Hand Surg. 2009;34(5):928–9.

Ilyas AM, Ast M, Schaffer A, Thoder J. De quervain tenosynovitis of the wrist. J Am Acad Orthop Surg. 2007;15(12):757–64.

Inoue G, Tamura Y. Recurrent dislocation of the extensor carpi ulnaris tendon. Br J Sports Med. 1998;32:172–4.

Inoue G, Tamura Y. Surgical treatment for recurrent dislocation of the extensor carpi ulnaris tendon. J Hand Surg Br. 2001;26(6):556–9.

INRS, Institut National de Recherche et de Sécurité. Les troubles musculosquelettiques du membre supérieur (TMS-MS). Guide pour les préventeurs [En ligne]. Disponible sur: http://www.inrs.fr/media.html?refINRS=ED%20957. Consulté le 3 janv 2022a.

INRS, Institut National de Recherche et de Sécurité. Tableaux des maladies professionnelles - Régime général 57 - Affections périarticulaires provoquées par certains gestes et postures de travail [En ligne]. Disponible sur: http://www.inrs.fr/publications/bdd/mp/tableau.html?refINRS=RG%2057. Consulté le 3 janv 2022b.

Iorio ML, Huang JI. Extensor carpi ulnaris subluxation. J Hand Surg juill. 2014;39(7):1400–2.

Iorio ML, Bayomy AF, Huang JI. Morphology of the extensor carpi ulnaris groove and tendon. J Hand Surg déc. 2014;39(12):2412–6.

Iwamoto A, Morris RP, Andersen C, et al. An anatomic and biomechanic study of the wrist extensor retinaculum septa and tendon compartments. J Hand Surg Am. 2006;31:896–903.

Jackson WT, Viegas SF, Coon TM, Stimpson KD, Frogameni AD, Simpson JM. Anatomical variations in the first extensor compartment of the wrist. A clinical and anatomical study. J Bone Joint Surg Am. 1986;68(6):923–6.

Jaworski CA, Krause M, Brown J. Rehabilitation of the wrist and hand following sports injury. Clin Sports Med. 2010;29(1):61–80.

Jeyapalan K, Choudhary S. Ultrasound-guided injection of triamcinolone and bupivacaine in the management of de Quervain's disease. Skelet Radiol. 2009;38(11):1099–103.

Jirarattanaphochai K, Saengnipanthkul S, Vipulakorn K, Jianmongkol S, Chatuparisute P, Jung S. Treatment of de Quervain disease with triamcinolone injection with or without nimesulide. A randomized, double-blind, placebo-controlled trial. J Bone Joint Surg Am. 2004;86:2700–6.

Johanson ME, James MA, Skinner SR. Forearm muscles activation during power grip and release. J Hand Surg. 1998;23(5):938–44.

Kang HJ, Koh IH, Jang JW, Choi YR. Endoscopic versus open release in patients with de Quervain's tenosynovitis: a randomised trial. Bone Jt J. 2013;95-B(7):947–51.

Kataoka T, Moritomo H, Omori S, Iida A, Omokawa S, Suzuki D, et al. Pressure and tendon strain in the sixth extensor compartment of the wrist during simulated provocative maneuvers for diagnosing extensor carpi ulnaris tendinitis. J Orthop Sci Off J Jpn Orthop Assoc. 2015;20(6):993–8.

Kauer JMG. The distal radio-ulnar joint. Anatomic and functional considerations. Clin Orthop Relat Res. 1992;275:37–45.

Kay NR. De Quervain's disease. Changing pathology or changing perception? J Hand Surg (Br). 2000;25:65–9.

Khan KM, Cook JL, Taunton JE, Bonar F. Overuse tendinosis, not tendinitis part 1: a new paradigm for a difficult clinical problem. Phys Sportsmed. 2000;28(5):38–48.

Kim BS, Yoon HG, Kim HT, Park KH, Kim CG, Song HS. Subluxation of the extensor carpi ulnaris tendon associated with the extensor digitorum tendon subluxation of the long finger. Clin Orthop Surg. 2013;5(1):82–6.

Kim S, Ahmed M, Avins A, Ioannidis J. A genetic marker associated with De Quervain's tenosynovitis. Int J Sports Med. 2017;38(12):942–8.
Kohyama S, Tanaka T, Okano E, Naoyuki O. Anatomical variations of the extensor carpi Ulnaris groove: a new computed tomography-based evaluation. J Hand Surg Asian-Pac. 2017;22(3):281–5.
Kollitz KM, Iorio ML, Huang JI. Assessment and treatment of extensor carpi Ulnaris tendon pathology: a critical analysis review. JBJS Rev. 2015;3(6):e3.
Kulthanan T, Chareonwat B. Variations in abductor pollicis longus and extensor pollicis brevis tendons in de Quervain syndrome: a surgical and anatomical study. Scand J Plast Reconstr Surg Hand Surg. 2007;41:36–8.
Kume K, Amano K, Yamada S, Amano K, Kuwaba N, Ohta H. In de Quervain's with a separate EPB compartment, ultrasound-guided steroid injection is more effective than a clinical injection technique: a prospective open-label study. J Hand Surg Eur. 2012;37:523–7.
Kurppa K, Viikari-Juntura E, Kuosma E, Huuskonen M, Kivi P. Incidence of tenosynovitis or peritendinitis and epicondylitis in a meat-processing factory. Scand J Work Env Hea. 1991;17(1):32–7.
Kutsumi K, Amadio PC, Zhao C, Zobitz ME, Tanaka T, An KN. Finkelstein's test: a biomechanical analysis. J Hand Surg. 2005;30(1):130–5.
Kwon BC, Choi SJ, Koh SH, Shin DJ, Baek GH. Sonographic identification of the intracompartmental septum in de Quervain's disease. Clin Orthop Relat Res. 2010;468:2129–34.
Lane LB, Boretz RS, Stuchin SA. Treatment of De Quervain's disease: role of conservative management. J Hand Surg. 2001;26(3):258–60.
Laoopugsin N, Laoopugsin S. The study of work behaviours and risks for occupational overuse syndrome. Hand Surg. 2012;17(2):205–12.
Lapidus PW, Fenton R. Stenosing tenovaginitis at the wrist and fingers: report of 423 cases in 369 patients with 354 operations. AMA Arch Surg. 1952;64:475–87.
Le Viet D. Les tendinites du poignet. Concours Méd. 1997;119:2221–6.
Le Viet D. Ténosynovite de De Quervain. Maîtrise Orthopédique. 2002;114:10–1.
Lee KH, Kang CN, Lee BG, Jung WS, Kim DY, Lee CH. Ultrasonographic evaluation of the first extensor compartment of the wrist in de Quervain's disease. J Orthop Sci. 2014a;19(1):49–54.
Lee YM, Song SW, Sur YJ, Ahn CY. Flexor carpi radialis brevis: an unusual anomalous muscle of the wrist. Clin Orthop Surg sept. 2014b;6(3):361–4.
Lee ZH, Stranix JT, Anzai L, Sharma S. Surgical anatomy of the first extensor compartment: A systematic review and comparison of normal cadavers vs. De Quervain syndrome patients. J Plast Reconstr Aesthet Surg. 2017;70(1):127–31.
Lillegraven S, Bøyesen P, Hammer HB, Østergaard M, Uhlig T, Sesseng S, et al. Tenosynovitis of the extensor carpi ulnaris tendon predicts erosive progression in early rheumatoid arthritis. Ann Rheum Dis. 2011;70(11):2049–50.
Loomis LK. Variations of stenosing tenosynovitis at the radial styloid process. J Bone Joint Surg Am. 1951;33-A(2):340–6.
Lopes RV, Furtado RN, Parmigiani L, et al. Accuracy of intra-articular injections in peripheral joints performed blindly in patients with rheumatoid arthritis. Rheumatology. 2008;47(12):1792–4.
Low TH, Hales PF. High incidence and treatment of flexor carpi radialis tendinitis after trapeziectomy and abductor pollicis longus suspensionplasty for basal joint arthritis. J Hand Surg Eur. 2014;39(8):838–44.
Lunsford D, Dolislager C, Krenselewski B, Oosting K, Beasley J, Phillips T, et al. Effective conservative treatments for De Quervain's tenosynovitis: A retrospective study. J Hand Ther 1 juill 2016;29(3), 379.
Luong DH, Smith J, Bianchi S. Flexor carpi radialis tendon ultrasound pictorial essay. Skeletal Radiol. 2014;43(6):745–60.
Ma T, Song L, Ning S, Wang H, Zhang G, Wu Z. Relationship between the incidence of de Quervain's disease among teenagers and mobile gaming. Int Orthop. 2019;43(11):2587–92.
MacLennan AJ, Nemechek NM, Waitayawinyu T, Trumble TE. Diagnosis and anatomic reconstruction of extensor carpi ulnaris subluxation. J Hand Surg Am. 2008;33(1):59–64.
Mahakkanukrauh P, Mahakkanukrauh C. Incidence of a septum in the first dorsal compartment and its effects on therapy of de Quervain's disease. Clin Anat. 2000;13:195–8.
Mantovani G, Lino W Jr, Fukushima WY, Cho AB, Aita MA. Anomalous presentation of flexor carpi radialis brevis: a report of six cases. J Hand Surg Eur. 2010;35(3):234–5.
Mardani-Kivi M, Karimi Mobarakeh M, Bahrami F, Hashemi-Motlagh K, Saheb-Ekhtiari K, Akhoondzadeh N. Corticosteroid injection with or without thumb Spica cast for de Quervain tenosynovitis. J Hand Surg. 2014;39(1):37–41.
Martinoli C, Bianchi S, Dahmane M, Pugliese F, Bianchi-Zamorani MP, Valle M. Ultrasound of tendons and nerves. Eur Radiol. 2002;12(1):44–55.
Matzon JL, Graham JG, Lutsky KF, Takei TR, Gallant GG, Beredjiklian PK. A prospective evaluation of the anatomy of the first dorsal compartment in patients requiring surgery for De Quervain's tenosynovitis. J Wrist Surg. 2019;08(05):380–3.
McAuliffe JA. Tendon disorders of the hand and wrist. J Hand Surg. 2010;35(5):846–53.
McCann PA, Amirfeyz R, Wakeley C, Bhatia R. The volar anatomy of the distal radius—an MRI study of the FCR approach. Injury. 2010;41(10):1012–4.
Meachim G, Roberts C. The histopathology of stenosing tendovaginitis. J Pathol. 1969;98:187–92.
Mehdinasab SA, Alemohammad SA. Methylprednisolone acetate injection plus casting versus casting alone for the treatment of de Quervain's tenosynovitis. Arch Iran Med. 2010;13(4):270–4.
Melone PJ Jr, Polatsch DB, Pallotta A, et al. Traumatic extensor carpi ulnaris disruption: subluxation, dis-

location, rupture. In: Slutsky DJ, editor. Principles and practice of wrist surgery. Philadelphia: Springer; 2010. p. 185–97.
Menendez ME, Ring D. de Quervain tendinopathy: "success" and other subtleties. J Hand Surg. 2014;39(6):1232–3.
Menendez ME, Thornton E, Kent S, Kalajian T, Ring D. A prospective randomized clinical trial of prescription of full-time versus as-desired splint wear for de Quervain tendinopathy. Int Orthop. 2015;39(8):1563–9.
Michaelides M, Drakonaki E, Petridou E, Pantziara M, Ioannides C. Osteoid osteoma of the scaphoid bone associated with flexor carpi radialis calcific tendinitis and treated with CT-guided RF ablation. Skelet Radiol. 2018;47(10):1449–53.
Middleton P, Montero C. Le travail musculaire excentrique : intérêts dans la prise en charge thérapeutique du sportif. Ann Réadapt Médecine Phys août. 2004;47(6):282–9.
Mirzanli C, Ozturk K, Esenyel CZ, Ayanoglu S, Imren Y, Aliustaoglu S. Accuracy of intrasheath injection techniques for de Quervain's disease: a cadaveric study. J Hand Surg Eur. 2012;37:155–60.
Monaco JE. Orthopedic considerations in pregnancy. Prim Care Update Ob/Gyns. 1996;3:197–200.
Montalvan B, Parier J, Brasseur JL, et al. Extensor carpi ulnaris injuries in tennis players: a study of 28 cases. Br J Sports Med. 2006;40:424–9. discussion 429
Moore JS. De Quervain's tenosynovitis. Stenosing tenosynovitis of the first dorsal compartment. J Occup Environ Med. 1997;39:990–1002.
Muckart RD. Stenosing tendovaginitis of abductor pollicis longus and extensor pollicis brevis at the radial styloid (de Quervain's disease). Clin Orthop. 1964;33:201–8.
Nagaoka M, Matsuzaki H, Suzuki T. Ultrasonographic examination of de Quervain's disease. J Orthop Sci. 2000;5:96–9.
Naredo E, D'Agostino MA, Wakefield RJ, Moller I, Balint PV, Filippucci E, et al. Reliability of a consensus-based ultrasound score for tenosynovitis in rheumatoid arthritis. Ann Rheum Dis. 2012;
Nayak SR, Hussein M, Krishnamurthy A, Mansur DI, Prabhu LV, et al. Variation and clinical significance of extensor pollicis brevis: a study in south Indian cadavers. Chang Gung Med J. 2009;32:600–4.
Neustadt DH. Local corticosteroid injection therapy in soft tissue rheumatic conditions of the hand and wrist. Arthritis Rheum. 1991;34:923–6.
Nguyen ML, Jones NF. Rupture of both the abductor pollicis longus and extensor Pollicis brevis tendons after steroid injection for de Quervain tenosynovitis. Plast Reconstr Surg. 2012;129(5):883e–6e.
Nguyen A, Jousse-Joulin S, Saraux A. Ténosynovite de De Quervain. Rev Rhum Monogr. 2012;79(2):78–84.
Niumsawatt V, Soliman BA, Rozen WM. The aberrant flexor carpi ulnaris and its clinical implications. J Plast Reconstr Aesthetic Surg JPRAS juin. 2013;66(6):172–4.
Ohberg L, Alfredson H. Effects on neovascularisation behind the good results with eccentric training in chronic mid-portion Achilles tendinosis? Knee Surg Sports Traumatol Arthrosc Off J ESSKA. 2004;12(5):465–70.
Oka Y, Handa A. Recurrent dislocation of the ECU tendon in a golf player: release of the extensor retinaculum and partial resection of the ulno-dorsal ridge of the ulnar head. Hand Surg. 2001;6(2):227–30.
Parellada AJ, Morrison WB, Reiter SB, Carrino JA, Kloss LA, Glickman PL, et al. Flexor carpi radialis tendinopathy: spectrum of imaging findings and association with triscaphe arthritis. Skelet Radiol. 2006;35(8):572–8.
Park JW, Lee KH, Lee JI. Osteoid osteoma of the distal pole of the scaphoid mimicking flexor carpi radialis tendinitis. J Hand Surg Eur Vol juin. 2016;41(5):556–7.
Patel KR, Tadisina KK, Gonzalez MH. De Quervain's disease. Eplasty. 2013;13:ic52.
Patry L, Rossignol M, Baillargeon M, Costa MJ, Institut de recherche en santé et en sécurité du travail du Québec, Régie régionale de la santé et des services sociaux, et al. Guide pour le diagnostic des lésions musculo-squellettiques attribuables au travail répétitif, vol. 2. Sainte-Foy: Editions MultiMondes; 1997.
Petit Le Manac'h A, Roquelaure Y, Ha C, Bodin J, Meyer G, Bigot F, et al. Risk factors for de Quervain's disease in a French working population. Scand J Work Environ Health. 2011;37(5):394–401.
Plotkin B, Sampath SC, Sampath SC, Motamedi K. MR imaging and US of the wrist tendons. Radiographics. 2016;36(6):1688–700.
Pressney I, Upadhyay B, Dewlett S, Khoo M, Fotiadou A, Saifuddin A. Accessory flexor carpi ulnaris: case report and review of the literature. BJR Case Rep. 2020;6(3):20200010.
Ranney D, Wells R, Moore A. Upper limb musculoskeletal disorders in highly repetitive industries: precise anatomical physical findings. Ergonomics. 1995;38:1408–23.
Read HS, Hooper G, Davie R. Histological appearances in post-partum de Quervain's disease. J Hand Surg Br. 2000;25:70–2.
Reddy RS, Compson J. Examination of the wrist soft tissue, joints and special tests. Curr Orthop. 2005;19(3):180–9.
Redvers-Chubb K. De Quervain's syndrome: it may not be an isolated pathology. Hand Ther. 2016;21(1):25–32.
Rettig AC. Athletic injuries of the wrist and hand: part II: overuse injuries of the wrist and traumatic injuries to the hand. Am J Sports Med. 2004;32(1):262–73.
Revue médicale suisse. Diagnostic différentiel des ténosynovites [En ligne]. Disponible sur : https://www.revmed.ch/RMS/2011/RMS-286/Diagnosticdifferentiel-des-tenosynovites. Consulté le 12 mai 2022.
Richie CA, Briner WW Jr. Corticosteroid injection for treatment of de Quervain's tenosynovitis: a pooled quantitative literature evaluation. J Am Board Fam Pract. 2003;16:102–6.
Robinson BS. Rehabilitation of a cellist after surgery for de Quervain's tenosynovitis and intersection syndrome. Med Probl Performing Artists. 2003;18(3):106–12.

Rodineau J. Les tendinites et ténosynovites du poignet. Rev Prat (Paris). 1991;41:2699–706.

Roquelaure Y, Ha C, Leclerc A, Touranchet A, Sauteron M, Melchior M, et al. Epidemiologic surveillance of upper-extremity musculoskeletal disorders in the working population. Arthritis Rheum. 2006;55(5):765–78.

Rosen A, Weiland AJ. Rheumatoid arthritis of the wrist and hand. Rheum Dis Clin N Am. 1998;24(1):101–28.

Rossi C, Cellocco P, Margaritondo E, Bizzarri F, Costanzo G. De Quervain disease in volleyball players. Am J Sports Med. 2005;33(3):424–7.

Roulot E. L'extenseur ulnaire du carpe et sa pathologie. Main Coude Poignet - Prem Partie. 2012;79(2):72–7.

Rousset P, Vuillemin-Bodaghi V, Laredo JD, Parlier-Cuau C. Anatomic variations in the first extensor compartment of the wrist: accuracy of US. Radiology. 2010;257(2):427–33.

Rowland P, Phelan N, Gardiner S, Linton KN, Galvin R. The effectiveness of corticosteroid injection for De Quervain's Stenosing tenosynovitis (DQST): a systematic review and meta-analysis. Open Orthop J. 2015;9(1):437–44.

Ruchelsman DE, Vitale MA. Extensor carpi ulnaris subsheath reconstruction. J Hand Surg. 2016;41(11):433–9.

Ruland RT, Hogan CJ. The ECU synergy test: an aid to diagnose ECU tendonitis. J Hand Surg Am. 2008;33(10):1777–82.

Salva-Coll G, Garcia-Elias M, Leon-Lopez MM, Llusa-Perez M, Rodríguez-Baeza A. Role of the extensor carpi ulnaris and its sheath on dynamic carpal stability. J Hand Surg Eur. 2012;37(6):544–8.

Sampson SP, Wisch D, Badalamente MA. Complications of conservative and surgical treatment of de Quervain's disease and trigger fingers. Hand Clin. 1994;10:73–82.

Sato J, Ishii Y, Noguchi H. Diagnostic performance of the extensor carpi ulnaris (ECU) synergy test to detect sonographic ECU abnormalities in chronic dorsal ulnar-sided wrist pain. J Ultrasound Med Off J Am Inst Ultrasound Med. 2016;35(1):7–14.

Scheller A, Schuh R, Hönle W, Schuh A. Longterm results of surgical release of de Quervain's stenosing tenosynovitis. Int Orthop. 2009;33(5):1301–3.

Shaaban H, Giakas G, Bolton M, et al. The loadbearing characteristics of the forearm: pattern of axial and bending force transmitted through ulna and radius. J Hand Surg Br. 2006;31:274–9.

Shen PC, Wang PH, Wu PT, Wu KC, Hsieh JL, Jou IM. The estrogen receptor-β expression in De Quervain's disease. Int J Mol Sci. 2015;16(11):26452–62.

Shen PC, Chang PC, Jou IM, Chen CH, Lee FH, Hsieh JL. Hand tendinopathy risk factors in Taiwan: a population-based cohort study. Medicine (Baltimore). 2019;98(1):e13795.

Shin AY, Deitch MA, Sachar K, Boyer MI. Ulnarsided wrist pain. Diagnosis and treatment. J Bone Joint Surg. 2004;86A:1560–74.

Shiraishi N, Matsumura G. Anatomical variations of the extensor pollicis brevis tendon and abductor pollicis longus tendon: relation to tenosynovectomy. Okajimas Folia Anat Jpn. 2005;82(1):25–9.

Sibbitt WL Jr, Peisajovich A, Michael AA, Park KS, Sibbitt RR, Band PA, et al. Does sonographic needle guidance affect the clinical outcome of intraarticular injections? J Rheumatol. 2009;36(9):1892–902.

Singh R, Patel A, Roulohamin N, Turner R. A classification for extensor carpi Ulnaris groove morphology as an aid for ulnar sided wrist pain. J Hand Surg Asian-Pac. 2016;21(2):246–52.

Skoff H. Postpartum/newborn De Quervain's tenosynovitis of the wrist. Am J Orthop. 2001;30:428–30.

Soejima O, Iida H, Naito M. Flexor carpi radialis tendinitis caused by malunited trapezial ridge fracture in a professional baseball player. J Orthop Sci. 2002;7(1):151–3.

Sookur PA, Naraghi AM, Bleakney RR, Jalan R, Chan O, White LM. Accessory muscles: anatomy, symptoms, and radiologic evaluation. Radiographics. 2008;28:481–99.

Spinner M, Kaplan EB. Extensor carpi ulnaris. Its relationship to the stability of the distal radio-ulnar joint. Clin Orthop Relat Res. 1970;68:124–9.

Stahl S, Vida D, Meisner C, Lotter O, Rothenberger J, Schaller HE, et al. Systematic review and metaanalysis on the work-related etiology of de Quervaińs tenosynovitis: a critical appraisal of its recognition as an occupational disease. Plast Reconstr Surg. 2013;132:1.

Stahl S, Vida D, Meisner C, Stahl AS, Schaller HE, Held M. Work related etiology of de Quervain's tenosynovitis: a case-control study with prospectively collected data. BMC Musculoskelet Disord. 2015;16(1):126.

Ta KT, Eidelman D, Thomson JG. Patient satisfaction and outcomes of surgery for de Quervain's tenosynovitis. J Hand Surg Am. 1999;24(5):1071–7.

Tagliafico AS, Ameri P, Michaud J, Derchi LE, Sormani MP, Martinoli C. Wrist injuries in nonprofessional tennis players: relationships with different grips. Am J Sports Med. 2009;37(4):760–7.

Topper SM, Wood MB, Cooney WP. Athletic injuries of the wrist. In: Cooney WP, Linscheid RL, Dobyns JH, editors. The wrist: diagnosis and operative treatment. St Louis: Mosby; 1998. p. 1031–74.

Van Oudenaarde E, Brandsma JW, Oostendorp RAB. The influence of forearm, hand and thumb positions on extensor carpi ulnaris and abductor pollicis longus activity. Acta Anat. 1997;158:296–302.

Verhiel SHWL, Özkan S, Chen NC, Jupiter JB. Long-term outcomes after extensor carpi ulnaris subsheath reconstruction with extensor retinaculum. Tech Hand Up Extrem Surg. 2020;24(1):2–6.

Vollala VR, Kumar PB. Additional belly of flexor carpi ulnaris muscle found in a south Indian male cadaver. Internet J Orthop Surg. 2007;5(1):13.

Volpe A, Pavoni M, Marchetta A, et al. Ultrasound differentiation of two types of de Quervain's disease: the role of retinaculum. Ann Rheum Dis. 2010;69:938–9.

Vuillemin V, Guerini H, Bard H, Morvan G. Stenosing tenosynovitis. J Ultrasound févr. 2012;15(1):20–8.

Waldman SD. Flexor carpi Ulnaris tendinitis. In: Atlas of common pain syndromes. 4h ed. Philadelphia: Elsevier; 2019. p. 200–3.

Walker-Bone K, Palmer KT, Reading I, Coggon D, Cooper C. Prevalence and impact of musculoskeletal disorders of the upper limb in the general population. Arthritis Care Res. 2004;51(4):642–51.

Waseem M, Khan M, Hussain N, Giannoudis PV, Fischer J, Smith RM. Eponyms: errors in clinical practice and scientific writing. Acta Orthop Belg. 2005;71(1):1–8.

Watson J, Gonzalez M, Romero A, Kerns J. Neuromas of the hand and upper extremity. J Hand Surg. 2010;35:499–510.

Wharton R, Thaya M, Eckersley R. The dangers of injecting blind: abductor pollicis longus tendon rupture in de Quervain's disease. J Hand Surg Eur. 2015;40(3):322–3.

White GM, Weiland AJ. Symptomatic palmar tendon subluxation after surgical release for De Quervain's disease: a case report. J Hand Surg Am. 1984;9:704–6.

Wick MC, Weiss RJ, Arora R, Gabl M, Gruber J, Jaschke W, et al. Enthesiopathy of the flexor carpi ulnaris at the pisiform: findings of high-frequency sonography. Eur J Radiol févr. 2011;77(2):240–4.

Witt J, Pess G, Gelberman RH. Treatment of de Quervain's tenosynovitis. A prospective study of the results of injection of steroids and immobilization in a splint. J Bone Joint Surg Am. 1991;73:219–22.

Wolf JM, Sturdivant RX, Owens BD. Incidence of de Quervain's tenosynovitis in a young, active population. J Hand Surg. 2009;34(1):112–5.

Wolfe SW. Green's operative hand surgery. 6th ed. Philadelphia: Elsevier Churchill Livingstone; 2011.

Wolfe SW, Hotchkiss RN, Pederson WC, Kozin SH. Green's operative hand surgery. 6th ed. Philadelphia: PA: Elsevier; 2010.

Yamabe E, Nakamura T, Pham P, et al. The athlete's wrist: ulnar-sided pain. Semin Musculoskelet Radiol. 2012;16:331–7.

Yoshida T. Ulnar-side wrist pain. J Jpn Soc Surg Hand. 2010;26(3):383–6.

Zarin M, Ahmad I. Surgical treatment of de Quervain's disease. J Coll Physicians Surg Pak. 2003;13:157–8.

Zingas C, Failla JM, Van Holsbeeck M. Injection accuracy and clinical relief of de Quervain's tendinitis. J Hand Surg Am. 1998;23:89–96.